T0383922

Healing Knowledge in Atlantic Africa

In this ambitious analysis of medical encounters in Central and West Africa during the era of the Atlantic slave trade, Kalle Kananoja focuses on African and European perceptions of health, disease and healing. Arguing that the period was characterised by continuous knowledge exchange, he shows that indigenous natural medicine was used by locals and non-Africans alike. The mobility and circulation of healing techniques and materials was an important feature of the early modern Black Atlantic world. African healing specialists not only crossed the Atlantic to the Americas, but also moved within and between African regions to offer their services. At times, patients, Europeans included, travelled relatively long distances in Africa to receive treatment. Highlighting cross-cultural medical exchanges, Kananoja shows that local African knowledge was central to shaping responses to illness, providing a fresh, global perspective on African medicine and vernacular science in the early modern world.

KALLE KANANOJA is a senior researcher at the University of Oulu. He is an expert in early modern Atlantic history and has published articles on Angolan and Afro-Brazilian religious and medical culture. Kananoja is the co-editor of *Healers and Empires: Healing as Hybrid and Contested Knowledge in Global History, 1700s–1900s* (2019).

Global Health Histories

Series editor
Sanjoy Bhattacharya, *University of York*

Global Health Histories aims to publish outstanding and innovative scholarship on the history of public health, medicine and science world-wide. By studying the many ways in which the impact of ideas of health and well-being on society were measured and described in different global, international, regional, national and local contexts, books in the series reconceptualise the nature of empire, the nation state, extra-state actors and different forms of globalisation. The series showcases new approaches to writing about the connected histories of health and medicine, humanitarianism, and global economic and social development.

Healing Knowledge in Atlantic Africa

Medical Encounters, 1500–1850

Kalle Kananoja

University of Oulu

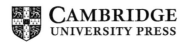

CAMBRIDGE
UNIVERSITY PRESS

University Printing House, Cambridge CB2 8BS, United Kingdom

One Liberty Plaza, 20th Floor, New York, NY 10006, USA

477 Williamstown Road, Port Melbourne, VIC 3207, Australia

314–321, 3rd Floor, Plot 3, Splendor Forum, Jasola District Centre,
New Delhi – 110025, India

79 Anson Road, #06–04/06, Singapore 079906

Cambridge University Press is part of the University of Cambridge.

It furthers the University's mission by disseminating knowledge in the pursuit of
education, learning, and research at the highest international levels of excellence.

www.cambridge.org
Information on this title: www.cambridge.org/9781108491259
DOI: 10.1017/9781108868020

First published 2021

A catalogue record for this publication is available from the British Library.

Library of Congress Cataloging-in-Publication Data
Names: Kananoja, Kalle, author.
Title: Healing knowledge in Atlantic Africa : medical encounters, 1500–1850 /
 Kalle Kananoja, University of Oulu, Finland.
Description: 1[st. edition]. | New York : Cambridge University Press, 2021. |
 Series: Global health histories | Includes bibliographical references and index.
Identifiers: LCCN 2020034141 (print) | LCCN 2020034142 (ebook) |
 ISBN 9781108491259 (hardback) | ISBN 9781108811781 (paperback) |
 ISBN 9781108868020 (epub)
Subjects: LCSH: Medicine–Africa. | Traditional medicine–Africa.
Classification: LCC R651 .K37 2021 (print) | LCC R651 (ebook) |
 DDC 610.96–dc23
LC record available at https://lccn.loc.gov/2020034141
LC ebook record available at https://lccn.loc.gov/2020034142

ISBN 978-1-108-49125-9 Hardback

For Holger

Contents

Figures

Tables

Acknowledgements

This book would not exist without Holger Weiss, who has guided and supported me since day one of my pursuits in African and Atlantic histories. His tireless efforts in advancing African and global historical studies in Finland remain, after over two decades, a constant source of inspiration. Holger was the first to read my full manuscript and made numerous helpful suggestions along the way. I dedicate this book to him, with gratitude and in friendship.

Markku Hokkanen has supported this project from its inception. He commented on earlier versions of my manuscript chapters, and has provided impeccable support mostly over the telephone. Markku is one of the few who understood my aims with this book, for which I remain in his debt. Large parts of the book were conceived during joint projects with Markku and Lauri Tähtinen, who both taught invaluable lessons in argumentation and helped me sharpen my analytical tools. It has been a joy and an honour to work with them. I am also most obliged to Toby Green and Jan Kuhanen, who read the complete manuscript and spurred me on.

Studying African history in Finland would not have been possible without the pioneers who paved the way. I thank Matti Peltola, Juhani Koponen, Harri Siiskonen, Martti Eirola, Seppo Sivonen, Holger Weiss, Pekka Masonen and Risto Marjomaa for clearing the path, providing inspiration and encouraging me onward. The late Raimo Harjula had a lasting effect on my early scholarly formation, and unknowingly planted many seeds for this project. I gratefully cherish his memory.

I thank the anonymous reviewers from the bottom of my heart for their critical but constructive feedback, which made me rethink and revise the manuscript. Their generosity touched me profoundly and helped me raise the bar. I remain responsible for any errors that remain.

José Curto, Linda Heywood and John Thornton mentored my work on Angolan and Atlantic history, and I remain grateful for their kindness over the years. Along with the rest of the Angola Resgate network, they provided hard-to-find primary and secondary sources by selflessly sharing their digital collections. Daniel Domingues and Roquinaldo Ferreira likewise shared their knowledge and transcriptions of primary sources. Mariana Candido's questions at the ASAUK conference in 2014 in Brighton sparked two chapters in the book. Hugh Cagle helped immensely in keeping this project on the track. *Obrigado à tod@s!*

While working on this book, I was blessed with opportunities to travel and interact with scholars in numerous conferences and workshops. From Rio de Janeiro to Paris, from Cambridge to Toronto, and from Lisbon to New York, I have not only enjoyed the camaraderie but also sought to learn from the critical feedback and suggestions provided by Carlos Almeida, Cátia Antunes, Francisco Bethencourt, Kristen Block, Dorit Brixius, Samuël Coghe, Richard Drayton, João Figueiredo, Jorge Flores, Madalina Florescu, Pablo Gómez, Philip Havik, Eric Herschtal, José da Silva Horta, Frank Luce, André Machado, Timo McGregor, André Nogueira, Vanessa Oliveira, Eduardo França Paiva, Luis Nicolau Parés, Vanicleia Santos, Filipa Ribeiro da Silva, Hugo Ribeiro da Silva, Estevam Thompson, David Treece, Jorge Varanda, Megan Vaughan, Jelmer Vos, Tim Walker and Case Watkins. Still others corresponded by email, answered my queries and shared material, including Marc Hertzman, Adam Jones, Carolyn Roberts and the late Joseph Miller and Jan Vansina. *Obrigado mais uma vez!*

In Finland, this project was supported by wonderful colleagues in Åbo, Helsinki, Jyväskylä, Oulu and Tampere who shared the joys of academic freedom and the pressing demands of impending deadlines and administrative duties. I remain grateful and say *kiitos* to Sylvia Akar, Rani-Henrik Andersson, Lotta Aunio, Daniel Blackie, Jari Eilola, Axel Fleisch, Heini Hakosalo, Kaisa Harju, Liban Ali Hersi, Patrik Hettula, Laura Hollsten, Marja-Liisa Honkasalo, Marko Juntunen, Hannu Juusola, Jonna Katto, Leila Koivunen, Saara-Maija Kontturi, Ritva Kylli, Tuomas Laine-Frigrén, Matti La Mela, Ilkka Lindstedt, Stefan Norrgård, Johanna Nurmi, Stefan Nygård, Jussi Pakkasvirta, Esa Ruuskanen, Riikka Tuori, Mikko Viitamäki, Pia Vuolanto, Victor Wilson, Kaarle Wirta and Aleksi Ylönen. A special thank you to my students at the University of Helsinki, who were often the first to hear about and to comment on my archival discoveries, and also to question my lines of argumentation. I hope I have been able to give in return as much as I have received from you.

In a culture of quick fixes, I am grateful for the funding agencies and institutions that still value and understand the somewhat longer incubation period needed in humanistic projects. The archival research and initial writing were made possible by a three-year Academy of Finland postdoctoral fellowship (grant no. 267280). I am especially grateful to the external evaluators who supported this project in its planning stage. A one-year fellowship at the Collegium for Advanced Studies at the University of Helsinki helped me in turning several conference presentations into book chapters. I thank director Minna Palander-Collin and deputy director Katja Ritari for their invaluable support. I am also grateful to the Oskar Öflund Foundation for a small grant for language editing in the final stages of revising the manuscript. As this project was nearing its end, an Almeida Family Fellowship at the John Carter Brown Library provided an opportunity to tie up loose ends. Sincerest thanks go to Neil Safier, Tara Kingsley, Val Andrews and Guillaume Candela.

Tremendous respect to the archives and libraries that preserve our cultural heritage and make the work of historians possible. I owe a debt of gratitude to the archivist and librarians at the Arquivo Histórico Ultramarino, Arquivo Nacional da Torre do Tombo and Biblioteca Nacional de Portugal, where I have always felt welcome. I also want to thank librarians and the long-distance loan services at the Finnish National Library and the universities of Helsinki, Turku and Åbo Akademi. At Cambridge University Press, I want to thank Lucy Rhymer and Emily Sharp for their patience and guidance throughout the review and publication process.

Musical collaborators, neighbours and friends in Turku and Helsinki provided opportunities for escape and much-needed time away from 'the project'. I would like to thank Joakim Stolpe and Lotta Green, Marko Syrjäläinen, Mirosol, RTQ, Oskari and Milla Forstén, Mika and Pia Martikainen, Johannes and Elisa Huhtinen, Miia and Matti Koivu, Jussi Mellin, Jukka Vaajoensuu, Lasse and Marke Kiukas, Timo Mansikka-aho, Martti Viljainen, Sakari Lähdetie, Timo Saario, and my brothers Vesku L. and Jupe P.

My father Leif Gustafsson (1948–2017) sadly passed away before the completion of this book. I thank his spirit and my mother Taru-Maija Gustafsson for letting me follow my own paths and for backing me when those paths turned narrow. I am thankful as well to my sisters Jenni Vire and Milla Gustafsson, and to Markku and Sinikka Kananoja. Sanna has followed this and other projects with an open heart and lovingly tolerated my absences during research trips and intensive writing periods. My greatest debt is to her and our daughters, Rauha and Kerttu, for their love and laughter that keep me warm, now and always.

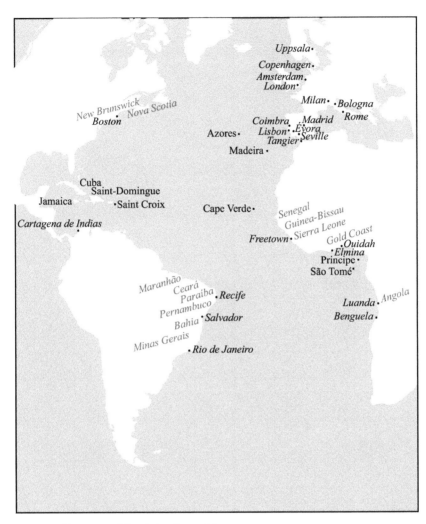

Figure 0.1 The Atlantic world.
Source: Map by Victor Wilson

Introduction

In March of 1628, a Kongolese man named João Alvares Vieira denounced a healer he identified as Domingos Ambundo. This Mbundu healer resided in Luvo, some 60 kilometres north of Mbanza Kongo. Vieira described how he and his wife, Dona Maria Afonso (as well as other family members), had twice taken their ailing daughter to Domingos's hut in order to cure her illness. Domingos had prepared his home remedies by adding herbs and pieces from the *takula* tree to boiling water. He had also thrown a wooden male figure into the concoction. João Alvares Vieira, a Kongo Christian, claimed that he knew that this figure was not God and, hence, neither believed in nor respected it. Neither did he believe that it could improve a person's health. In his testimony, he labelled Domingos's healing as silliness and deception. However, he did admit to believing in the efficacy of the herbal and *takula* concoction that the healer had prepared. Why else would he have taken his daughter to Domingos? After all, similar remedies were widely used to cure people in Kongo at the time.[1]

Altogether, three witnesses testified against the Mbundu healer Domingos, corroborating João Alvares Vieira's deposition, which remains remarkable in many ways. It was one of over seventy denunciations culled in Luanda and Mbanza Kongo in the 1620s. Although only a few of these denunciations concerned African healers, diviners and sorcerers, this documentation provides a rare first-hand African account of popular healing. It shows how Kongolese Christians reflected upon the limits of acceptable religiosity over a century after Catholicism became an integral feature of the Kongo's religious landscape. Since many witnesses in these and subsequent Inquisition proceedings were local Africans, their voices offer a unique view of Mbundu and Kongo understandings of health, illness and healing. Depositions by individuals like

---

[1] Arquivo Nacional da Torre do Tombo (subsequently ANTT), Tribunal do Santo Ofício, Inquisição de Lisboa (subsequently TSO/IL), Diversos, Denunciações do reino do Congo e Angola, 73r, 82r.

1

João Alvares Vieira complement the sources produced by European missionaries and colonial officials. Certainly, Vieira's testimony has to be placed within the context of the Inquisition as part of what Toby Green has termed 'the reign of fear'.[2] When João Alvares Vieira denounced the Mbundu healer Domingos, it was not only the healer whose activity was being investigated – the denouncer's faith was similarly being questioned because of his presence at an autochthonous ritual.

João Alvares Vieira's deposition reveals many common elements that can be observed in numerous other cases discussed in this book. The first is the presence of a Mbundu healer in what was obviously Kikongo-speaking territory north of Mbanza Kongo. This reflects the mobility of the medical practice and of practitioners in West-Central Africa. The Inquisition documentation from later periods reveals that healers were highly mobile, and it is not surprising to find itinerant healers, whose mobility was regarded as a sign of their spiritual power. But this mobility also applied to patients, who would sometimes travel considerable distances to reach a famed healer, as Vieira and his family obviously did. It can also be observed that João Alvares Vieira's daughter was cared for by a therapy management group, consisting of parents and relatives but also slaves, who accompanied the patient to the healer.[3]

Second, João Alvares Vieira testified to the healing power of the *takula* tree, which was widely used and traded in West-Central Africa in this period. It was sought by Portuguese and Dutch merchants in the port of Mayumbe and exchanged for slaves in the kingdom of Ndongo as well as shipped to Brazil and Europe as a textile dye.[4] Vieira probably mentioned the name *takula* because he knew that Europeans also used it for healing purposes. He expected the investigating priests to regard it as a natural rather than diabolical ingredient in the healing ritual. Third, Domingos Ambundo, João Alvares Vieira and other witnesses who testified in the case were all Catholics. For example, one of the witnesses was identified as Dom Pedro, the son of Dom Ambrosio de Mendes and Dona Estefana, certainly members of the Kongolese Christian elite.[5] They

---

[2] Toby Green, *Inquisition: The Reign of Fear* (Basingstoke: Macmillan, 2007).

[3] John M. Janzen, *The Quest for Therapy: Medical Pluralism in Lower Zaire* (Berkeley: University of California Press, 1978). Chapter 1 provides further information on therapy management groups as well.

[4] Kalle Kananoja, 'Bioprospecting and European Uses of African Natural Medicine in Early Modern Angola', *Portuguese Studies Review* 23 (2016): 45–69.

[5] ANTT, TSO/IL, Diversos, Denunciações do reino do Congo e Angola, 61r, 69r, 82v. On Kongo elites, see, e.g., Linda Heywood and John Thornton, 'Central African Leadership and the Appropriation of European Culture', in *The Atlantic World and Virginia, 1550–1624*, edited by Peter C. Mancall (Chapel Hill: University of North Carolina

obviously knew that the healing ritual contained suspicious elements. Similar to Capuchin missionaries who wrote at length about Kongolese rituals, João Alvares Vieira acknowledged that natural medicinals were potent cures, whereas the local deities used in the ritual had lost their potency for Kongolese Christians. They were part of a show put on by Domingos. Vieira sought to convince his interrogators that it was the healer's Catholic conviction that was questionable, not his search for a medicine to cure his daughter.

This book places João Alvares Vieira's experience in the larger context of cross-cultural medical interaction in Atlantic Africa in the early modern period. This interaction was characterised by continuous knowledge exchange between Africans and Europeans. In *Civilization and Capitalism*, Fernand Braudel commented on European expansion, pointing out that humans had already explored and exploited the whole world for centuries or millennia before the rise of Europe. Arguing that Europe neither discovered nor first explored America and Africa, Braudel wrote about the nineteenth-century explorers of central Africa, whom black Africans carried around on their backs while Europeans claimed that they were discovering a sort of New World. But in Africa, as in America, Europeans were merely rediscovering old tracks and rivers used by the indigenous inhabitants of these continents. In short, 'Europeans very often rediscovered the world using other people's eyes, legs and brains.'[6]

The following chapters reveal the ways in which Europeans depended on other people's eyes and brains in Atlantic Africa. Braudel's insight has come under increasing scrutiny as scholars have begun to examine how practical knowledge was embedded in local experiences.[7] Preserving health was a central concern in foreign environments. On their voyages through the Atlantic and Indian Oceans, Europeans faced a practical problem of preserving fresh, plant-based medicinals. One of the solutions to this dilemma was medical interaction with the peoples of Asia and the Americas. These cross-cultural exchanges were overlooked for a long time, perhaps because they were not seen as part of European medicine's

Press, 2007), 194–224; Cécile Fromont, *The Art of Conversion: Christian Visual Culture in the Kingdom of Kongo* (Chapel Hill: University of North Carolina Press, 2014).

[6] Fernand Braudel, *Civilization and Capitalism, 15th–18th Centuries, Vol. I: The Structures of Everyday Life: The Limits of the Possible*, translated by Siân Reynolds (London: Collins, 1981), 62–63.

[7] Clifford Geertz, *Local Knowledge: Further Essays in Interpretive Anthropology* (New York: Basic Books, 1983); Walter D. Mignolo, 'The Geopolitics of Knowledge and the Colonial Difference', *South Atlantic Quarterly* 101 (2002): 56–96; Jan Golinski, *Making Natural Knowledge: Constructivism and the History of Science* (Chicago: University of Chicago Press, 2005).

slow development during the early modern period. However, for the Europeans travelling into new worlds, the significance of locally produced and available medicinals was undoubtedly great. Historians of science and medicine have increasingly noted these cross-cultural exchanges and highlighted their impact on 'Western' medicine. Yet, they have had very little to say about medical interaction in Atlantic Africa.[8] It is symptomatic of this historiography that we know much more about African healers and medical practices in the Americas than about public health in precolonial Africa.[9]

Medicine and natural history developed hand in hand with European colonial expansion in the Atlantic and Indian Oceans. In the Portuguese colonial world, a network of Portuguese physicians and apothecaries debated and inquired about the unfamiliar nature and debilitating fevers. As Hugh Cagle has demonstrated, encounters with new types of nature and disease led to a range of geographical imaginings. In the vast and internally differentiated intertropical world, nature and disease varied greatly.[10] The local knowledge of American and Asian peoples was an

---

[8] Michael N. Pearson, 'First Contacts between Indian and European Medical Systems: Goa in the Sixteenth Century', in *Warm Climates and Western Medicine: The Emergence of Tropical Medicine, 1500–1900*, edited by David Arnold (Amsterdam: Rodopi, 1996), 20–41; Harold J. Cook, *Matters of Exchange: Commerce, Medicine, and Science in the Dutch Golden Age* (New Haven, CT: Yale University Press, 2007); Mark Harrison, *Medicine in an Age of Commerce and Empire: Britain and Its Tropical Colonies, 1660–1830* (Oxford: Oxford University Press, 2010); Pratik Chakrabarti, *Medicine and Empire 1600–1960* (Basingstoke: Palgrave Macmillan, 2014). In a 2015 overview, Mark Harrison blamed the absence of documentation on the lack of research on African medical history prior to 1800. See Mark Harrison, 'A Global Perspective: Reframing the History of Health, Medicine, and Disease', *Bulletin of the History of Medicine* 89 (2015): 650.

[9] Pablo F. Gómez, *The Experiential Caribbean: Creating Knowledge and Healing in the Early Modern Atlantic* (Chapel Hill: University of North Carolina Press, 2017); Londa Schiebinger, *Secret Cures of Slaves: People, Plants, and Medicine in the Eighteenth-Century Atlantic World* (Stanford, CA: Stanford University Press, 2017). Besides the Caribbean, much of this scholarship has concentrated on Brazil, with several case studies on individual healers: Luiz Mott, 'O calundu-angola de Luzia Pinta: Sabará, 1739', *Revista do Instituto de Arte e cultura*, Ouro Preto 10 (1994): 73–82; Alexandre Almeida Marcussi, 'Estratégias de mediação simbólica em um calundu colonial', *Revista de História* 155 (2006): 97–124; André Nogueira, 'Relações sociais e práticas mágicas na capitania do ouro: o caso do negro angola Pai Caetano (Vila Rica – 1791)', *Estudos Afro-Asiáticos* 27 (2005): 181–203; Kalle Kananoja, 'Pai Caetano Angola, Afro-Brazilian Magico-Religious Practices, and Cultural Resistance in Minas Gerais in the Late Eighteenth Century', *Journal of African Diaspora Archaeology and Heritage* 2 (2013): 19–39; Ramon Fernandes Grossi, 'O caso de Ignácio Mina: tensões sociais e práticas "mágicas" nas minas', *Varia Historia* 20 (1999): 118–131; James H. Sweet, *Domingos Álvares, African Healing, and the Intellectual History of the Atlantic World* (Chapel Hill: University of North Carolina Press, 2011); João José Reis, *Domingos Sodré, um sacerdote africano: Escravidão, liberdade e candomblé na Bahia do século XIX* (São Paulo: Companhia das Letras, 2008).

[10] Hugh Cagle, *Assembling the Tropics: Science and Medicine in Portugal's Empire, 1450–1700* (Cambridge: Cambridge University Press, 2018), 10–11.

integral part of medical reciprocity and botanical collection.[11] This book argues that Atlantic Africa was not exceptional in this regard.[12]

Natural history was meant to serve the state and the ruling class. A typical travelling scientist was an upper-class male, who travelled from the known towards the unknown and returned relatively quickly to Europe. His successful journey was made possible by a large group of

---

[11] Richard Grove, *Green Imperialism: Colonial Expansion, Tropical Island Edens and the Origins of Environmentalism, 1600–1860* (Cambridge: Cambridge University Press, 1995); Richard Drayton, *Nature's Government: Science, Imperial Britain, and the 'Improvement' of the World* (New Haven, CT: Yale University Press, 2000); Londa Schiebinger, *Plants and Empire: Colonial Bioprospecting in the Atlantic World* (Cambridge, MA: Harvard University Press, 2004); Antonio Barrera-Osorio, *Experiencing Nature: The Spanish American Empire and the Early Scientific Revolution* (Austin: University of Texas Press, 2006); Júnia Ferreira Furtado, 'Tropical Empiricism: Making Medical Knowledge in Colonial Brazil', in *Science and Empire in the Atlantic World*, edited by James Delbourgo and Nicholas Dew (London: Routledge, 2007), 127–151; Timothy D. Walker, 'Acquisition and Circulation of Medical Knowledge within the Early Modern Portuguese Colonial Empire', in *Science in the Spanish and Portuguese Empires*, edited by Daniela Bleichmar, Paula de Vos, Kristin Huffine and Kevin Sheehan (Stanford, CA: Stanford University Press, 2009), 247–270; Timothy D. Walker, 'The Medicines Trade in the Portuguese Atlantic World: Acquisition and Dissemination of Healing Knowledge from Brazil (c. 1580–1800)', *Social History of Medicine* 26 (2013): 403–431. On the role of Africans in transmitting knowledge in the Americas, see, e.g., Susan Scott Parrish, 'Diasporic African Sources of Enlightenment Knowledge', in *Science and Empire in the Atlantic World*, edited by James Delbourgo and Nicholas Dew (London: Routledge, 2007), 281–310; Londa Schiebinger, 'Scientific Exchange in the Eighteenth-Century Atlantic World', in *Soundings in Atlantic History: Latent Structures and Intellectual Currents, 1500–1830*, edited by Bernard Bailyn (Cambridge, MA: Harvard University Press, 2009), 294–328; Pablo F. Gómez, 'The Circulation of Bodily Knowledge in the Seventeenth-Century Black Spanish Caribbean', *Social History of Medicine* 26:3 (2013): 383–402. For an Indian Ocean perspective, see Dorit Brixius, 'From Ethnobotany to Emancipation: Slaves, Plant Knowledge, and Gardens on Eighteenth-Century Isle de France', *History of Science* 58 (2019): 51–75.

[12] Earlier forays into medicine in Atlantic Africa include, e.g., Luis de Pina, 'Notas para a medicina indígena angolana no século XVIII', *Boletim Geral das Colónias* 151 (1938): 12–26; William Simon, 'A Luso-African Formulary of the Late Eighteenth Century: Some Notes on Angolan Contributions to European Knowledge of Materia Medica', *Pharmacy in History* 18 (1976): 103–114; Heinrich Loth, *Altafrikanische Heilkunst* (Leipzig: Verlag Philipp Reclam, 1984); José Pedro Sousa Dias, 'Índice de drogas medicinais angolanas em documentos dos séculos XVI a XVIII', *Revista Portuguesa de Farmácia* 45 (1995): 174–184; Daniel Hopkins, 'Danish Natural History and African Colonialism at the Close of the Eighteenth Century: Peter Thonning's "Scientific Journey" to the Guinea Coast, 1799–1803', *Archives of Natural History* 26 (1999): 369–418; Judith A. Carney and Richard Nicholas Rosomoff, *In the Shadow of Slavery: Africa's Botanical Legacy in the Atlantic World* (Berkeley: University of California Press, 2009); Jonathan Roberts, 'Medical Exchange on the Gold Coast during the Seventeenth and Eighteenth Centuries', *Canadian Journal of African Studies* 45 (2011): 480–523; Abena Dove Osseo-Asare, *Bitter Roots: The Search for Healing Plants in Africa* (Chicago: University of Chicago Press, 2014); Hugh Cagle, 'Beyond the Senegal: Inventing the Tropics in the Late Middle Ages', *Journal of Medieval Iberian Studies* 7 (2015): 1–21; John Rankin, *Healing the African Body: British Medicine in West Africa 1800–1860* (Columbia: University of Missouri Press, 2015); Kananoja, 'Bioprospecting and European Uses'; Tom C. McCaskie, '"The Art or Mystery of Physick" – Asante Medicinal Plants and the Western Ordering of Botanical Knowledge', *History in Africa* 44 (2017): 27–62.

assistants, who carried the supplies, collected specimens and participated in cataloguing them. Yet, the contributions of these assistants, including Africans on both sides of the Atlantic, have largely been overlooked until recently. In the intellectual order of European colonists, the role of non-European men and women in the production of knowledge was downplayed or ignored completely. However, the contributions of local informants can be traced in the published works, private notes and journals of European surgeons and natural historians.[13]

While earlier scholarship on Africa during the era of the trans-Atlantic slave trade largely focused on violence and patterns of trade,[14] this book takes a road less travelled. It concentrates on health, disease and medical knowledge in Atlantic Africa from roughly the early sixteenth to the early nineteenth century. The book focuses on African and European perceptions of health, disease and healing in tropical Africa. The research highlights cross-cultural medical exchanges and argues that local African knowledge was central to shaping European responses to illness. Medical interaction between Africans, Europeans residing in Africa for extended periods and Eurafricans[15] in turn shaped natural history collections in European centres of learning, but the true value of medico-

---

[13] Schiebinger, *Plants and Empire*, 46; Hugh Cagle, 'The Botany of Colonial Medicine: Gender, Authority, and Natural History across Iberian Empires', in *Women of the Iberian Atlantic*, edited by Sarah E. Owens and Jane E. Mangan (Baton Rouge: Louisiana State University Press, 2012), 174–195.

[14] Paul E. Lovejoy, *Transformations in Slavery: A History of Slavery in Africa* (Cambridge: Cambridge University Press, 1983); Joseph C. Miller, *Way of Death: Merchant Capitalism and the Angolan Slave Trade 1730–1830* (Madison: University of Wisconsin Press, 1988); Luiz Felipe de Alencastro, *O Trato dos viventes: Formação do Brasil no Atlântico Sul* (São Paulo: Companhia das Letras, 2000); José C. Curto, *Enslaving Spirits: The Portuguese-Brazilian Alcohol Trade at Luanda and Its Hinterland, c. 1550–1830* (Leiden: Brill, 2004); Marcus Rediker, *The Slave Ship: A Human History* (New York: Penguin, 2007); Roquinaldo Ferreira, *Cross-Cultural Exchange in the Atlantic World: Angola and Brazil during the Era of the Slave Trade* (Cambridge: Cambridge University Press, 2012); Toby Green, *The Rise of the Trans-Atlantic Slave Trade in Western Africa, 1300–1589* (Cambridge: Cambridge University Press, 2012); Mariana P. Candido, *An African Slaving Port and the Atlantic World: Benguela and Its Hinterland* (Cambridge: Cambridge University Press, 2013); Randy J. Sparks, *Where the Negroes Are Masters: An African Port in the Era of the Slave Trade* (Cambridge, MA: Harvard University Press, 2014); Arlindo Manuel Caldeira, 'Angola and the Seventeenth-Century South Atlantic Slave Trade', in *Networks and Trans-cultural Exchange: Slave Trading in the South Atlantic, 1590–1867*, edited by David Richardson and Filipa Ribeiro da Silva (Leiden: Brill, 2015), 101–142; Linda M. Heywood, *Njinga of Angola: Africa's Warrior Queen* (Cambridge, MA: Harvard University Press, 2017); Daniel B. Domingues da Silva, *The Atlantic Slave Trade from West Central Africa, 1780–1867* (Cambridge: Cambridge University Press, 2017).

[15] George E. Brooks, *Eurafricans in Western Africa: Commerce, Social Status, Gender, and Religious Observance from the Sixteenth to the Eighteenth Century* (Athens: Ohio University Press, 2003).

botanical knowledge lay in its applicability to frequent health concerns among those who lived and settled in Atlantic Africa.

Early modern Africa has often been characterised as a 'white man's grave'. Until advances in tropical medicine in the late nineteenth century, a hostile disease environment hampered European colonisation of Africa.[16] Yet, before that Europeans had been active on the Atlantic and Indian Ocean coasts of Africa for over four centuries. West-Central Africa, in particular, served as a major source of slaves for the Portuguese in the southern Atlantic. In comparison to India and Brazil, however, the Portuguese presence in Angola was demographically small. Some came in service of the crown or the Church. Others sought quick profits from the slave trade, while the colony also served as a penal colony to which criminals were forcefully transported.[17] All these men – and considerably fewer women – had to find ways to recreate their lives in Africa, including finding efficacious remedies for foreign diseases.

Following Hippocratic environmentalism rather than Galenic humoural theory, Europeans often explained disease in Africa, and elsewhere in the Atlantic world, by referencing environmental and climatic factors.[18] African disease causation, in turn, was divided into natural and social aspects, with Africans making a distinction between so-called diseases of God and diseases of man. While the social dimension – diseases thought to be caused by human action, witchcraft or the breaking of taboos – has gained wide currency among scholars of African religions, this book contends that Africans and Europeans found common ground in natural explanations for disease. The search for remedies in Africa led many Europeans to rely upon local Africans who had knowledge of healing plants. Therefore, the answer to the dilemma of healing tropical diseases required a turn to systematic bioprospecting to learn the uses of African natural medicine. Although the term bioprospecting was not coined until 1992, it refers to an old practice, namely drug development based on medicinal plants and traditional knowledge from the 'biodiversity-rich' regions of the globe.[19]

---

[16] Philip D. Curtin, 'The White Man's Grave: Image and Reality, 1780–1850', *Journal of British Studies* 1 (1961): 94–110; Philip D. Curtin, *Disease and Empire: The Health of European Troops in the Conquest of Africa* (Cambridge: Cambridge University Press, 1998).

[17] Gerald J. Bender, *Angola under the Portuguese: The Myth and the Reality* (Berkeley and Los Angeles: University of California Press, 1978), 59–64; A. J. R. Russell-Wood, *The Portuguese Empire, 1415–1808: A World on the Move* (Baltimore and London: Johns Hopkins University Press, 1998), 58–64.

[18] Suman Seth, *Difference and Disease: Medicine, Race, and the Eighteenth-Century British Empire* (Cambridge: Cambridge University Press, 2018).

[19] Cori Hayden, *When Nature Goes Public: The Making and Unmaking of Bioprospecting in Mexico* (Princeton, NJ: Princeton University Press, 2003), 1.

The commercial search for exotic medicines, dyestuffs and foods outside Europe was common in the early modern era, and many Europeans valued the knowledge of indigenous Africans, Americans and Asians.[20] Yet, European interest in African medicine has often been treated as a phenomenon that only began in earnest in the second half of the nineteenth century.[21] Although historians have long recognised the pioneering contributions of Portuguese physicians in the understanding of tropical diseases, Atlantic African natural medicine, especially in the early modern period, has received scant attention compared to India and Brazil.[22] Yet, similar to what took place in India and Brazil, the Portuguese had been interested in local medical practices and ingredients in Angola ever since they first settled there.[23] Moreover, as the third and fourth chapters of this book argue, the Portuguese were not the only ones interested in African healing knowledge; the same also applies to other Europeans who were active in Atlantic Africa.

[20] Grove, *Green Imperialism*; Drayton, *Nature's Government*; Schiebinger, *Plants and Empire*; Cook, *Matters of Exchange*; Cagle, 'The Botany of Colonial Medicine'.
[21] Helen Tilley, *Africa as a Living Laboratory: Empire, Development, and the Problem of Scientific Knowledge, 1870–1950* (Chicago: University of Chicago Press, 2011); Helen Tilley, 'Global Histories, Vernacular Science, and African Genealogies; or, Is the History of Science Ready for the World', *Isis* 101 (2010): 110–119; Deborah Neill, *Networks in Tropical Medicine: Internationalism, Colonialism, and the Rise of a Medical Specialty, 1890–1930* (Stanford, CA: Stanford University Press, 2012); Markku Hokkanen, 'Imperial Networks, Colonial Bioprospecting and Burroughs Wellcome & Co.: The Case of *Strophanthus Kombe* from Malawi (1859–1915)', *Social History of Medicine* 25 (2012): 589–607; Osseo-Asare, *Bitter Roots*.
[22] Charles R. Boxer, *Two Pioneers of Tropical Medicine: Garcia d'Orta and Nicolás Monardes* (London: The Hispanic & Luso-Brazilian Councils, 1963). For a comprehensive bibliography up to the mid-1990s, see José Pedro Sousa Dias, 'Bibliografia sobre a farmácia e a material médica da expansão e da colonização portuguesa (séculos XVI a XVIII)', *Mare Liberum* 11–12 (1996): 165–207; Walker, 'Acquisition and Circulation' and 'The Medicines Trade'; Márcia Moisés Ribeiro, *A ciência dos trópicos: A arte médica no Brasil do século XVIII* (São Paulo: Editora HUCITEC, 1997); Vera Regina Beltrão Marques, *Natureza em Boiões: Medicina e boticários no Brasil setecentista* (Campinas: Editora da UNICAMP, 2000); Cagle, *Assembling the Tropics*.
[23] Among the few English-language contributions discussing West-Central African medicine and medical practices in the early modern period are Simon, 'A Luso-African Formulary'; Miller, *Way of Death*; James H. Sweet, *Recreating Africa: Culture, Kinship, and Religion in the African-Portuguese World, 1441–1770* (Chapel Hill: University of North Carolina Press, 2003); Kalle Kananoja, 'Healers, Idolaters and Good Christians: A Case Study of Creolization and Popular Religion in Mid-Eighteenth Century Angola', *International Journal of African Historical Studies* 43 (2010), 443–465; Kalle Kananoja, *Central African Identities and Religiosity in Colonial Minas Gerais* (Unpublished Ph.D. thesis, Åbo Akademi University, 2012). For a modern ethnographic perspective, see Eric Bossard, *La medecine traditionnelle chez les Ovimbundu* (Neuchâtel: Institut d'Ethnologie, Université de Neuchâtel, 1987); Eric Bossard, *La medecine traditionnelle au centre et a l'ouest de l'Angola* (Lisbon: Instituto de Investigação Científica Tropical, 1996).

The reasons for the acceptance and adoption of natural medicine in different parts of Atlantic Africa were pragmatic. Pharmaceuticals imported from Europe were expensive and their supply was never sufficient to quench the demand for medical drugs in the tropics. Curiosity also played a part, as physicians as well as ordinary European men and women experimented with local products. After all, natural medicine in Africa did not differ significantly from early modern European medicine, with both consisting of the use of various plants and mineral products. Furthermore, from the mid-eighteenth century onwards, scientific and economic interests started to play a greater role in African medical history.[24] Ultimately, as Suman Seth has demonstrated for the British Empire, the crucial question was one of local knowledge and medical expertise versus academic learning: 'The debate between those who claimed a kind of universal, or at least easily transferrable, medical knowledge, and those claiming superior, locally based empirical and experiential skills was one that shaped medical practice and socio-professional life throughout the growing [British] empire.'[25] By emphasising day-to-day cross-cultural medical interaction rather than medical theorising, especially in Chapters 1 through 5, I demonstrate the importance of local knowledge in shaping healing knowledge in Atlantic Africa.

Linda Heywood and John Thornton have argued that Portuguese settlement in West-Central Africa led to processes of cultural creolisation between Europeans and Africans.[26] One of the areas affected by creolisation, which has not been hitherto studied, was health and medicine. For Atlantic Africa as a whole, I argue that, in medical matters, Europeans learned and willingly borrowed more from locals than they gave in return or contributed to the African population's health. Early modern European medical thought was dominated by Hippocratic and Galenic ideas of disease and the body. Restoring the patient to health relied on purging the body of 'bad humours' by using strong laxatives as well as

---

[24] On Portuguese scientific expeditions, see William J. Simon, *Scientific Expeditions in the Portuguese Overseas Territories (1783–1808) and the Role of Lisbon in the Intellectual-Scientific Community of the Late Eighteenth Century* (Lisbon: Instituto de Investigação Científica Tropical, 1983).

[25] Seth, *Difference and Disease*, 51. As Schiebinger, *Secret Cures of Slaves*, 5, put it: 'Fine educations in Europe could not guarantee success on the ground in the tropics.'

[26] Linda M. Heywood, 'Portuguese into African: The Eighteenth-Century Central African Background to Atlantic Creole Cultures', edited by Linda M. Heywood, *Central Africans and Cultural Transformations in the American Diaspora* (Cambridge: Cambridge University Press, 2002), 91–113; Linda M. Heywood and John K. Thornton, *Central Africans, Atlantic Creoles, and the Foundation of the Americas, 1585–1660* (Cambridge: Cambridge University Press, 2007).

bleedings to reduce the volume of blood.[27] These were also common indigenous methods in Atlantic Africa. Moreover, an idea that illness was caused by spiritual forces still prevailed in Portuguese popular culture.[28] Thus, in many ways early modern European and African medical practices resembled one another and, as Timothy D. Walker has noted, the Portuguese were far more receptive to the adoption and dissemination of indigenous medical practices than has generally been appreciated.[29]

Health and Healing in African and Atlantic History

Healing and medicine in Africa are significant not only for their therapeutic effects, but also because they have long been implicated in the organisation and transformation of social and communal life on the continent. In most African societies, several kinds of healers have worked and continue to work side by side. No single healer decides the cause or cure of illnesses because multiple authorities coexist and negotiate the course of treatment in coordination with the patient and his relatives and neighbours. The history of therapeutics therefore needs to take account of all the forces affecting community and domestic organisations to the greatest extent possible given the sources at hand. One must also recognise the ambiguity of a healer's practice in assessing the physical signs and the totality of the patient's social situation.[30]

In an early interpretation, Robin Horton argued that African traditional thought forms a tight system from which escape is impossible. He contrasted it with Western scientific thought, which constantly tests its assumptions against experience.[31] In a critique of Horton's thesis, Steven Feierman argued that European medicine is not a fully open system, nor is African medicine closed.[32] This book agrees with Feierman and contends that Atlantic African healing systems were open

27 Georgina Silva dos Santos, 'A Arte de Sangrar na Lisboa do Antigo Regime', *Tempo* 10 (2005): 43–60.
28 Jose Pedro Paiva, *Bruxaria e superstição num país sem "caça às bruxas" 1600–1774* (Lisbon: Notícias Editorial, 1997), passim.
29 Walker, 'Acquisition and Circulation'; Timothy D. Walker, 'Global Cross-Cultural Dissemination of Indigenous Medical Practices through the Portuguese Colonial System: Evidence from Sixteenth to Eighteenth-Century Ethno-Botanical Manuscripts', in *The Globalization of Knowledge in the Iberian Colonial World*, edited by Helge Wendt (Berlin: Max Planck Institute for the History of Science, 2016), 161–192.
30 Steven Feierman, 'Struggles for Control: The Social Roots of Health and Healing in Modern Africa', *African Studies Review* 28 (1985): 73–147.
31 Robin Horton, 'African Traditional Thought and Western Science', *Africa* 37 (1967): 50–71, 155–187.
32 Steven Feierman, 'Change in African Therapeutic Systems', *Social Science and Medicine* 13:4 (1979): 277–284.

to creative modification and experiment and that medical pluralism already characterised African healing in the precolonial period. Africans observed, studied and selectively adopted European medicines and therapeutic practices, and they visited European doctors whose remedies they regarded as potent. Alternatives for medical intervention should not be seen as mutually exclusive but as representing a spectrum of valid therapeutic options.[33]

The precolonial period has rarely been featured in studies of health and healing in Africa. John Janzen's study of the *Lemba* cult of healing is a rare exception in the field. *Lemba* came into being in the seventeenth century in Equatorial Africa. Its illness has been described as possession by *Lemba*'s ancestors; as any illness affecting the head, heart, abdomen and sides; as difficulty breathing, which is a typical witchcraft symptom; as miraculous recovery from a deadly disease, and more. The individuals afflicted and directed towards membership in *Lemba* were normally the region's elite, prominent healers, chiefs and judges. Their engagement in mercantile networks and ability to succeed in commerce made them vulnerable to the envy of their kinsmen, and therefore marginal in society, 'sick' with the *Lemba* affliction. Following Victor Turner, Janzen described *Lemba* as a 'drum of affliction' (*ngoma* or *nkonko*). In Equatorial Africa, it was considered an extraordinary institution, the most important of the consecrated medicines (*min'kisi*) among those that achieved corporate status.[34]

Healers and diviners were highly regarded religious specialists in Central African societies, whose professional status was acquired through individual initiation conducted by older members of the profession. The method of historical linguistics has revealed that such ritual/ medical specialists have been present in Bantu societies since times immemorial. The Njila languages spoken in nearly all the countries of West-Central Africa stem from a single ancestral tongue labelled 'proto-Njila'. The word denoting these specialists, **-ganga* in proto-Njila, survived in languages spoken in West-Central Africa, although religious

---

[33] William C. Olsen and Carolyn Sargent, 'Introduction', in *African Medical Pluralism*, edited by William C. Olsen and Carolyn Sargent (Bloomington: Indiana University Press, 2017), 1–27.

[34] John M. Janzen, *Lemba, 1650–1930: A Drum of Affliction in Africa and the New World* (New York: Garland Publishing, 1982), 3–4; Victor W. Turner, *The Drums of Affliction: A Study of Religious Processes among the Ndembu of Zambia* (Oxford: Oxford University Press, 1968), 15. Turner adopted the term 'drums of affliction' for Ndembu rituals because the Ndembu often use the term 'drum' (*ng'oma*) as a synonym for a type and actual performance of a ritual. Rituals were performed by cult associations on behalf of persons believed to be afflicted with an illness of misfortune caused by ancestor-spirits, witches or sorcerers.

vocabulary underwent a great many changes as speakers of Njila languages dispersed throughout the region. Male and female diviners, who operated via spirit possession, were, according to Jan Vansina, 'the most spectacular professionals' in Central Africa. They used trances to directly relay the wishes and observations of the spirits who entered into them. Divination by spirit possession gave them an unchallengeable authority in society.[35]

While this book is more concerned with the healing register, harming has often been paired with healing in African political discourse. In some cases, Portuguese settlers were accused of taking advantage of African sorcerers' powers to eliminate their enemies. Anthropologists have pointed to the ambivalence of medicinal charms and power objects and their ability to heal or harm. In the early modern period, this can be observed in cases where African ritual specialists in Angola were accused of using medicines for their therapeutic effects and to hurt and harm as well as eliminate their enemies. Most early modern Europeans, the Portuguese included, shared a belief in witchcraft and magic as real phenomena, although witchcraft trials declined in number and witchcraft was decriminalised across Europe between the late seventeenth and late eighteenth centuries. The African terms for powerful physical substances were often translated into European languages as 'poison'. In the Portuguese southern Atlantic world, *feitiço* was the most common term to denote all kinds of power objects used by Africans, including physical substances, which were sometimes referred to as poison (*veneno*). What is significant, however, is that a belief that harm could be done to people through spiritual or occult means was widely shared by people of different continental origins in the Atlantic world. They also shared a sense

---

[35] Jan Vansina, *How Societies Are Born: Governance in West Central Africa before 1600* (Charlottesville and London: University of Virginia Press, 2004), 51, 167–168. The societies in the Great Lakes Region of East-Central Africa gave recognition to the powers of healers very early on. Social innovations led to the separation of the powers of healer-diviners (*mufŪmŪ) and other healers (*mugàngà), who could use the power of 'seeing' but who did not have a similar role as communal leaders. Although the power of *muganga* healers became separate from the power of *mufumu* leaders, the role of healers and midwives cannot be considered as socially less important. The men and women attending to people's health were experts in herbal knowledge, bonesetting and giving birth. They were also subject to witchcraft accusations because of their constant contact with the powers guiding life, death and nature, which could be harnessed for social good in giving health as well as for antisocial ends in terms of causing misfortune and taking life. David Lee Schoenbrun, *A Green Place, A Good Place: Agrarian Change, Gender, and Social Identity in the Great Lakes Region to the 15th Century* (Oxford: James Currey, 1998), 108–112.

that poisons could be involved in harming people and that spiritual power could also protect and heal.[36]

Healing and harming knowledge travelled from Africa throughout the Black Atlantic. The slave trade made the Americas a cultural melting pot with medical pluralism a norm, not an exception. Pluralism has been regarded as the central feature of Latin American and Caribbean medical cultures. In the slave societies of the New World, African healing knowledge was highly sought after because the number of European and university-trained doctors was minuscule and their services often inaccessible for economic or geographic reasons, but also because of physicians' desire to develop new cures, underpinned by the political and economic ambitions of European states.[37] As Pablo Gómez has shown, African healers took root in the early modern Caribbean and began to form authoritative knowledge and truth about the natural world, particularly that of the body, by creating sensorial landscapes based on experiential phenomena.[38] Similarly, the medical culture of eighteenth-century Saint Domingue was dominated by Africans as healers of people and animals. Hybridisation of European, African and Caribbean healing systems was regarded as a normal course of events.[39]

In the British West Indian colonies, African healing often went by the name obeah and healers were called obeah men and obeah women. Obeah men were respected for their healing knowledge but feared because of the magical powers associated with them. In the colonial Caribbean, the English denounced obeah as superstition and actively persecuted practitioners as charlatans who led the slaves astray. In the early nineteenth century, Africans were still punished harshly for practising obeah. It remained punishable for a long time and has only in recent decades become more tolerated.[40] This was also true in non-British

---

[36] On the harming register, see Nancy Rose Hunt, 'Health and Healing', in *The Oxford Handbook of Modern African History*, edited by John Parker and Richard Reid (Oxford: Oxford University Press, 2013), 384–386. On shared approaches to spiritual power and witchcraft in the early modern Caribbean, see Diana Paton, *The Cultural Politics of Obeah: Religion, Colonialism and Modernity in the Caribbean World* (Cambridge: Cambridge University Press, 2015), 22–27.

[37] Kalle Kananoja, 'Infected by the Devil, Cured by Calundu: African Healers in Eighteenth-Century Minas Gerais, Brazil', *Social History of Medicine* 29 (2016): 490–511; Schiebinger, *Secret Cures of Slaves*, 5.

[38] Gómez, *The Experiential Caribbean*.

[39] Karol K. Weaver, *Medical Revolutionaries: The Enslaved Healers of Eighteenth-Century Saint Domingue* (Urbana and Chicago: University of Illinois Press, 2006).

[40] Paton, *The Cultural Politics of Obeah*; John Savage, 'Slave Poison/Slave Medicine: The Persistence of Obeah in Early Nineteenth-Century Martinique', in *Obeah and Other Powers: The Politics of Caribbean Religion and Healing*, edited by Diana Paton and Maarit Forde (Durham, NC and London: Duke University Press, 2012), 149–171; Kenneth M. Bilby and Jerome S. Handler, 'Obeah: Healing and Protection in West Indian Slave Life', *The Journal of Caribbean History* 38 (2004): 153–183; Jerome

possessions in the Caribbean, such as the Danish-held Saint Croix, where obeah men accused of poisoning people received death sentences. Obeah men were feared among the whites because they were respected by blacks and were seen as potential leaders of slave rebellions. However, from a medical perspective practising obeah and using herbal remedies was not seen as unacceptable in the Danish colonial context. Slave owners accepted that slaves treated each other, occasionally with more success than the doctors on Saint Croix, who sought to understand why Afro-Caribbean remedies were effective.[41]

It could be assumed that there was little room for African healing knowledge in the American South. However, before the American Civil War the medical culture was characterised by experimentation, scepticism and competing visions of scientific legitimacy. Perhaps the best-known example of the transmission of African healing knowledge to North America is the use of variolation in Boston in the early eighteenth century, when Cotton Mather learned the practice from his Senegambian slave Onesimus. Despite popular resistance, variolation was employed to stave off a smallpox epidemic.[42] In the slave societies of the American South, medical interaction led to cross-cultural experimentation, in which the medical systems of American Indians and African slaves spread far and wide. As in other New World slave societies, views regarding black healers were contradictory and conflicting. While slave owners might have recorded recipes of the herbal remedies used by the enslaved in their private notebooks, they at the same time outlawed the activities of black healers. Despite this, African healing knowledge remained vibrant in North America for a long time, eventually hybridising with other forms of healing.[43]

The Atlantic slave trade was a dehumanising experience for the enslaved. Compared to the so-called numbers game, the medical

Handler, 'Slave Medicine and Obeah in Barbados, circa 1650 to 1834', *New West Indian Guide–Nieuwe West-Indische Gids* 74 (2000): 57–60.

[41] Niklas Thode Jensen, *For the Health of the Enslaved: Slaves, Medicine and Power in the Danish West Indies, 1803–1848* (Copenhagen: Museum Tusculanum Press, 2012), 70–72. See also Gunvor Simonsen, 'Magic, Obeah and Law in the Danish West Indies, 1750–1840s', in *Ports of Globalisation, Places of Creolisation: Nordic Possessions in the Atlantic World during the Era of the Slave Trade*, edited by Holger Weiss (Leiden: Brill, 2016), 245–279.

[42] Mark A. Peterson, '*Theopolis Americana*: The City-State of Boston, the Republic of Letters, and the Protestant International, 1689–1739', in *Soundings in Atlantic History: Latent Structures and Intellectual Currents, 1500–1830*, edited by Bernard Bailyn and Patricia L. Denault (Cambridge, MA and London: Harvard University Press, 2009), 357–359.

[43] Sharla M. Fett, *Working Cures: Healing, Health, and Power on Southern Slave Plantations* (Chapel Hill: University of North Carolina Press, 2002).

dimensions of the Atlantic slave trade and slavery in the New World have
received scant attention in the historiography.[44] Joseph Miller wrote
extensively about diseases of West-Central Africa and how the high rate
of mortality affected the profitability of the slave trade. Together with
Dauril Alden, he also analysed the transmission of smallpox to Brazil.
Epidemic diseases held a central role in Miller's analyses as well as in the
work done by Jill Dias and Douglas Wheeler concerning Angola.[45] The
biological experience of enslaved Africans has also been studied by
tracing slave ancestors from Atlantic Africa to the West Indies.
Nutritional and disease environments shaped the health of the enslaved
in their homelands, and the Middle Passage had devastating epidemiological and pathological consequences for blacks. In slavery in the
Americas, nutrition was to play an important role in the development
of diseases. Caribbean slaves fared poorly from a demographic standpoint because of high rates of infant and child mortality caused by poor
nutrition.[46]

Few studies have considered issues related to mental health in slavery
and the slave trade, although they were certainly part of the early modern
Atlantic medical landscape.[47] A study on slave health in the Danish West
Indies concluded that while a few cases of mental illness were mentioned
from various plantations and at the public hospital near Christiansted, it

[44] David L. Chandler, 'Health Conditions in the Slave Trade of Colonial New Granada', in
Slavery and Race Relations in Latin America, edited by Robert B. Toplin (Westport, CT:
Greenwood Press, 1974), 51–88; David L. Chandler, *Health and Slavery in Colonial
Colombia* (New York: Arno Press, 1981); Todd L. Savitt, *Medicine and Slavery: The
Diseases and Health Care of Blacks in Antebellum Virginia* (Urbana and Chicago:
University of Illinois Press, 1978); Marie Jenkins Schwartz, *Birthing a Slave:
Motherhood and Medicine in the Antebellum South* (Cambridge, MA: Harvard University
Press, 2006); Sowande' M. Mustakeem, *Slavery at Sea: Terror, Sex, and Sickness in the
Middle Passage* (Urbana, Chicago and Springfield: University of Illinois Press, 2016).
[45] Miller, *Way of Death*; Dauril Alden and Joseph C. Miller, 'Out of Africa: The Slave
Trade and the Transmission of Smallpox to Brazil, 1560–1831', *The Journal of
Interdisciplinary History* 18 (1987): 195–224; Jill R. Dias, 'Famine and Disease in the
History of Angola, c. 1830–1930', *Journal of African History* 22 (1981): 349–378;
Douglas L. Wheeler, 'A Note on Smallpox in Angola, 1670–1875', *Studia* 13/14
(1964): 351–362.
[46] Kenneth F. Kiple, *The Caribbean Slave: A Biological History* (Cambridge: Cambridge
University Press, 1984). See also Richard B. Sheridan, *Doctors and Slaves: A Medical and
Demographic History of Slavery in the British West Indies, 1680–1834* (Cambridge:
Cambridge University Press, 1985).
[47] William Dosite Postell, 'Mental Health among the Slave Population on Southern
Plantations', *The American Journal of Psychiatry* 110 (1953): 52–54; William
D. Pierson, 'White Cannibals, Black Martyrs: Fear, Depression, and Religious Faith
as Causes of Suicide among New Slaves', *Journal of Negro History* 62 (1977): 147–159;
Terri L. Snyder, *The Power to Die: Slavery and Suicide in British North America* (Chicago
and London: University of Chicago Press, 2015).

does not seem to have been a great problem. However, the study also acknowledged that it is worth 'considering if the cases of fatal accidents points to depressions or other psychological illnesses among the enslaved workers'.[48] In the southern Atlantic, mental illness was most commonly conceptualised as *banzo*, which was encountered in Angola and Brazil in the eighteenth and nineteenth centuries.[49] Elsewhere in the Black Atlantic, a similar ailment was observed in late eighteenth-century Cuba, where a Spanish surgeon named Francisco Barrera y Domingo wrote an extensive treatise on slave medicine. Barrera's views on melancholy were partly rooted in the writings of other physicians and partly in his own innovations based on observation and experience in the Caribbean.[50]

A Global Framework for Studying Health and Medicine in Atlantic Africa

When studying contemporary societies, medical anthropologists have increasingly begun to look at Africa as a continent where global flows of capital, technologies, information and people originate and circulate within and beyond national and continental boundaries. Public health policies and practices in sub-Saharan Africa have become globally inflected by the practice of biomedicine, which, like other modalities of healing, is inexplicably intertwined with politics, religion and community and family life. While transnational entanglements and networks shape biomedicine in Africa, affective and material resources are not allocated equally across space. Despite the global circulation of international standards of medical education, research, practice and policy, local realities of resource-poor settings produce effects that do not resemble their ostensible aims. Transnational capitalism and neoliberal reform have put further economic strains on inadequate healthcare services.[51]

---

[48] Jensen, *For the Health of the Enslaved*, 109.
[49] The discourse and experience of *banzo*, conceptualised as melancholy or nostalgia, in the late eighteenth-century and early nineteenth-century Brazil has been analysed in several articles by Ana Maria Oda, who has examined historical representations of *banzo* primarily in Brazil. Ana Maria Galdini Raimundo Oda, 'O banzo e outros males: o pathos dos negros escravos na Memória de Oliveira Mendes', *Revista Latinoamericana de Psicopatologia Fundamental* 10 (2007): 346–361; Ana Maria Galdini Raimundo Oda, 'Escravidão e nostalgia no Brasil: o banzo', *Revista Latinoamericana de Psicopatologia Fundamental* 11 (2008): 735–761. See also Chirly dos Santos-Stubbe, 'Banzo: Uma nostalgia afro-brasileira', *Journal of Psychology in Africa* 1 (1989): 8–14.
[50] Adrián López Denis, 'Melancholy, Slavery, and Racial Pathology in Eighteenth-Century Cuba', *Science in Context* 18 (2005): 179–199.
[51] Kathryn Rhine, 'Introduction', in *Medical Anthropology in Global Africa*, edited by Kathryn Rhine et al. (Lawrence: University of Kansas, 2014), 5; Randall M. Packard, *A History of Global Health: Interventions into the Lives of Other Peoples* (Baltimore: Johns

Folk healing, therefore, continues to play an important role in Africa. Medical anthropologists and historians have pointed out that 'traditional'[52] African therapies and medicinal products often move across vast regional distances, with healers travelling from afar claiming heightened potency.[53] This book shows that the mobility and circulation of healing techniques and materials was an important feature of the early modern Black Atlantic world and not something that began in the nineteenth century or later. African healing specialists not only crossed the Atlantic to the Americas and Europe – where Lisbon remained the most important centre of African healing from the sixteenth to perhaps the nineteenth century[54] – but also moved within and between regions to offer their services. At times, patients, Europeans included, travelled relatively long distances in Africa to receive treatment from a certain healer.

How does the global historical framework fit precolonial Atlantic Africa, and how does it relate to the social and cultural history of medicine in the region? While some Africanist scholars have warned about hopping on the global history bandwagon and have duly emphasised a focus on the mechanisms of connection and their limits, others have pointed out that Africans lived, not isolated, but in broader historical contexts long before colonial rule in the twentieth century.[55] Interaction with the Islamic world, Indian Ocean and Mediterranean regions are the most obvious examples of contacts that predated links with the Atlantic economy. Islam, especially, was significant for the development of medical practices in Muslim Africa.[56] Moreover,

Hopkins University Press, 2016); Stacey A. Langwick, *Bodies, Politics, and African Healing: The Matter of Maladies in Tanzania* (Bloomington: Indiana University Press, 2011).

[52] Given the transformations in African healing over centuries, I use the term 'traditional medicine' cautiously.

[53] Stacey A. Langwick, Hansbjörg Dilger and Abdoulaye Kane, 'Introduction: Transnational Medicine, Mobile Experts', in *Medicine, Mobility, and Power in Global Africa: Transnational Health and Healing*, edited by Hansbjörg Dilger, Abdoulaye Kane and Stacey A. Langwick (Bloomington: Indiana University Press, 2012), 1–27. For a critique of the term 'traditional medicine', see Sjaak van der Geest, 'Is There a Role for Traditional Medicine in Basic Health Services in Africa? A Plea for Community Perspective', *Tropical Medicine and International Health* 2 (1997): 903–911.

[54] Daniela Buono Calainho, *Metrópole das Mandingas: Religiosidade negra e inquisição portuguesa no Antigo Regime* (Rio de Janeiro: Garamond, 2008).

[55] Robert Harms, *Africa in Global History with Sources* (New York: W. W. Norton, 2018); Toby Green, *A Fistful of Shells: West Africa from the Rise of the Slave Trade to the Age of Revolution* (London: Allen Lane, 2019).

[56] Ismail H. Abdalla, 'The Ulama of Sokoto in the Nineteenth Century: A Medical View', in *African Healing Strategies*, edited by Brian M. du Toit and Ismail H. Abdalla (Owerri: Trado-Medic Books, 1985), 8–19; Ismail H. Abdalla, 'Diffusion of Islamic Medicine

Africans' experience of global historical processes can direct attention to changes occurring on the fringes of 'civilisations' instead of concentrating on their relatively stable centres as distortedly narrow regional fields are increasingly becoming 'globalised'.[57]

Circulation of knowledge was central to the shaping of what Londa Schiebinger has called the Atlantic world medical complex. Multidirectional trade in people, disease, plants and knowledges linked Europe, Africa and the Americas along interconnected nexuses, where the West Indies served as a 'centre of calculation' and doctors and healers of all types as 'knowledge brokers'. The slave trade nexus joined Africa and the Americas, but in Schiebinger's formulation knowledge was only carried from Africa to the Caribbean.[58] Highlighting the Africans' Atlantic experience just in the Americas, however, leaves Africa disconnected from the rest of the world, as if it was impossible for European and American medical knowledge to circulate to Africa. Although they probably had little to do with the fate of Africa during the era of the slave trade, Central Africans practised phlebotomy and sought surgical knowledge from the Portuguese, as demonstrated in Chapter 5. Some of the Angolan slaves taken to Brazil continued to practise as barbers on the other side of the Atlantic. European and American medicinals were spreading to the interior of Central Africa by the seventeenth century, and quina was used as an antimalarial medicine in Central and West Africa in the eighteenth century. To fully appreciate the Atlantic world medical complex, these connections as well as the linkages between the Atlantic and Indian Oceans must be taken into account.

This book contends that global history can provide a complementary interpretive layer when thinking about African medicine and vernacular science in the early modern world. While the Atlantic can be conceptualised as the primary arena of interaction for West and West-Central Africans and the Indian Ocean for East Africans, I argue that the Atlantic served as a passageway to the world beyond it. This can be discerned in the movement of people, commodities and plants between the Indian and Atlantic Oceans, with West-Central African slaves providing labour not only in the Americas, but also working in South and South East Asia; Asian textiles and cowries flooding the local markets in

into Hausaland', in *The Social Basis of Health and Healing in Africa*, edited by Steven Feierman and John M. Janzen (Berkeley: University of California Press, 1992), 177–194.

[57] Frederick Cooper, 'African History/Global History', *Perspectives on History* 50 (December 2012); Joseph C. Miller, 'History and Africa/Africa and History', *American Historical Review* 104 (1999): 1–32, especially 29–31.

[58] Schiebinger, *Secret Cures of Slaves*, 13–14, 153–156.

Atlantic Africa; and the movement and circulation of plants between continents.

The last example is the most relevant for the purposes of the present work. Historians and archaeologists have long acknowledged that tropical Africa participated in the global migration of crops.[59] Edible bananas (genus *Musa*) are perhaps the best-known example of an Indian Ocean crop that spread into Africa, although the origins and dating of their domestication have been brought into question.[60] Undoubtedly, many plants spread across cultural borders in Atlantic Africa without external agency but, starting from the fifteenth century, the Portuguese also played a major role as carriers in the global dissemination of cultivated plants. In seventeenth-century Dutch Brazil, naturalists Georg Marcgraf and Willem Piso documented plants of commercial importance and with medicinal qualities, both indigenous and those imported from Africa and Asia. In the eighteenth century, Dom João V (1706–1750) ordered the cultivation of Asian plants in West Africa and Brazil. Pepper seeds and cuttings from India were also regularly sent to Brazil and Angola. Several plants of American origin – sweet potatoes, peanuts, manioc and maize corn, to name just a few – were introduced to Atlantic Africa in the sixteenth century. Maize became a popular crop throughout Atlantic Africa, and manioc spread rapidly throughout Central Africa and the Upper Guinea coast.[61]

Similarly to other plants, medicinals circulated between regions and continents and multiple innovators participated in the shaping of drug knowledge across vast geographic regions and over long periods of time. One of the best-known African plant medicines to have had an impact outside of Africa in the early modern period was the grains of paradise or guinea grains (*Aframomum melegueta*), also referred to as melegueta

---

[59] See, e.g., John W. Purseglove, 'The Origins and Migrations of Crops in Tropical Africa', in *Origins of African Plant Domestication*, edited by Jack R. Harlan, Jan M. J. de Wet and Ann B. L. Stemler (The Hague and Paris: Mouton Publishers, 1976), 291–309; Ilaria Maria Grimaldi, 'Taro across the Oceans: Journeys of One of Our Oldest Crops', in *News from the Past: Progress in African Archaeobotany*, edited by Ursula Thanheiser (Groningen: Barkhuis, 2016), 67–82; Dorian Q. Fuller and Chris J. Stevens, 'Sorghum Domestication and Diversification: A Current Archaeobotanical Perspective', in *Plants and People in the African Past: Progress in African Archaeobotany*, edited by Anna Maria Mercuri et al. (New York: Springer, 2018), 427–452.

[60] The debates are summarised in Katharina Neumann and Elisabeth Hildebrand, 'Early Bananas in Africa: The State of the Art', *Ethnobotany Research & Applications* 7 (2009): 353–362.

[61] Russell-Wood, *The Portuguese Empire*, 148–150, 154, 164–168. In the second half of the seventeenth century, Duarte Ribeiro de Macedo proposed a concerted imperial effort to transfer the most profitably traded plants from the East Indies to Brazil. On this plan, see Cagle, *Assembling the Tropics*, 254–270.

pepper, which enjoyed widespread popularity among African folk remedies in the Americas. Of the Asian plants with medical value, Indian pennywort (*Centella asiatica*) spread widely throughout West and East Africa. African 'traditional' medicine has changed and moved over time both within and without the continent as many people in many places shared and elaborated on plant medicine recipes over a span of years and centuries. 'Traditional' medicine has rarely been purely local, as knowledge about healing plants has spread widely across continents when plants, people and information have migrated.[62] Although early modern sources are not rich enough to write extensive biographies of medicinals in the same way that Guillaume Lachenal has so magisterially done for a twentieth-century pharmaceutical product,[63] or to explore the ethos of medical research and drug development in Africa,[64] they allow us, at least, to reconstruct the great variety of these materials and their movement over time and space.

The world, and therefore global history, was present in Atlantic Africa's medical thought in many other ways. A mid-seventeenth-century Portuguese soldier serving in Angola, when writing a catalogue of the region's medicinal plants, began his manuscript by pointing out that he wanted to imitate Monardes, a Sevillian physician best known for his study of medicinals imported to Spain from the West Indies. In West Africa, a Danish physician named Paul Erdmann Isert, wanting to make a scientific contribution to global natural history, sought patronage from Sir Joseph Banks. Although he failed to get attention from London, Isert's fellow Scandinavian, Adam Afzelius, was more successful. He joined Banks's network of collectors and travelled to Sierra Leone in the 1790s.[65] Their attempts at seeing African natural resources in a global perspective will be discussed in Chapters 3 and 4, respectively.

---

[62] Osseo-Asare, *Bitter Roots*.

[63] Guillaume Lachenal, *The Lomidine Files: The Untold Story of a Medical Disaster in Colonial Africa*, translated by Noémi Tousignant (Baltimore: Johns Hopkins University Press, 2017).

[64] P. Wenzel Geissler, 'Studying Trial Communities: Anthropological and Historical Inquiries into Ethos, Politics and Economy of Medical Research in Africa', in *Evidence, Ethos and Experiment: The Anthropology and History of Medical Research in Africa*, edited by P. Wenzel Geissler and Catherine Molyneux (New York: Berghahn Books, 2011), 1–28; Paul Wenzel Geissler, Guillaume Lachenal, John Manton and Noémi Tousignant, eds., *Traces of the Future: An Archaeology of Medical Science in Africa* (Bristol: Intellect, 2016).

[65] Hanna Hodacs, 'Local, Universal, and Embodied Knowledge: Anglo-Swedish Contacts and Linnaean Natural History', in *Global Scientific Practice in an Age of Revolutions, 1750–1850*, edited by Patrick Manning and Daniel Rood (Pittsburgh: University of Pittsburgh Press, 2016), 90–104.

Africa, and African medicine, was therefore clearly present in early modern medical thought outside the continent. For example, a central figure in the early eighteenth-century Portuguese popularisation of medical prescriptions from the tropics, João Curvo Semedo, published African treatments alongside Asian and Brazilian ingredients in his books. In other parts of Europe, a German doctor writing about global medical geographical knowledge in the late eighteenth century included Africa in it, although, like Curvo, he had never visited the continent (see Chapter 7). Drawing upon published European sources, he thought it was important to include and deal with Atlantic Africa in detail and place it in a global, comparative framework.

Sources and Methodology

By analysing a variety of written sources, this book argues that, in Angola, along the Gold Coast and in Sierra Leone, indigenous natural medicine was used by and enjoyed widespread popularity among locals and non-Africans alike. Based on the early contacts and long-standing acknowledgements of African natural medicine, knowledge began to be systematised in the latter half of the seventeenth century by slave traders, military officials and missionaries. European attitudes towards African natural medicine were generally positive, although indigenous medical practitioners were occasionally criticised on religious grounds because of their ritual proceedings. Another source of criticism was the arbitrary dosages of medicine used by popular healers.

Like in most studies of Atlantic Africa in the precolonial period, the sources for this book present an asymmetry in that they contain much more information on Europeans than on Africans. Despite this limitation, it would be erroneous to suggest that precolonial African medical practices cannot be studied in the light of European written sources. Although African informants and assistants were rarely put in the spotlight and almost always remained anonymous, their voices can be discerned through a close reading of European sources. While unpublished manuscripts might give clearer hints on how knowledge about African medical practices was constructed, in published works this often has to be read between the lines.

The book surveys mostly Portuguese but also Danish, Dutch and English printed and archival sources. The foremost archival research has taken place in Portugal, and it is strongly present in Chapters 1 and 2 as well as Chapters 5 through 7. At the overseas archive (*Arquivo Histórico Ultramarino*, AHU), the documentation on medical issues includes the governors' and the bishops' reports on health conditions in the colonies of Angola and Benguela, decisions by Luanda's municipal council touching upon hygiene and the nomination of doctors, and occasional letters from Angola's chief physicians. There are also nomination letters of physicians and surgeons, correspondence from the *Misericórdia* brotherhood concerning hospitals and leave requests by soldiers wanting to travel to Brazil or Portugal to treat their illnesses. Accounts of military campaigns also include sporadic references to health and disease in the interior.

Besides the AHU, I have made use of the documentation produced by the Lisbon Inquisition, which had commissioners in Angola. The denunciations received by the Inquisition include information on African healing practices, including notes on the use of medicinal plants and ritual practices. Relatively few denunciations from Angola proceeded to full-scale *processos* or trials. The trial records provide even more detailed accounts of the healing rituals and remedies used in curing illness. The Inquisition sources also reveal the proclivity of Portuguese settlers in Angola to turn to local folk healers when seeking medical assistance.

The Portuguese National Library includes further valuable sources on West-Central African medical history. At least two manuscripts were compiled by Portuguese soldiers on herbal remedies in seventeenth- and eighteenth-century Angola. These texts provide not only listings of the most popular ingredients used in the region, but also information on how diseases were conceptualised by laypeople. The manuscripts are essential for discussing how disease was understood by Central Africans and the Portuguese in this period. They provide clues to studying everyday forms of herbal healing that did not necessarily take place in a highly ritualised setting. They also show that African medical knowledge was circulating, at least to some extent, openly. Although everyday plant remedies were occasionally well-kept secrets, mostly they were freely available to anyone.

Besides the archival documentation, this book relies on published sources such as missionary accounts. Italian Capuchin missionary records are worth underlining for the detailed information they provide on specialist healers and plant remedies. While some missionaries were clearly open to experimenting with African medicinals, others were afraid of the healers' and diviners' powers to heal and harm. When ill, they often suspected that someone had used poison against them. In addition to the Capuchin accounts, the documents compiled by Padre António Brásio in the *Monumenta Missionaria Africana* (*MMA*) series are essential for any scholar of precolonial Atlantic Africa. They provide a wealth of information on issues related to health, disease and medicine.

A few physicians and surgeons also wrote longer treatises on their experiences of treating illnesses in Atlantic Africa. Unlike many amateur botanists, physicians like Aleixo de Abreu, Francisco Damião Cosme and José Pinto de Azeredo were less interested in African healing practices, or at least they did not demonstrate this interest in their writings. Beyond the longer treatises, the documents signed by physicians and surgeons contain very little material on the practice of medicine in Africa. For the most part, these specialists of European medicine remained silent on everyday experiences of health and illness. While this can signify many things, I have interpreted it as powerlessness in the face of disease and death. Until the late nineteenth century, Portuguese physicians simply did not understand or have the means to cure diseases that prevailed in Atlantic Africa. Rather than admitting this in writing to their superiors in European metropoles, they chose to remain silent, employing their therapeutic tools in the best way they could. European doctors stationed in Africa simply did not have an advantage. They fumbled around bleeding and purging patients, which often did more harm than good. This must have been a demoralising experience for many men of medicine, who firmly believed they could help their countrymen and alleviate suffering in a foreign environment. Seeing their fellow Europeans turn to African healers certainly did not raise their spirits.

For other parts of Atlantic Africa, namely the Gold Coast and Sierra Leone, I have mostly drawn upon published sources. Chapter 3 deals with the Gold Coast by concentrating on Dutch and Danish documentation. For Sierra Leone, in Chapter 4, the focus is on the journal of the Swedish botanist Adam Afzelius and the work of an English physician named Thomas Winterbottom. These sources clearly reveal that the Portuguese in West-Central Africa were not the only ones interested in African healing knowledge.

Structure of the Book

The book consists of seven chapters. Chapter 1 discusses medical pluralism and the multiplicity of healing (and harming) specialists. It begins by focusing on conceptions of disease and bodily health in Central African communities. Relying on Inquisitional sources, the chapter then concentrates on ritual practitioners who attracted more attention than those practising everyday acts of herbal healing. At best, these sources provide us with a glimpse into a healer's hut. They also demonstrate that the careers of Angolan healers were characterised by great mobility, meaning that spirit entities could also move from place to place.

In Chapter 2, the focus turns from healing specialists to the materiality of medicine in Angola and Kongo. It delves into substances that gained popularity as medicinals among Europeans and Africans, and it points to the existence of regional and Atlantic markets for medical plants, minerals and animal parts, which were regarded as potent cures. In other words, not only healers but also healing substances were mobile and traversed the Atlantic in addition to being traded locally. Although rare sources, pharmacopoeias compiled by Portuguese officers document the wide variety of substances that were used by healers and common people for self-medication. When used in different cultural settings, the beliefs connected to certain substances changed. Perhaps the most remarkable cross-cultural experiments concerned a plant called *enkasa*, which was used in poison ordeals, but, in the popular Catholicism of the Kingdom of Kongo, became transformed into a sacred tree. In the eighteenth century, the plant turned up as a multipurpose drug in Portugal, where it was also used by a lay exorcist to chase away the Devil.

Chapters 3 and 4 turn from West-Central Africa to the Gold Coast and Sierra Leone. Focusing largely on Dutch, Danish and Swedish documentation, they open with the question of the uniqueness of cross-cultural medical encounters in Portuguese Angola. The evidence is strong that similar processes of medical interaction were taking place in West Africa, where the minuscule European settler population was in constant contact with local go-betweens. For many Europeans, African healers became the first choice when their lives were in danger. Even when African healers were not necessarily the first choice, the medical pluralism of Atlantic African trading communities ensured that there were several possibilities for obtaining a cure, ranging from self-help to European physicians, surgeons and pharmacists or to African herbalists and spirit healers. Finally, these chapters point to the important role of African women in providing access to local sources of healing knowledge.

Chapter 5 returns to West-Central Africa to discuss European healers and medical practices. It demonstrates the state of European healthcare in Luanda and its hinterland, where access to Portuguese doctors was limited and hospitals operated with extremely scant resources. The transfer of European medical knowledge was restricted to the training of African barbers, who had become common in most Portuguese settlements by the end of the eighteenth century. European medical substances enjoyed limited popularity in Angola. However, an American import, cinchona or Peruvian bark, was brought to Angola in substantial quantities. The first documented instances of the use of this antimalarial agent, which was later commercialised as quinine, were recorded in Angola and are analysed here.

Illness and disease are the central foci of Chapter 6, which argues that early modern European and African ways of understanding health and disease were not fundamentally different; rather, there was a great deal of common ground and similarities between the two. This was a prerequisite for meaningful cross-cultural exchanges in the field of health and healing. The chapter explores early modern social diagnoses of diseases. It shows that humoural theory had relatively little influence and only a minor place in West-Central Africa, where physicians were rare. Instead, lay diagnoses and self-medication were common. The chapter closes with a discussion of mental afflictions among West-Central Africans and the Portuguese settlers in Angola, showing that the Atlantic slave trade gave rise to a new disease category that also spread trans-Atlantically to the Americas. The experiences of enslavement and the horrors of the Middle Passage gave rise to a disease called *banzo*, an affliction likened to melancholia by the Portuguese, but perhaps best translated literally as a longing for home.

Chapter 7 focuses on medical geography in the southern Atlantic. It discusses early modern European conceptions of environment and climate in connection to health and disease, showing that both environment and climate were integral components in conceptualising disease patterns in West-Central Africa. Travelling for health, or moving to a more salubrious climate, was a regular feature of migrant experiences in this world. This could mean moving within Africa or travelling from Africa to Brazil or Portugal to seek treatment and recovery from tropical illnesses.

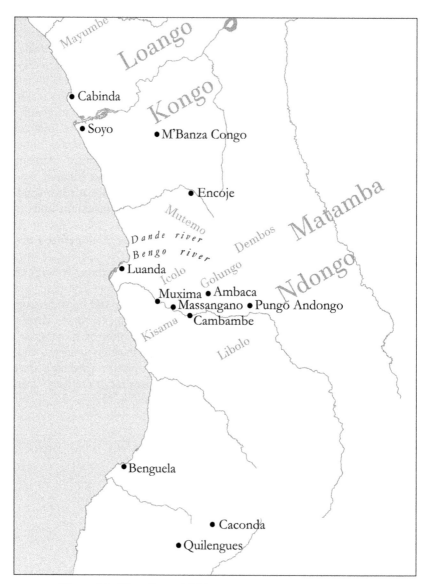

Figure 1.1 West-Central Africa.
Source: Map by Victor Wilson

1   Healing (and Harming) Specialists
Plural Medicine in Angola and Kongo

In 1750, several people were called to testify against Dona Ana Maria Antunes de Almeida and Manoel da Silva Vieira. The couple lived in a consensual union in Icolo, having formerly resided in Golungo. Most of the witnesses, including two priests, hailed from these interior districts in the colony of Angola. Dona Ana Maria was accused of invoking the Devil with pagan rites for an 'illness of her ancestors, which she had inherited'. According to the witnesses, Dona Ana Maria and Vieira had invited black sorcerers (*magicos*) to bring fortune for themselves and to harm their enemies. Among the people who Vieira was accused of harming was Manoel de Souza Manaya, whose murder Vieira had allegedly caused by witchcraft with the help of African witches. Dona Ana Maria, a widow who had been married twice, was claimed to have murdered her two husbands by 'diabolic arts' and to have used magic in order to make Vieira fall in love with her.[1]

The witnesses, all of whom claimed that Dona Ana Maria's and Vieira's infringements were 'public and notorious' throughout the districts of Golungo and Icolo, named several Africans as the accomplices of the accused. They were Francisco de Porto, Antonio Mendes, Antonio Martins, Baxi or Sebastião á Dacala, Sebastião Vicente (also known as Lemba or Calemba),[2] Dom João and Jeronimo. Many of these Africans were designated by the witnesses as *quimbares*, referring to free or freed blacks who lived with whites and usually worked as itinerant traders.[3] From the outset, it was evident that these accusations concerned both healing and harming, with no clear distinction being made between these specialised roles. Markedly, many witnesses referred to these men not only as *magicos*, or sorcerers, but also as surgeons (*cirurgião*), pointing to

---

[1] ANTT, TSO/IL, Processo 13834, Denúncias contra Manuel da Silva Vieira e Ana Antunes de Almeida, passim.
[2] This is possibly a reference to an individual initiated into the *Lemba* healing cult. See Janzen, *Lemba, 1650–1930*.
[3] See Ferreira, *Cross-Cultural Exchange*, 59.

27

their role as healers. One of the religious specialists, Sebastião Vicente, was referred to as a hermaphrodite, and he was also known as Sebastiana. Cross-dressing healer-diviners were known by the title *kimbanda*. They formed a discrete group of religious specialists in Angola and were mentioned in several documentary sources. Choosing to live together in bands, they formed a respected healing society offering a wide variety of spiritual services.[4]

In addition to the male religious specialists, four of Dona Ana Maria's slaves were named as being dedicated to spirits and playing an active role in their adoration. Witnesses pointed to several 'idols' or spirits adored by the accused, explaining that these were the same spirits invoked by pagan Angolans (*gentio deste Reino*). The spirits were Macongo, Kiteri, Muta, Kibuku, Casuto, Ginxi and Sucu. Some of the witnesses also named the spirits Dom Petello and Dom Pedro. Some of these spirits were well known in the interior of Angola. Many witnesses must have implicitly been referring to the spirit Kibuku when claiming that Vieira used black magic to rise in the colonial military hierarchy. Kibuku was known in Mbundu areas as a spirit of good fortune and wealth. Casuto was another well-known spirit in the interior of Angola, which was claimed to cause illness. Macongo was alternately referred to as Muene Congo, implying that it was a spirit of an ancestral ruler. According to one of the witnesses, Captain-Major Lope de Carvalho Fogaça, Sucu was a spirit that brought fortune and wealth.[5]

Music was a central element in the rituals, a way to venerate the spirits. Participants played hand drums (*atabailes*) and other percussion instruments, they sang and they clapped their hands. In possession ceremonies, spirits entered into Dona Ana Maria Almeida, speaking through her mouth while she appeared like a ghost with deformed eyes. They could also enter any of the four female slaves, who would then speak with an altered voice a secret language understood only by other participants. A further element that raised suspicions against Vieira was that he wore string bracelets on his wrists as protective magic.[6]

According to Father Antonio de Sousa Benevides, Dona Ana Maria and Vieira also believed in Zumbi, 'because their understanding is that souls of the other world come to this one, and cause illness and infirmity in living bodies'. Benevides denounced Almeida for consulting the spirits

---

[4] Sweet, *Recreating Africa*, 54–57.
[5] ANTT, TSO/IL, Processo 13834, f. 14v. The folios in this processo have been numbered twice. I am referring to the newer foliation, which includes the first three folios that are not originally numbered.
[6] ANTT, TSO/IL, Processo 13834, passim.

to find out what caused her partner's illness.[7] Another priest, Domingos de Lemos Terra, claimed that Vieira suffered from hearing problems, which, according to the African healer Baxi á Dacala, was caused by the Zumbi of Manoel de Souza Manaya, the man allegedly murdered by Vieira.[8]

Denunciations against Dona Ana Maria and Vieira demonstrate the entanglements of healing and harming spiritual powers in Atlantic Africa. Although these rituals were dramatic, curing did not always entail super-natural elements. This chapter begins with a discussion of concepts related to health and illness in West-Central African societies. It then focuses on the plurality of African healing specialists in the region. Some of the African healers treated everyday occurrences of illness with natural remedies and could be referred to as herbalists. Other healer-diviners focused on treating social ills or so-called diseases of man. Besides offering herbal remedies, their methods often included religious rituals and ceremonial practices similar to the ones allegedly employed by Dona Ana Maria Antunes de Almeida and Manoel da Silva Vieira. Such activities were often scrutinised and investigated by the Inquisitional commissioners in Luanda. The activities of herbalists, on the contrary, rarely led to denunciations to the Portuguese religious or secular author-ities. Methodologically, therefore, the activities and ritual practices of healer-diviners are over-represented in the Inquisition sources, which mostly remain silent on everyday herbalism in Angola.

Health and Illness in West-Central African Societies

Historical linguistics help elucidate ancestral concepts related to health and illness. Many terms pertaining to health and healing are assumed to have been part of the earliest Bantu-speaking societies several thousand years ago. These concepts remained relatively unchanged as populations migrated from their original homelands in West Africa to populate Central, Southern and East African environments. Cognate terms per-taining to therapeutic concepts that appear in one or several major West-Central African language groups – Kikongo, Kimbundu and Umbundu – include, for example:[9]

---

[7] ANTT, TSO/IL, Processo 13834, ff. 4v–5r.

[8] ANTT, TSO/IL, Processo 13834, f. 7r.

[9] John M. Janzen, *Ngoma: Discourses of Healing in Central and Southern Africa* (Berkeley: University of California Press, 1992), 190–210. Asterisks and numbers indicate Guthrie's *Comparative Series* (C.S.) of cognate reconstructions. Malcolm Guthrie, *Comparative Bantu: An Introduction to the Comparative Linguistics and Prehistory of the Bantu Languages*, 4 vols. (Farnborough: Gregg Press, 1967–1971).

C.S. 677 * -dúád- to become ill; C.S. 678 * -dúádì- illness;
C.S. 679 *-dúáídé- illness

C.S. 786 * -gàngà- / * -ngàngà- medicine man, doctor; C.S. 787
* -ganga- medicine

C.S. 1564 * -pód- to become cold, to cool down; C.S. 1565 * -
pód- to become cured, to get well

C.S. 1730 * -tí- medicine; C.S. 990 * -kàg- to protect with
medicine

C.S. 412 * -cúkù- cupping horn; C.S. 440 * -cúmo- cupping
horn; C.S. 439 * -cumik- bleed by cupping; C.S. 700 * -dumik-
bleed by cupping

C.S. 1072 * -kìtì- fetish, charm; C.S. 1073 * -kítì-, or -kíci- spirit

C.S. 1474 * -pémbà- white clay; C.S. 1477 * pémbé- white clay

Recognition of sickness is signalled by the cognate term dúád, or dúádì, whose verb form luala in Kikongo expresses the existential quality of suffering, injury or misfortune. This is differentiated from physical injury or soreness, for which pútá or púté is used. Numerous metaphors are used to refer to health, including 'balance' and 'purity'. The cognate pód, signifying 'to become cool, or cool down' or to 'become well, healthy', stands in contrast to the heat of disease or witchcraft. In Kikongo and Kimbundu, this is related to the action of the cupping horn (mpodì); the cupping horn 'sucks out' (hola mpoka) the impurity. Terms for the cupping horn and for the process of bleeding by cupping in Eastern and Western Bantu dialects suggest that this is an ancient therapy system, although there may have been an even older cognate that is now lost. Sickness and misfortune are also related to the concept of interdiction, prohibition or abstinence. It emerges in the context of ritual activities, initiations or naming, but also with abstinence from specified foods in connection with an ailment or an affliction.[10]

In West-Central Africa and elsewhere on the continent, misfortunes or afflictions stemming from 'natural' or God-given causes are distinguished from those stemming from human involvement. Terms for God are associated with illness and misfortunes that are 'in the order of things', or 'of God'. Unnatural or inauspicious misfortunes are, by contrast, said to be caused by 'people'. In Kikongo, this is expressed as [kimbevo] kia muntu. Human-caused misfortunes could be described by terms related to the use of powerful words and the intentions behind them. In Kikongo, loka signifies the use of powerful words in an oath or curse, and kindoki their imputed use, which is believed to cause sickness

---

[10] Janzen, Ngoma, 64–65.

and misfortune.[11] It is worth noting that the interpretation of illness might change as the illness itself changes through time. Illness episodes interpreted as 'natural' at an early stage might later be explained in terms of sorcery or spirit causes.[12] From the patient's perspective, this meant that in many quotidian occurrences of illness, a herbalist would be sought first, but if the sickness persisted, a different diagnostician would be consulted.

If the use of sorcery was imputed, these diagnostic encounters had to consider the harming register prevalent in Central African societies. In contrast to helpful and beneficent sorcery idioms, witchcraft anxieties and spiritual insecurities were all part of the negative register of vernacular therapeutic practice. Medicines, medicinal charms and power objects were used to curse and harm enemies in politics and everyday life.[13] Further, in many African languages the term for medicine refers to wholesome as well as harmful substances.[14] The attempts to abolish witchcraft by legal means, which were part of the colonial state apparatus in the twentieth century, were still absent (except for the Inquisition) in the early modern period, when the Portuguese and other European settlers in Atlantic Africa commonly shared a belief in magic and sorcery. The ambivalence of 'medicines', broadly defined, to heal and harm is notable in some Inquisitional cases. This ambivalence made healing specialists suspect in the eyes of Portuguese officials and European priests, but it must have been a cause of distrust also for many of the patients. Healers needed to build a reputation as benign, yet powerful, experts in the use of medicinal herbs and charms.

Among the Kongo, in the colonial period common and simple problems like headache, stomach ache, cold, fever or accidental wounds were generally categorised as mild and benign afflictions, and therefore, as 'natural'. They were only suspected to be caused by spiritual beings or living humans if they did not respond to systematic treatment. Minor ailments such as these were typically treated at home or by a specialist called *nganga mbuki*. Perhaps the best English translation for this title would be 'herbalist'. *Nganga mbuki* used medicine (*bilongo*) not connected to *nkisi* objects and spirits. Their curing methods also included scarifications, incisions, bonesetting, steam baths, massage and headpack applications. In contrast to specialists who dealt with problems of

---

[11] Janzen, *Ngoma*, 65. See also David Westerlund, *African Indigenous Religions and Disease Causation: From Spiritual Beings to Living Humans* (Leiden: Brill, 2006).
[12] Feierman, 'Struggles for Control', 77.   [13] Hunt, 'Health and Healing', 385–386.
[14] Susan Reynolds Whyte, 'The Power of Medicines in East Africa', in *The Context of Medicines in Developing Countries: Studies in Pharmaceutical Anthropology*, edited by Sjaak van der Geest and Susan Reynolds Whyte (Dordrecht: Kluwer, 1988), 218.

nkisi and *kindoki, nganga mbuki* were usually tolerated by missions and colonial rulers.[15]

When the Portuguese first encountered foreign medical systems in Atlantic Africa, they immediately found overlaps with Hippocratic-Galenic medicine. The hot/cold distinction of diseases was especially important for cultural translation. Conceptual convergence between African and Hippocratic-Galenic medicine was made possible by the concept of *pód* (to become cold, to cool down or to become cured, to get well), because humouralism recognised excess heat, caused by yellow bile, as a cause of illness. Bloodletting as medical technology was practised in Portugal and elsewhere in Europe not only by the cutting of a vein, but also by cupping. This was done by scratching the surface of the skin and applying a cup to it. A sucking force was introduced either by directly sucking air out of a hole in the base of the cup or by first heating the cup and then letting it cool while attached to the body. But bloodletting was not limited to Europe. On the island of São Tomé, the Portuguese witnessed how the locals used cupping horns to relieve symptoms of fever, which afflicted them especially when cold winds began to blow from the south in June. They applied cupping horns on the forehead and temples and occasionally on the shoulders.[16]

Cupping was also widely used on the other side of the southern Atlantic in Brazil. João Ferreira da Rosa's *Trattado unico da constituiçam pestilencial de Pernambuco* (1694), the first published vernacular medical treatise on colonial Brazil, points to the different kinds of cupping horns used in Recife. Bull's horns were the most widely used. Obviously, this therapeutic practice was used both by surgeons and folk healers. Although he did not specify the ethnic origins of folk practitioners, Rosa specifically referred to female folk healers (*curandeiras*), who operated within a humoural framework and told their patients that the humour drawn out with the cupping horns was the one that had caused the illness. However, Rosa then criticised them for using bull's horns. According to him, surgeons using glass horns performed cupping with much more precision.[17]

Early modern European illness causation resembled African medicine in that disease aetiologies were divided into natural and magical causes. Natural factors, such as the imbalance in the four bodily humours, were

---

[15] Westerlund, *African Indigenous Religions*, 213.

[16] 'Notícias das terras de Guiné', in António Brásio, ed., *Monumenta Missionaria Africana* (subsequently *MMA*), IV: 630–631. On bloodletting in Portugal, see Santos, 'A Arte de Sangrar'.

[17] João Ferreira da Rosa, *Trattado unico da constituiçam pestilencial de Pernambuco* (Lisboa: n. p., 1694), 111.

linked to factors like diet, evacuations, exercise, air, sleep and strong emotions. Hippocratic-Galenic medical knowledge was confronted with social illness causation and popular healing forms. Social illness causation in Europe was intellectually linked to the African idea of 'diseases of man' and was based on the use of spells to harm other people, or in other words, on expressions of antagonism and tension within the community. Magical charms and spells were regarded as potent because the Devil gave them power to work.[18]

Herein lay the common ground between precolonial West-Central African and early modern European concepts of illness, health and healing. When Portuguese and other Europeans fell ill, they turned to indigenous Africans for help in order to obtain local cures. Eventually, this led to compilations of pharmacopoeias in manuscript form. Herbal knowledge also found its way into missionary and travel accounts. The composition of these works was simple and followed a general outline. The African name for the medicinal was followed by instructions on how to use it, for which illnesses it was used and occasionally information on where it could be found. Pharmacopoeias provide copious information on illness and disease in West-Central Africa.[19]

Evidence on the social diagnosis of diseases can be found in pharmacopoeias and travel accounts, which listed local medicines that enjoyed widespread use. These medicinals have been identified and classified by José Pedro Sousa Dias, who listed 124 different drugs based on their composition – animal, vegetable or mineral. In West-Central Africa, these were used to treat almost 100 diseases and injured body parts. Yet, Dias's schematic listing does not address which were the most common afflictions among the local population and European settlers. Neither does it analyse regional or chronological variations in disease prevalence. Most afflictions named in pharmacopoeias and missionary accounts referred to genital-urinary afflictions, venereal and gastrointestinal illnesses, skin diseases and fevers. Antidotes were an important category of herbal remedies, and they were used to cure poisoning and snake bites.[20]

Individual pharmacopoeias compiled by Portuguese officers in the seventeenth and eighteenth centuries (see Chapter 2) could include as many as fifty medicinal substances. They were compiled with the help of

---

[18] David Gentilcore, *Healers and Healing in Early Modern Italy* (Manchester: Manchester University Press, 1998), 6, 21–23.

[19] Although ignoring some primary sources and providing a minimal interpretation, a useful summary of this data can be found in Dias, 'Índice de drogas medicinais'.

[20] Dias, 'Índice de drogas medicinais'.

local herbalists, and although written down by Europeans, the African input weighed heavily in listing the diseases that could be cured with these natural medicines. It is noteworthy that trained physicians for the most part disregarded African healing practices, and the collecting of household remedies was left in the hands of laypersons. The widespread use of plants as antidotes demonstrates that remedies for animal bites were extremely important in local societies. Diseases that abound in Francisco Buitrago's pharmacopeia, composed in the early eighteenth century, include fevers, eye diseases, epilepsy and kidney stones, but more commonly it lists bodily symptoms quite generally: swellings, pain in the stomach or womb, internal sores and headaches. A large percentage of African household medicines clearly concentrated on treating easily definable symptoms.[21]

While most diseases could clearly affect anyone regardless of sex, West-Central Africans acknowledged a gendered aspect of medicine by pointing to medicinals that were especially useful in treating women's health complaints. These were generally related to menstruation, childbirth and abortions. West-Central African women were known to use abortifacients. The best-known case concerns the Kongo prophet Dona Beatriz Kimpa Vita, whose position as a leader of a religious movement was undermined by her pregnancy in 1705. She had formed a close relationship with a man named João Barro, and twice had recourse to abortive medicine. On the third occasion, however, it failed to work.[22] In the late eighteenth century, the Portuguese recognised one of the local abortifacients as a plant called *matangas suesue*. According to a contemporary description, this powerful and forceful remedy caused an immediate abortion.[23]

The question is, to what extent did cross-cultural interaction lead to convergence in African and European medicine during the era of the Atlantic slave trade? Linguistic changes give some indication of the translations and adaptations that resulted from medical encounters. Cannecattim's early nineteenth-century Kimbundu dictionary indicates that the Portuguese word for fever (*febre*) had become a loan word (*febele*)

---

[21] For a detailed listing of remedies in Buitrago's pharmacopeia, see Appendix A.

[22] John K. Thornton, *The Kongolese Saint Anthony: Dona Beatriz Kimpa Vita and the Antonian Movement, 1684–1706* (Cambridge: Cambridge University Press, 1998), 166.

[23] Simon, 'A Luso-African Formulary', 113–114. The original document, which I have consulted to confirm Simon's mistranscription of *Matangas Suesue*, is in Arquivo Histórico Ultramarino, Conselho Ultramarino (subsequently AHU, CU), Angola, Cx. 68, Doc. 56 [Doc. 5937], Oficio do capitão de granadeiros de Luanda, Álvaro Carvalho Matoso ao secretário de Estado do da Marinha e Ultramar, Martinho de Melo e Castro, 24 March 1784.

in Kimbundu. Fevers were further divided into malign, continuous, small and intermittent types.[24] Assis Junior's twentieth-century dictionary offers another clue to the transformations that had taken place. He defined the Kimbundu word *ndúa* as diseases caused by excess blood.[25] The proto-Bantu term C.S. 677 * -*dúád*- signifies 'to become ill', but it acquired a new connotation as a result of therapeutic interaction. In a European humoural framework, illness was treated primarily by bloodletting and purging. As Cannecattim's and Assis Junior's dictionaries show, there were numerous Kimbundu expressions for different illnesses. Cannecattim distinguished only between illness (*uh'achi* or *mah'achi*), headache, sore throat, pain in the womb and an ache in the legs. Assis Junior's dictionary demonstrates a larger variety and more precise (biomedical) translations of the names of diseases. The same applies to Bentley's late nineteenth-century dictionary of Kikongo, which lists thirty-nine different diseases.[26]

Inside a Healer's Hut

Much like Dona Ana Maria's and Vieira's case, another Inquisition trial preceding theirs contained the same dramatic elements: harming by witchcraft, healing by spirit possession. Captain-major of Ambaca, João Pereira da Cunha, his Angolan concubine, Catarina Juliana, and the couple's slaves were taken to Lisbon for trial in 1750.[27] Cunha was accused of adoring the spirits Muta, Gangazumba and Kibuku. He had allegedly killed his predecessor by poisoning or witchcraft and hired local sorcerers to protect him from misfortune. Cunha passed away soon after arriving in Lisbon, and his trial never really commenced. However, following lengthy investigations in Angola, he was posthumously deemed innocent.

João Pereira da Cunha's partner, Catarina Juliana, was given her own trial. Her confession from 1758 included a detailed description of a *xinguila*'s ritual practice in the interior of Angola. Catarina related how, in the mid-1740s, while living in Ambaca, she had suffered from a swelling and had gone to visit a free black named Matheus Capichi.

---

[24] Bernardo Maria de Cannecattim, *Diccionario da lingua bunda, ou angolense, explicada na portugueza, e Latina* (Lisbon: Impressão Regia, 1804), 411. Cf. W. Holman Bentley, *Dictionary and Grammar of the Kongo Language* (London: Baptist Missionary Society, 1887), 82, which translates ague fever to *mvuka* in Kikongo.

[25] A. de Assis Junior, *Dicionário Kimbundu-Português: Linguístico, Botânico, Histórico e Corográfico* (Luanda: Argente, Santos & C.ª, n.d.), 35.

[26] Bentley, *Dictionary and Grammar*, 501.

[27] These trials are studied in detail in Kananoja, 'Healers, Idolaters, and Good Christians'.

Matheus directed Catarina to the house of Esperança, who was a *xinguila*
by profession. Esperança told Catarina that her sickness was caused by
two spirits, Kibuku and Muta. The healer called on people to gather in
her house, and they began a spirit possession ceremony. Esperança,
entranced, performed a dance Catarina called the *calandúz* and called
on the spirits Kibuku and Muta. After the dance, she killed a chicken and
mixed its blood with some herbal powders. She applied this potion to
Catarina, who did not immediately experience any improvement in her
condition. The treatment was continued, however, and Esperança made
four visits to Catarina's home, bringing her herbal medicine, which she
mixed with castor oil and applied.[28]

In connection with João Pereira da Cunha's and Catarina Juliana's
trials, several African sorcerers were arrested in or near Ambaca and sent
to Lisbon, where their trials never progressed. However, their houses
were searched at the time of the arrest and their wealth was confiscated.
Three of the sorcerers had significant collections of religious items and
natural medicines (Table 1.1). These inventories provide an invaluable
glimpse inside a healer's hut and into the everyday life of popular healers
in Ambaca.

As is clear, Muta was the spirit that connected the three men, as they
all had items dedicated to it. However, none of them mentioned items
dedicated to Kibuku. Muta, or Muta Kalombo, was venerated in the
interior of Angola as a personal spirit related to hunting, warfare and
fire.[29] Macongo, which was mentioned as one of the spirits adored by
Dona Ana Maria and Vieira, was apparently also adored by João Pedro. It
may well have been one of the seventeenth-century ancestors and may
refer to a person who was once an Umbundu lord, or a spirit of the
hunt.[30] João Pedro had a special connection to this spirit, as objects
pertaining to Macongo were the most numerous. He also adored Vunji,
which might have referred to an ancestral spirit from Matamba.[31]

[28] Kananoja, 'Healers, Idolaters, and Good Christians', 460. Giovanni Antonio Cavazzi da
Montecuccolo, *Istorica descrizione de tre regni Congo, Matamba et Angola* (Bologna:
Giacomo Monti, 1687), 221–223, noted that any man or woman could become a
xinguila, but usually spirit possession was manifested in 'important persons'. In
Kongo, Luca da Caltanisetta described a similar spirit medium, called *nganga ngombo*.
Luca da Caltanisetta, *Diaire Congolais (1690–1701)*, translated from Italian by François
Bontinck (Louvain: Éditions Nauwelaerts, 1970), 103.
[29] Defined, however, as a 'god of aquatic animals' in Oscar Ribas, *Ilundo: Divindades e ritos
angolas* (Luanda: Museu de Angola, 1958), 69.
[30] Jan Vansina, personal communication, 5 and 13 November 2009.
[31] Jan Vansina, personal communication, 13 November 2009. Ribas, *Ilundo*, 82, defines
Vunji as a 'goddess of justice'.

Table 1.1 *Items confiscated from three African healers in 1750 and the spirits they pertained to*[1]

João Pedro Macollo	*Macongo*	• *gonguinha* filled with a black feather, five bones, a rosary of shells, pale brown powder and a piece of wood Dedicated to no particular spirit • *pemba* reserved for his prayers
Muta Kalombo • *macua* (calabash shell) • buffalo tail	• three charm packages in pots (*basouras*) with red and white legs • *gonguinha* (small clapperless bell) filled with pale brown powder and five bones and shells • *gonguinha* filled with feathers and a shell, rosary made of shells, nine small bones and packs of red and brown powder	
Vunji • buffalo horn filled with black powder, with two skins and a shell encircled by pieces of bark from a *mulemba* tree		
Felipe Dias Chaves *Muta Kalombo* • belt with a leather pouch attached, containing black powder, two small horns, three iron rings and two bones (all *mandingas*, according to Chaves)	• *macua* • buffalo tail Dedicated to no particular spirit • two pouches containing cards with drawings of 'demons' • a monkey's skull for curing headaches	• black, pale brown and red powders for curing sores on feet • *pemba* reserved for his prayers
Danla á Tango *Muta* • horn of *quihoé* and in it tied two skins, one of *cabindo* and another of *caxingia*, which are mandingas and in it a belt of skin of *sengui* Dedicated to no particular spirit • a bell with red powders, which he said were *quilembas* against paralysis • a *Luanda* and two skins of *caxingia* and an amulet of *sengui* and a hummingbird, which he said were all for women giving birth to twins and called it *cacullo e cabassa*	• a human tooth • an amulet (*xillo*) of *inta*, which he said was from *sonna Kibundo* • four *mocotes* of antelope that he said was medicine for *huene huene* • a jaguar's nail of *gombo*, used when performing spirit possession (*xinguilão*) • six small pieces of wood, which are '*banzes*' for a successful march (trip) • a cord attached to a piece of wood • a twisted straw meant to protect children from the wind • an egg of *perdir* for protection	• a small pack of powder to apply on eyebrows • two knots of wood, which he said were worn to cover his body • two beaks of *cossa* called *bambis*, whistles used to scare away birds from their fields by virtue of the Devil • two small whistles to prevent children from dying • two small bones from a cripple to cure diphtheria • a bone from a jaguar and an antelope to cure diphtheria • *mucollos* or cables, which he said were his

Table 1.1 (*cont.*)

• a pack of yellow powders 'for lunch' • a pack of black powders to apply on eyebrows • another pack of black powders 'for lunch'	• four pegs of wood, two with feathers, one red and the other white, which he said were of Lufaco	• a piece of *hucuso* to be used when beginning his devilries • five pieces of *curida* said to heal neck pain

[1] ANTT, TSO/IL, Processo 10120, Processo de João Pedro Macollo, 9r–10r; ANTT, TSO/IL, Processo 14150, Processo de Felipe Dias Chaves, 4r–4v; ANTT, TSO/IL, Processo 14150, Processo de Danla á Tango, 7r–8r.

Of the three arrested healers, most items were confiscated from Danla á Tango. Only one of them was identified as being dedicated to Muta, but the rest were not connected to any particular spirit, or at least such connections were not documented. Some items, such as the whistles to prevent children from dying or the jaguar's nail used in spirit possession ceremonies, clearly had magical uses. Others were part of Angola's rich folk pharmacopoeia (see Chapter 2) and used to treat specific bodily disorders. Powders to apply on eyebrows were possibly used to cure fevers and headaches. While it is clear that Danla á Tango relied on magical rituals to heal and divine, he could perhaps best be referred to as a healer-herbalist, who also offered everyday remedies to ailing people. All three arrested healers were versed in local idioms of healing and practised in local circumstances. Despite their contact with Portuguese settlers, the items inventoried in their huts demonstrate no global medical influences, unless one counts the rosary of shells confiscated from João Pedro Macollo as a hybrid item.

The term *pemba*,[32] which the witnesses in the Inquisition trials referred to as white clay, had several meanings in Central Africa. It played an important role in West-Central African spirit possession ceremonies. Several of the witnesses who denounced Dona Ana Maria and Vieira said that participants in spirit possession rituals smeared their bodies with *pemba* and put it on their tongue.[33] Similarly, *pemba* was confiscated

---

[32] In Kikongo, *pemba* signifies 'to become white', whereas *mpemba* signifies 'marks of pipe-clay' and *mpembe* 'whiteness, pallor'. *Pemba* is also used for drawing the lines that identify the areas of vibration of the spiritual entities. See Victor Turner, *The Forest of Symbols: Aspects of Ndembu Ritual* (Ithaca, NY and London: Cornell University Press, 1967), 65–66; William W. Megenney, 'Sub-Saharan Lexicon in Afro-Brazilian Cantigas de Pretos Velhos (Umbanda) as Clues to Slave Demography', *Iberoromania* 45 (1997): 32.

[33] ANTT, TSO/IL, Processo 13834, passim.

from the three men who were accused of sorcery and of being João Pereira da Cunha's accomplices in Ambaca. It referred not only to white clay, but also to kaolin and manioc flour. Significantly, the German naturalist Friedrich Welwitsch mentions stone material known as *pedra pemba* found in several mountainous districts of Angola, including Golungo, where Dona Ana Maria and Vieira lived. According to Welwitsch, who was active in Angola in the 1850s, the powder ground from this mineral had a very important social and domestic role in the lives of Angolans. It was mixed into the majority of remedies used by blacks and used in various types of fetishes buried in the ground or exposed in caverns. It was also used for painting bodies and houses.[34]

In West-Central Africa, the colour white was a conspicuous feature in most rituals of healing. It was either employed as the only colour element or else in combination with red. In early twentieth-century Kongo, *nkisi* (pl. *minkisi*) spirits were the objects of domination and manipulation by humans, which was made possible through their material incarnation in man-made objects. They were mainly used to treat illness. Rituals that contained white as the only colour element were used to treat diseases that were in some way connected with the *simbi* spirits. The white *minkisi* of healing were all classified as water *minkisi*, or in other words, as *minkisi* containing a *simbi* spirit from the water. There were five *minkisi* in this category: Mbwanga, Nsonde, Musansi bitutu, Nkita and Mukisi nsi. These water *minkisi* were believed to cure headache, depression and madness, epilepsy, leprosy, swellings and boils all over the body, stomach complaints and swollen eyes and legs. These white *minkisi* contained chalk among the ingredients, but not the colours red or black.[35]

White and red could also be used concurrently in connection with the curing of certain diseases. The illnesses thought to have been caused by witches or wizards (*bandoki*), or by the most powerful spirits of the most distant ancestral origin, were always cured by rituals or *minkisi* in which white and red were found together, mixed with the medicine. A common procedure in curing illnesses caused by witches was to consult the healer of a certain *nkisi* specialising in these types of diseases. *Nkisi Kula* was the most common *nkisi* used in connection with the treatment. *Kula* consisted of a large bundle containing many small bags of cloth filled with chalk, yellow or red ochre, and medicines. Some of the bags also

[34] Frederico (Friedrich) Welwitsch, *Synopse explicative das amostras de madeiras e drogas medicinaes e de outros objectos mormente ethnographicos* (Lisbon: Imprensa Nacional, 1862), 25–26.
[35] Anita Jacobson-Widding, *Red–White–Black as a Mode of Thought: A Study of Triadic Classification by Colours in the Ritual Symbolism and Cognitive Thought of the Peoples of the Lower Congo* (Uppsala: Acta Universitatis Upsaliensis, 1979), 199–203.

contained pungent red pepper. The ill body was struck or massaged with the bags of cloth, so that the burning pepper penetrated into the skin and disturbed the spirit that had taken possession of the ill person. The treatment of a person thought to have been attacked by a witch began with the healer giving the sick person medicine to drink and to smear on his or her body. Relatives and other participants in the ritual then began to sing, make invocations and fall into ecstasy while the sick person was massaged with banana stalks. This was done in order to squeeze out the spirit possessing the body.[36]

The use of a white substance in a spirit possession ceremony was observed by eight soldiers sent on an errand by the captain-major of the *presídio* of Massangano in 1719. On the estate owned by Dona Catherina Correa, the soldiers heard noise generated by a large gathering of people. They encircled the place and saw that the people were 'invoking the demon'. When they were detected, most of the participants managed to run away, including the 'master' in charge of the ceremony. The soldiers arrested a free black woman named Domingas de João and a slave named José Correa, who belonged to the owner of the estate. She told the soldiers that the ritual was arranged to cure her son, who had been caught by a *zumbi*. The soldiers found a bag of medicine left by the healer. They also saw that an abundance of food and drink had been prepared for the ritual.

For the purposes of the ritual, Domingas and other people were 'smeared with various things' and covered with flour.[37] Although *pemba* was not specifically mentioned in this case, it is likely that the white flour would have been designated as *pemba* by the locals who witnessed the ritual. In form, the ritual followed the rule that the chief participants were made to appear white, in this case by using manioc flour. Although the ritual was led by a healer, the 'master' who managed to run away, it seems that Domingas had an equally important role in it. Both she and José Correa, who seems to have been a mere onlooker present at the ceremony, were sent to a prison in Luanda. The jailer was baffled by his new prisoners, writing to the Inquisition and wanting to know what he was supposed to do with the two and 'so many other blacks, who have been arrested during recent years for the same reason'.[38]

---

[36] Jacobson-Widding, *Red–White–Black*, 232–238.

[37] ANTT, TSO/IL, Caderno do Promotor 94, ff. 375r–387r.

[38] ANTT, TSO/IL, Caderno do Promotor 94, ff. 387. An earlier provision in the year 1703 decreed that prisoners whose cases pertained to ecclesiastical jurisdiction were to be placed in public jail in Luanda. See 'Provisão determinando que, emquanto se não fizesse o Aljube, os presos da Jurisdição Eclesiastica fossem internados nas Cadêas

After returning to Lisbon, the Capuchin missionary Frei Joseph de Modena gave his deposition of this case to the Inquisition in 1721. When asked to explain the term *zumbi* to the Inquisitors, he answered that it was a belief that a sickness, which had 'come naturally', was caused by 'a soul of one of the ancestors' of the sick person. In other words, that is what the healers told their patients in order to extract payment in kind from them. The patients duly offered a banquet to appease the *zumbi*, but in Modena's view the only purpose of the ritual was to invoke the demon. Modena also noted that despite the remedies applied by the healers, the patients often died. Although Modena had not encountered another ritual in which the participants would have been covered with flour, he did mention that 'on some occasions the blacks paint their throat, chests, and backs' with something called 'Mono-Mono'.[39]

Attributing sickness to spiritual forces – a so-called disease of man – was a common explanation for illness in West-Central Africa and elsewhere on the continent among speakers of the Bantu languages. In a medical context, *zumbi* generally referred to unsatisfied ancestral spirits. Already in the seventeenth century, chronicler António de Oliveira de Cadornega recorded that sick people commonly expressed their malady by saying that a *zumbi* had entered them or infected them. People were often very cautious of all signs referring to *zumbi*, for example the appearance of their ancestors or any other dead people in their dreams. If the dead appeared in dreams, it was taken as a sign that they had come to fetch the person into the Other World. To avert this, a sacrificial offering was made at the grave of the ancestor.[40]

In the denunciations made to the Inquisition from Angola, it was often said that people suffered from *zumbi*. A number of cases from the 1710s and 1720s concerned people who the healers had 'diagnosed' with *zumbi*. One of the best-known cases is that of a black soldier named Antônio de Freitas Galvão, who in 1720 sought a cure for a hernia, which had bothered him for several years. A healer from Dombe suggested that Galvão, who had already sought a variety of remedies in Benguela, heal himself by using local methods. The healer convinced Galvão that his hernia was caused by the *zumbi* of his deceased wife. In order to appease her spirit, Galvão organised a ceremony in his house with drummers and dancers. Along with his slaves and children, numerous people

Publicas, 20 de Maio de 1703', *Arquivos de Angola*, First Series, 2: 9–10 (1936): 145–146.

[39] ANTT, TSO/IL, Caderno do Promotor 94, ff. 371–373.

[40] António de Oliveira de Cadornega, *História geral das guerras angolanas* (Lisbon: Agência Geral das Colónias, 1940, 1942), I: 370 and III: 262.

participated in the ritual. He sacrificed a calf that was eaten by the participants. The priest in charge of the investigation noted in his conclusion that in all the *sertões* of Angola, both baptised and non-Christian blacks healed their infirmities with 'superstition and heathen rites', a practice that missionaries preaching in the *sertão* could not eradicate.[41]

Plurality and Mobility of African Healing Specialists

The primary responsibility of popular healers was safeguarding the health of communities and individuals. Besides their ritual expertise, they were esteemed for their knowledge of medicinal plants and herbal cures for illness and diseases. In addition to the already mentioned *xinguilas*, who specialised in spirit possession rituals, there were numerous other specialist healers with different titles. Some provided protective magic, others specialised in healing a certain illness and some merely predicted whether cures would be successful or not. As anthropologists have shown, societies across Africa continue to rely on generalists and specialists attending to internal medicine, broken bones, joint pains, fevers, childbirth complications, and an array of complex problems.[42]

According to Capuchin Father Giovanni Antonio Cavazzi (Table 1.2), among those offering protective magic were specialists with the title *ntinu-a-maza*, who were also known as 'kings of water'. They hid amulets in the bottom of rivers and made them reappear on the surface by throwing a gourd or another open container into the water. These amulets were then distributed to their followers as the most potent *nkisi* against all diseases. *Nconi* and *nzazi* were healers, who made their clients follow sets of taboos in order to regain health. *Nzazis* used four small statues and a bell in their ceremonies. Some healers focused only on certain ailments. For example, a *ngodi* was responsible for treating the deaf, but, according to Cavazzi, they never succeeded. Perhaps more important were healers titled *nsambi*, who treated a common disease resembling leprosy. They offered the sick a cup from which they drank first; then they said that the sick were cured thanks to their lips having made contact with the liquid. However, a more plausible reason for their success lay in their use of the bark of a certain tree, which, when ground and spread on the skin, produced a cure. Without specifying their specialties or methods, Cavazzi also listed healers titled *makuta*, *matamba*, *ngulungu* and *mbazi*.[43]

---

[41] ANTT, TSO/IL, Caderno do Promotor 92, ff. 235–285. See also Ferreira, *Cross-Cultural Exchange*, 182–184.
[42] Olsen and Sargent, 'Introduction', 5.   [43] Cavazzi, *Istorica descrizione*, 81–84.

Table 1.2 *Titles and functions of West-Central African healing specialists in Cavazzi*[1]

Title	Function(s)
nganga-ia-nzumbi	priest of the spirits
Xinguilas	spirit possession, healing
ntinu-a-maza (kings of water)	preparing amulets against all diseases
Nconi	healing, restoring patients to health by following prohibitions (taboos)
Nzazi	healing, restoring patients to health by following prohibitions (taboos)
Ngodi	treating the deaf
Nsambi	treating a disease resembling leprosy
Makuta	not specified
Matamba	not specified
Ngulungu	not specified
Mbazi	not specified
nganga-itiki	receiving offerings from the sick and placing them in shrines; collecting the first rain after the dry season and selling it as medicine

[1] Cavazzi, *Istorica descrizione*, 69–83.

Offerings to spirits were an integral part of healing an illness. According to Cavazzi, a religious specialist called a *nganga-itiki* was responsible for receiving the offerings from the sick and for placing them on altars in front of the statues of spirits. The statues included images of men and women, representing ancestral spirits, and of animals and monsters, depending on the traditions prevailing in the community. The *nganga-itiki* was responsible for establishing the days for the sacrifices. In addition, this religious specialist collected the first rainwater after the dry season and sold it as a remedy against misfortune.[44]

Among important West-Central African healing societies were the *Kimpasi*, which proliferated in Kongo in the seventeenth and eighteenth centuries. *Kimpasi* was a kind of social remedy, a secret society that sought to help a community or a group of communities suffering from calamities and problems. The initiates experienced ritual death, from which they emerged with a new identity.[45] In the 1660s, Christian Kongo elite took drastic measures to prevent the *Kimpasi* from spreading. They

[44] Cavazzi, *Istorica descrizione*, 71.
[45] See Anne Hilton, *The Kingdom of Kongo* (Oxford: Clarendon Press, 1985), 26–28; Thornton, *The Kongolese Saint Anthony*, 56–58.

ordered the seizure of *nkisi* and meted out severe penalties for *Kimpasi* initiates, and the Capuchins burned innumerable *nkisi* and *Kimpasi* enclosures. After the persecution, many former *Kimpasi* initiates affirmed their Christian faith.[46] During his eight-year stay in Kongo in the late eighteenth century, missionary Rafael de Castelo de Vide encountered *Kimpasi* houses that had never disappeared completely despite missionary efforts in the seventeenth century. According to Castelo de Vide, *Kimpasi* houses were places where many people, enticed by '*feiti-ceiros*' or sorcerers, went to seek cures for illness.[47]

Between those of Cavazzi and Castelo de Vide, one finds P. Giuseppe Monari da Modena's account of healers in the 1710s. Residing in West-Central Africa between 1711 and 1713, Monari recorded his reminiscences in 1723, possibly basing them on a manuscript he had written earlier. He noted that in each Kongo village (*libata*), there were male and female 'masters of medicine' who were very good doctors. Among the Mbundu, he reported three classes of 'surgeons' – the good, the wicked and the bad. Monari's use of the term 'surgeon' indicates that even Capuchin priests gave some credibility to African popular healers; they were not mere sorcerers and witches. However, it is clear from Monari's account that the 'surgeons' he described as good might better be termed herbalists. Their methods of using baths, herbs and roots were based on experience. They healed in the open without using secret words or ceremonies. Herbalists were above suspicion and did not constitute a threat to Catholic religion. The wicked ones, however, pretended to know what they did not know. They used superstitious words and actions, but the positive results of their healing activities were always based on the work of nature. They always carried a sack of various medicines with them, which they randomly mixed. According to Monari, the bad healers were the ones who invoked spirits and tried to keep their practice secret, although they also used natural remedies. Fearing arrest, they avoided being seen by white men and preferred lonely and hidden places to perform their rituals. They were often regarded as very powerful healer-diviners who had the gift of seeing into the future.[48]

Monari's moral taxonomy outlined the plurality of African popular healers from a Catholic perspective. Although motivated by the

---

[46] Hilton, *The Kingdom of Kongo*, 196.

[47] Academia das Ciências de Lisboa, Série Vermelha de Manuscritos, 396, *Viagem do Congolo, do Missionário Frei Rafael de Castello de Vide Hoje Bispo de S. Thomé*, 185–186, 190–191.

[48] P. Evaristo Gatti, ed., *Sulle terre e sui mari: Cavalieri di S. Francesco* (Parma: Cappuccini Prov. di Parma, 1931), 158–160.

Capuchin's religious fervour, it makes a clear distinction between everyday herbalism and secret spiritual practices. It also demonstrates that African popular healers could enjoy a status comparable to physicians and surgeons even in European eyes. It echoes an earlier textual source concerning Benguela. Its unidentified author insisted that among Africans living in Benguela were 'great herbalists and doctors, who possessed natural experience of the quality of the herbs'.[49] This is the only reference I have found in early modern Portuguese sources concerning Angola that employs the term herbalist (*erbolario*).

Beyond general descriptions and anecdotal evidence on the plurality of healers contained in Capuchin sources, information on the activities of healers and diviners in West-Central Africa can be gleaned from sporadic denunciations made to the Inquisition. Following an edict published by the Inquisition and distributed in Luanda, a batch of denunciations was collected in the town's Jesuit college in 1698 and 1699.[50] Of the eleven denunciations, seven dealt with healers or diviners. Six of the denouncers were slaves, with two of them being slaves of the Jesuits and the others owned by individual whites. Two of the denouncers were free blacks and only three were white.

Witnesses who had personally dealt with popular healers rarely wanted to admit that they had taken the initiative in seeking help from healers. This was the case with João Inácio, the first of the Jesuits' slaves, who had sought a healer to find a cure for his wife Izabel Inácio, also a slave at the college. João himself was occupied at the college as a *barbeiro*[51] and *sangrador*, or medical officer, who administered bloodletting to his patients. At his wife's request, he had called a Mbundu 'surgeon' to divine the cause of her illness. The healer had performed his ceremonies 'with his hands' and said that the infirmity was called *casuto*. He gave Izabel some herbs to cook in a pot filled with water. She then washed herself with the herbal medicine.[52]

---

[49] 'São grandes erbolarios e médicos, pela natural experiência que teem pela qualidade das hervas.' Luciano Cordeiro, ed., *1617–1622: Benguella e seu sertão por um anonymo* (Lisbon: Imprensa Nacional, 1881), 18.

[50] ANTT, TSO/IL, Caderno do Promotor 72, ff. 31r–58r, 296r–303v. Although I have not located this edict, one of the witnesses mentions that he had already witnessed and confessed to seeing some African religious ceremonies 'muito antes de se publicar o edital do Sancto Officio' (much before the publication of the edict by the Holy Office). ANTT, TSO/IL, Caderno do Promotor 72, f. 47v.

[51] *Barbeiro*, although translated as barber, was a slave with rudimentary training in European medical practice, which was often limited to bleeding the patients.

[52] ANTT, TSO/IL, Caderno do Promotor 72, ff. 43r–45v. See also Ferreira, *Cross-Cultural Exchange*, 182.

In his denunciation, João Inácio did not explain what *casuto* meant, or at least it was not recorded by the Jesuit scribe. However, *casuto* seems to have been a well-known spirit or deity in the Ganguela province of Matamba and was described by Cavazzi in the seventeenth century. In Ganguela, there was a healer-diviner (*xinguila*) devoted to the spirit Casuto. The *xinguila* had a large calabash called *iaco*, and one could pass a hand through its mouth. The *xinguila* first put small items on the bottom of the calabash and then added the bones, hooves and tails of sacrificial goats, chicken and dogs to it. These were mixed with olive oil and the juice of datura and distributed to the sick to be used as seasoning in their cooking. If the illness was serious, the bones were crushed and used as anointment on the painful parts of the body or as face paint.[53]

João Inácio revealed that the healer-diviner he had called for was a slave named Hieronimo, whose origins were not revealed. However, Cavazzi's account indicates that adoration of *casuto* had originated in Matamba. It would have spread to Luanda with slaves imported from the interior. João's statement also reveals that Central-African paradigms of therapeutic practice had remained dominant for baptised slaves owned by whites, even by Jesuit priests, in Luanda. The fact that João worked in medical practice as taught to him by Jesuits and still invited a popular healer to his house shows that he did not fully trust European medical practices. Furthermore, by adopting the Portuguese term 'surgeon' to designate the healer, he was placing Hieronimo's healing arts on equal standing with European practices.

Hieronimo's owner was Captain Manoel Simões Colaço, one of the richest and most influential merchants in Luanda. It is possible that he had purchased the healer on purpose to treat his slaves. This would have been a fairly common practice in the southern Atlantic world, where Brazilian slave owners often employed African healers as the primary medical specialists to take care of illnesses that slaves suffered from. This general trend began in the colonial period and persisted in imperial Brazil into the nineteenth century. For example, one of the best-known African healers in mid-nineteenth-century Bahia was Anacleto Urbano da Natividade, who was originally from Yorubaland. During a cholera epidemic in 1855, he treated people in their homes and also healed his owner's family members.[54]

Among the denounced, there were some slaves who had sought help from healers in order to cure their masters. Bernardino Correa da Gama,

[53] Cavazzi, *Istorica descrizione*, 233.
[54] Fayette Wimberly, 'The Expansion of Afro-Bahian Religious Practices in Nineteenth-Century Cachoeira', in *Afro-Brazilian Culture and Politics: Bahia, 1790s to 1990s*, edited by Hendrik Kraay (Armonk: M. E. Sharpe, 1998), 82–84. For colonial Brazil, see, e.g., Sweet, *Domingos Álvares*; Kananoja, 'Pai Caetano Angola'.

one of the white witnesses, denounced five of his slaves who had hired a Mbundu 'surgeon' named Thomé de Angonga from Massangano. Bernardino, however, had driven the healer away because he believed that Africans divined with 'diabolic arts'. Bernardino had inherited the five slaves from his father, Bernardo Correa, and it is reasonable to ask whether the slaves had similarly called a healer to treat their former master with his approval.[55] In a similar vein, the slaves of the widow Antonia de Sá sought to cure a child of their master. They were denounced by a slave named Domingas de Duarte, who related how she and other female slaves named Izabel, Mariana and Maria had sought out a healer. Either the slaves considered African therapeutic practices more potent than those brought to Luanda by the Portuguese or they could not afford to consult Portuguese medical practitioners. Izabel was nursing her master's daughter and called a '*feiticeiro* of the *sertão*' or a 'sorcerer from the backcountry' to divine the cause of the child's illness. The healer asked for a twined basket and maize flour and began a divination ceremony, speaking out words that Domingas did not understand. The diviner made the basket move in circles and, after the ceremony, gave herbal medicine to apply as a cure for the child.[56]

Following John Janzen, the slaves who were seeking help from healers for someone else's illness could be termed a 'therapy managing group'. In anthropological fieldwork carried out in the 1960s and 1970s, Janzen observed that '[t]he management of illness and therapy by a set of close kin is a central aspect of the medical scene in central Africa'. The therapy managing group of kinsmen or their advocates came into being whenever an individual or set of individuals became ill or was confronted with overwhelming problems.[57] Historical evidence from West-Central Africa suggests that therapy managing groups were meaningful in Angola throughout the seventeenth and eighteenth centuries. The therapy managing group exercised a brokerage function between the sufferer and the specialist, and for many Portuguese who fell ill in Angola they undoubtedly facilitated access to local healers.

Only one of the witnesses came to confess to having actually used the services of a healer to cure his own malady. Alexandre, a free black fisherman from Luanda, told how he had once been on a business trip in Libolo, which he called 'heathen lands'. He had hurt his leg and, being in great pain, decided to call for a local healer. The healer told Alexandre that he could not treat him before divining the cause of the illness, which

[55] ANTT, TSO/IL, Caderno do Promotor 72, ff. 31r–32v.
[56] ANTT, TSO/IL, Caderno do Promotor 72, ff. 298r–298v.
[57] Janzen, *The Quest for Therapy*, 4.

he commenced to do by conducting ceremonies 'with a pan'. The healer told Alexandre that his illness was 'inherited from his parents' and was called *miginga* in the language of the healer. However, the medicine did not have the desired effect because the pain in the leg continued to bother Alexandre. The healer was named Domingos and he was from the region of Ambaca, although Alexandre did not know the name of his village.[58]

Other slaves also confessed to being present at healing ceremonies. This was the case with Gregório de Pascoal, owned by a priest named João Rodrigues da Rocha. He confessed that a neighbour named Victoria had called him to participate in the sacrifice of a goat in service to and veneration of a dead ancestor. Gregorio called the diviners in charge of the ceremony 'Mbundu surgeons, who divine the cause of illness and other things'. He referred to Victoria as a 'surgeon' and a 'master of divination' who was consulted by many people seeking a cure for their illnesses. More than thirty people had watched the sacrifice of the goat, three of them also belonging to the same priest as Gregorio. All of them had eaten the sacrificed goat. Tellingly, Victoria's owner was identified as Sergeant-Major Inácio Matozo de Andrade. Here, then, is another case of a Portuguese officer owning an enslaved African healer.[59]

Finally, a similar sacrifice had taken place on one of the Jesuit estates in the district of Bengo. This was relayed by Matheos Sebastião, another slave of the college. He had seen how a free black healer named Paulo Cambundo, a resident in Bengo, and his diviner comrades, who lived in 'distant lands', had killed many chickens and a goat. They had also placed a pot over a fire. In the pot, Matheos observed blood, wild honey, red feathers and the bones of animals. Three men had danced around the fire, accompanied by musicians playing *maconzas*.[60] The purpose of the ceremony was to cure a sick black woman. Paulo, the master of the ceremony, invoked a spirit named Angola,[61] clearly a reference to the title *Ngola*, and in a ceremonial context to a former ruler's ancestral spirit.

These denunciations point to an important feature of the popular healers' sphere of operations in Angola in that they reveal their geographical mobility. In West-Central Africa, healers did not operate simply in their home villages but also travelled to serve their clients in different

---

[58] ANTT, TSO/IL, Caderno do Promotor 72, ff. 55r–57v.

[59] ANTT, TSO/IL, Caderno do Promotor 72, ff. 35r–37r. See also Ferreira, *Cross-Cultural Exchange*, 182.

[60] An instrument known as *güiro* in Latin America, except in Brazil, where it is called *reco-reco*. On musical connections between Angola and Brazil, see Gerhard Kubik, *Angolan Traits in Black Music, Games and Dances of Brazil: A Study of African Cultural Extensions Overseas* (Lisbon: Junta de Investigações Científicas do Ultramar, 1979).

[61] ANTT, TSO/IL, Caderno do Promotor 72, ff. 52r–53r.

locations, perhaps enjoying considerable fame and notoriety in so doing. In the first case, the healer Thomé de Angonga lived in the *presídio* of Massangano, not in the vicinity of Luanda, where he was invited to heal. In the second case, the unnamed healer hired by the slaves of Antonia de Sá did not live in Luanda but came from the *sertão* to offer his services. Similarly, Alexandre was treated in Libolo by a healer from Ambaca. Finally, Paulo Cambundo was joined in Bengo by a number of his healer-diviner colleagues from far and wide.[62]

Conclusion

This chapter has documented and identified the presence of several kinds of African healing specialists in West-Central Africa. Medical pluralism is a fitting term to describe the context of healing in this region in the seventeenth and eighteenth centuries. Ancient concepts related to health and illness point to widely shared and relatively unchanged therapeutic practices. There was room for many kinds of competing practitioners, from simple herbalists to powerful spiritual healers who operated in secret. Healers could specialise in the treatment of select afflictions or operate as 'generalists' treating a variety of maladies. Disease concepts changed slowly, but by the early nineteenth century there are indications that some Portuguese terms had been adopted to describe fevers.

From the point of view of cross-cultural medical interaction, the Portuguese shared a number of assumptions about illness causation and therapeutic practice. Among Europeans, this common ground led to widespread reliance on African healing and harming specialists. Not all medicines were beneficent, but accusations about the use of sorcery and poison occasionally emerged in the Inquisition documentation. This documentation points to the fact that even in and around Portuguese slaving ports in Luanda and Benguela, African idioms of healing remained a vibrant alternative for health seekers. In the hinterland of Luanda and *presídios* of the interior, African herbalists, healers and diviners were always the primary source of healing knowledge and power. The imagined powers of individual healers were made manifold by their mobility. Mobile healers offered the possibility of new cures, both spiritual and medicinal.

[62] On the mobility of healers in southern African history, see Markku Hokkanen, *Medicine, Mobility and the Empire: Nyasaland Networks, 1859–1960* (Manchester: Manchester University Press, 2017), 23–46.

2   Cross-Cultural Experiments
The Materiality of Medicine in West-Central Africa

Traversing the hinterland of Luanda in the 1830s, Italian doctor Tito Omboni and his entourage were ambushed one day. Omboni's domestic servant Antonio was injured on the left arm, which was pierced by a poisoned arrow and became extremely swollen. A black man in Omboni's company made Antonio swallow a large intake of a powder he carried with him, covered the wound and told the doctor to leave Antonio alone. The medicine was efficient against arrow poison. Omboni found out that it was the powder of a fruit called *angariari*. He had already encountered the same plant in Benguela upon his arrival in West-Central Africa and observed that locals used it to heal bites by poisonous reptiles. When later visiting the island of Príncipe, Omboni tested *angariari* on a monkey, first cutting it with a dagger dipped in a local poisonous plant called *pacopao*, then giving *angariari* as an antidote. The animal showed no signs of poisoning while Omboni stayed with it. After returning to Italy, Omboni introduced the plant at a scientific conference in Milan. A Catanian professor named Roberto Sava, who remembered that *angariari* was mentioned in Father Antonio Zucchelli's early eighteenth-century account of Angola, took charge of doing experiments to prove its usefulness. Omboni, who had witnessed a shepherd using the plant to heal a cow bitten by a snake in Africa, thought that *angariari* might prove a useful remedy against rabies.[1]

Tito Omboni was certainly not the first one to dream about finding effective and universal cures among Atlantic Africa's natural medicines. Experimenting with Central African plants, minerals and animal parts had been going on for more than three centuries before Omboni's encounter with *angariari*, and as Professor Sava acknowledged, Omboni was simply making a 'rediscovery' when he brought the plant to Milan. Named in many earlier accounts and pharmacopoeias as *engariaria*, the plant was one of the most important drugs to feature in

---

[1] Tito Omboni, *Viaggi nell' Africa Occidentale* (Milan: Civelli, 1846), 65, 139, 246.

50

lists of Angolan medicines. Around 1650, Afonso Mendes presented '*a gariária*' as a fruit imported to the colony of Angola from the Kingdom of Kongo. It could be cooked and the extracted liquid drunk, or else the fruit could be eaten to alleviate kidney stone pain.[2] Similarly, Father Girolamo Merolla claimed that *engariaria* was 'optimal' for curing kidney stone pain.[3] *Engariaria* had also found its way to England in the second half of the seventeenth century. In April of 1679, the philosopher John Locke noted in his journal that 'Mr. Toinard give [*sic*] me a peice [*sic*] of wood cald Angarian of Angola – the infusion is believed very good for the stone.'[4]

Engariaria was still in use in the late eighteenth century. The use of indigenous Angolan medicinals gained official support from Governor Dom Miguel Antonio de Melo, who in 1798 wrote about people's positive experiences with the medical uses of the *engariaria* fruit and other substances, namely *kikongo* wood, *enkasa* bark and *muriassangi* root. It was Melo's wish that these simples be analysed in Lisbon and made available to the whole of humanity. He was also clearly thinking about the profit that could be made by exporting and selling these drugs. Referring to *engariaria*, Melo wrote that 'in a few years, it would be possible to export the quantity needed to supply the pharmacies of Portugal'.[5]

Common to all these European observations, some of them based on personally experimenting with *engariaria*, was an appreciation for an African plant remedy. A shared trait in cross-cultural medical interaction during early modern European expansion was that local medicinals were regarded as the most suitable to cure diseases contracted in those places. This chapter focuses on remedies and the materiality of medicine in Angola. It discusses the exchange and transmission of medicinal knowledge between Africans and Europeans and the circulation of West-Central African medical ideas throughout the Atlantic world. This medical interaction started soon after Europeans made first contact with the

[2] Afonso Mendes, 'Caderno que trata das ervas, raízes e outras cousas que se tem descoberto no Sertão do Reino de Angola, com várias virtudes', edited by Ruela Pombo, *Diogo Cão*, II Série, No. 10 (1934), 298–304, and III Série, No. 1 (1935–1936), 41–48.

[3] P. Girolamo Merolla da Sorrento, *Breve, e succinta relazione del viaggio nel Regno di Congo Nell' Africa Meridionale* (Naples: F. Mollo, 1692), 188–189.

[4] Kenneth Dewhurst, *John Locke (1632–1704), Physician and Philosopher: A Medical Biography – with an Edition of the Medical Notes in His Journals* (London: Wellcome Historical Medical Library, 1963), 150–151.

[5] 'De Dom Miguel Antonio de Mello acerca do Breu, da Rezina, do Enxofre e dos Uzos Médicos que, por constantes e bem provadas experiencias têm determinados Simplices, 5 June 1798', *Arquivos de Angola*, First Series, 1:1 (1933), no page numbers.

Kingdom of Kongo, and the Portuguese eagerly began to learn healing methods from locals. African attempts to successfully acquire European medical knowledge will be returned to in Chapter 5, while this chapter concentrates on the better-documented Portuguese acquisitions of African natural products.

Natural Medicine and Amateur Botany

Medical knowledge played an important role in the early cultural exchanges between Europeans and Africans. In 1526, in a letter to King D. João III, D. Afonso I, the King of Kongo, requested Portuguese medical specialists. Pointing out that the Kongolese suffered from many and diverse infirmities, King Afonso argued that Kongolese Christians should benefit from Portuguese medical knowledge. Although in Kongo people cured themselves with plants and by traditional customs, Afonso argued that such drugs and ceremonies in which people put their faith were of little service to God, thus making a strong case for the eradication of indigenous healing practices. Afonso had a good sense of what the Portuguese could offer, for he specifically asked D. João III to send two physicians, two pharmacists and a surgeon.[6]

The King of Kongo was not the only African ruler interested in obtaining European healing knowledge. In 1621, as the Portuguese were making early attempts to improvise a colony in Benguela, Sumbe Ambuila requested that the governor of Angola supply soldiers, horses, a barber to offer medical treatment and a translator (*tendala*) to facilitate communication. Again, a local African ruler, who had been selling captives to European interlopers, was well aware of the kind of medical specialists the Portuguese could offer. The only problem was that the Portuguese in Benguela had enough difficulties in finding a surgeon to work in their own settlement. Simão Ferraz worked as a doctor and attended to the needs of the residents, but the quantity, and especially the quality, of available medicines in Angola was so poor that they were of little use.[7]

The great value African rulers put on certain medicinal plants is revealed by their inclusion among gifts offered to visiting Europeans. *Kikongo* wood (*Tarchonanthus camphoratus*, L.)[8] was one of the earliest

---

[6] 'Carta do Rei do Congo a D. João III, October 18, 1526', in Brásio, ed., *MMA*, I: 488–489.

[7] Candido, *An African Slaving Port*, 64.

[8] In early modern primary sources, *kikongo* was often referred to as sandalwood. In research literature I have consulted, including Simon, 'A Luso-African Formulary', and Bossard, *La medecine traditionnelle au centre et a l'ouest de l'Angola*, *kikongo* is identified as

wood exports to Portugal, as it was often included among the gifts offered
by African rulers to Portuguese kings. In 1565, for example, forty pieces
of *kikongo* were among the gifts sent by Ndongo's ruler to King
Sebastião. Father Francisco de Gouveia commented that the tree was
very valuable in Angola.[9] When Paulo Dias de Novais entered Angola in
1575, larger and smaller pieces of *kikongo* were again included among the
gifts to be sent to the king in Portugal.[10]

In their efforts to cure diseases contracted in Africa, the Portuguese
were eager to learn from the local population. Jesuit Father Garcia
Simões, who accompanied Paulo Dias de Novais in 1575, wrote about
a red dyewood known as *takula* (*Pterocarpus soyauxii*, Taub. and *P.
tinctorius*, Welw.). Local people used *takula* to paint their bodies from
head to toe, and it also had a medical use. *Takula* was used by Africans
and some Portuguese to cure fever and headaches. A white man who had
tried *takula* told Simões that it worked very well. Simões himself had
tried kola nuts but found them bitter like rhubarb. According to him,
kola nuts were used as a stimulant by blacks as well as whites.[11]

In the late sixteenth century, Duarte Lopes reported that in Kongo
fever was locally cured by mixing *takula* and *kikongo* wood with palm oil
and applying this to the body, from head to toe, twice or three times.
Kikongo was among the most appreciated medicines, and hence it was
expensive, with one piece costing a slave. He also noted that some trees
were effective as antidotes for snake bites, and that certain poisonous
snakes provided medicines to cure fever. To cure *kitanga* (yaws), the
Portuguese made an unguent of *kikongo* powder, but used vinegar
instead of palm oil.[12] The Portuguese willingness to use an African plant

Tarchonanthus camphoratus, L., but around Luanda a plant known as *kikongo* has been
referred to as belonging to the *Brachylaena* genus. John Gossweiler, *Flora exótica de
Angola: nomes vulgares e origem das plantas cultivadas ou subespontâneas* (Separata of
Agronomia Angolana, Luanda: Repartição Central dos Serviços de Agricultura de
Angola, 1950).

[9] 'Carta do padre Francisco de Gouveia para o Colégio das Artes, May 19, 1565', in
Brásio, ed., *MMA*, II: 530.

[10] 'História da residência dos padres da Companhia de Jesus em Angola, e cousas tocantes
ao Reino, e Conquista, May 1, 1594', in Brásio, ed., *MMA*, IV: 557.

[11] Gastão Sousa Dias, ed., *Relações de Angola (Primórdios da ocupação portuguesa)* (Coimbra:
Imprensa da Universidade, 1934), 55–56. *Takula* remained in use over the centuries. In
the 1920s, Father Wellens, a missionary and a botanical collector in Mayumbe, reported
that it was used as a plaster against several diseases, for example itching, irritations, skin
diseases and head parasites. É. de Wildeman, *Sur des plantes médicinales ou utiles du
Mayumbe (Congo Belge) d'apres des notes du R.P. Wellens* (Brussels: Institut Royal
Colonial Belge, 1938), 72.

[12] Filippo Pigafetta, *Relatione del reame di Congo et delle circonvicine contrade, tratta dalli scritti
e ragionamenti di Odoardo Lopez portoghese* (Rome: Appresso Bartolomeo Grassi, 1591),
14–15, 32–33, 69; Don R. Brothwell, 'Yaws', in *The Cambridge World History of Human*

product and mix it with something they were familiar with from home can be taken as an early indication of the emergence of hybrid medicinals.

The uses of *takula* and *kikongo* were also demonstrated by Barthélemy d'Espinchal de Massiac, who lived for eight years in Angola and Kongo in the 1640s. He wrote that, from time to time, the blacks covered their whole bodies with a red paste made of a mixture of *takula*, *kikongo* and palm oil. Besides its use for cosmetic and medicinal purposes, *takula* was used in Loango during female coming-of-age ceremonies. The widespread use of *takula* in West-Central Africa reflected the symbolic association between colour, the ancestral world and liminal states of initiation and rites of passage. According to Denbow, wood rather than rock-ochre was the only material available to produce the red pigment used for ritual purposes.[13]

Finding new drugs and an effective pharmacopoeia was partly fuelled by the vast fortunes to be made by selling exotic products in Europe. Yet, for Europeans living in Africa and elsewhere in the tropics, the most pressing motivation for experimenting with local natural medicines was survival. For them, the search for new remedies was a matter of necessity rather than profit or curiosity.[14] As Portuguese cultural interaction with West-Central Africans deepened, medicine chests also expanded. In West-Central Africa, this was well illustrated by Sergeant-Major Afonso Mendes, who around 1650 wrote one of the most remarkable works on seventeenth-century medicine in Africa. In his manuscript on medicinal plants he had found useful in the interior of Angola, Mendes listed over eighty treatments for various diseases and ailments. Citing the Sevillian physician Nicholas Monardes as an inspiration he sought to imitate, Mendes was clearly trying to attach himself to a global discourse on medical knowledge and natural history. Demonstrating that a geographically isolated outpost in Angola could be intellectually connected to the world beyond Africa, Mendes would certainly have earned a place in the global history of science had his manuscript been published. Instead, his service in Angola remains shrouded in obscurity.[15]

Mendes's pharmacopoeia demonstrates how certain drugs – such as *kikongo*, which Mendes singled out as an 'admirable' remedy against fevers and headaches – had remained in constant use since the sixteenth

---

Disease, edited by Kenneth F. Kiple (Cambridge: Cambridge University Press, 1993), 1096–1100.

[13] 'Relação de uma viagem a Angola, 1652', in Brásio, ed., *MMA*, XI: 261; James Denbow, *The Archaeology and Ethnography of Central Africa* (Cambridge: Cambridge University Press, 2013), 153.

[14] Schiebinger, *Plants and Empire*, 73–75.   [15] Mendes, 'Caderno que trata das ervas'.

century. One of the most versatile remedies mentioned by Mendes was cobra wood, or *kitenge*, which was used to cure fevers, stings, swellings, gout, snake bites, stomach ache, apoplexy and malaise. Only the root of the *kitenge* tree was used. It could be taken in powder form, drunk mixed with water or used as an unguent. According to Mendes, cobra wood was 'discovered' by whites in 1619, and it could be found in Mutemo, Hamba and Bango-Aquitamba. Mendes advised collecting *kitenge* only when the moon was waning, probably reflecting a local Central African custom.[16]

Mendes's list of treatments and remedies shows that the Portuguese in West-Central Africa had clearly adopted a number of local medical practices. Mendes did not specify who his informants were, but he had probably learned a great deal from African troops under his command and possibly from local popular healers. Some of his remedies could undoubtedly be classified as superstitious. For example, against fits of epilepsy, Mendes noted that 'an antelope claw, carried near the heart, is an admirable remedy, and many say that the left [claw] is better'.[17] One can also observe hybrid medicines among the remedies introduced by Mendes. For example, one could make an antidote by mixing the root of *malula* with wine. An unguent made by grating *malula* on a stone and mixing it in water was used by people who had stepped on *feitiços* or fetishes. Finally, ground *engala* (wild boar) tooth mixed with pure water or 'water of Almeirões' was used as a fever medicine.[18]

Similar to Mendes, Cadornega noted that indigenous medicine in West-Central Africa consisted mainly of drugs derived from plants. Africans knew their virtues and how to apply them. However, his opinion of local medical practices was more negative than Mendes's view. Basing his opinion on humoural theory, Cadornega argued that people using indigenous medicine did not recognise whether the drugs were 'hot' or 'cold', although, as shown in Chapter 1, the hot/cold distinction was conceptually part of framing disease in West-Central Africa. In many cases, the dosages were unclear, and in Cadornega's view people rather consulted the devil than developed a proper discourse on curing disease.[19]

In the Portuguese colonial world, missionary orders developed the foremost European body of expertise about indigenous medicine. Jesuits recognised the potential for profit from commercialising native

[16] Mendes, 'Caderno que trata das ervas', 298–300.
[17] Mendes, 'Caderno que trata das ervas', 300.
[18] Mendes, 'Caderno que trata das ervas', 42–43.
[19] Cadornega, *História geral*, III: 318.

drugs, and they quickly became the principal disseminators of these commodities.[20] While Jesuits in West-Central Africa undoubtedly experimented with local natural medicine, such medicines are best documented in Italian Capuchin sources. The Capuchins were by no means unified in their attitudes towards local medicinals; they demonstrate both positive and negative views towards them. Similar to Lopes and d'Espinchal, Cavazzi listed *kikongo* wood among the remedies used to combat the secondary symptoms of yaws. In addition, people used a plant called *pau da bata*, which was also exported to Italy.[21] Merolla was full of admiration for certain plant-derived drugs. For fever, he advised using *kiseko* wood in powder form mixed with water and spreading it on the temples or forehead of the patient. *Kikongo* wood had many virtues but, according to Merolla, it was most useful in purging the body. Finally, *mignamigna* (or *minhaminha*) produced both poison and antidote.[22]

Some Capuchins had obtained medical and herbal knowledge in Italy before commencing their sojourn in Central Africa (see Chapter 6). Some of them were also intimately connected to naturalists in Italy. Carlos Almeida has revealed the interconnections between Father Ambrogio Guattini and Giacomo Zanoni, one of the most prominent botanists in Bologna in the mid-seventeenth century. Guattini never hid his curiosity and extreme carefulness in observing nature. He wrote detailed descriptions of Central Africa's *naturalia*. According to Almeida, even when not directly connected to collectors in Europe, Capuchin accounts leave an impression of genuine interest in local nature, the qualities of plants and fruits, the behaviour of animals and the effects of 'air' on living beings in different latitudes.[23]

Although some Capuchins gave a glowing picture of the potentials of local natural medicine, not all missionaries shared this view. For example, Marcellino d'Atri and Luca da Caltanisetta lived in constant fear of poisoning and often blamed African healing specialists for their illness. This adversity to local African medicines and medical practices can partly be explained by the fear some missionaries felt towards local popular healers. On several occasions, d'Atri claimed that he and his companions had been poisoned. Similarly, Caltanisetta, when suddenly

---

[20] Walker, 'Acquisition and Circulation', 250.

[21] Cavazzi, *Istorica decrizione*, 142; Simon, 'A Luso-African Formulary', 108.

[22] Merolla, *Breve, e succinta relazione*, 188–189.

[23] Carlos José Duarte Almeida, *Uma infelicidade feliz: A imagem de África e dos Africanos na Literature Missionária sobre o Kongo e a região Mbundu (meados do séc. XVI – primeiro quartel do séc. XVIII)* (unpublished Ph.D. dissertation, Faculdade de Ciências Sociais e Humanas, Universidade de Lisboa, 2009), 209–214.

contracting diarrhoea or fever, recorded his suspicions that local sorcerers had added poison to the palm wine or fruits they offered to the missionaries. Capuchins employed theriac and other antidotes as well as bleedings to cure themselves when they felt that their lives were in danger on account of poisoned food or drink. Caltanisetta's opinion was that all missionaries to Central Africa should bring with them provisions of theriac, powder of Algaroth and manna and try not to be fooled by anyone, because everyone has to be prepared to act as 'one's own doctor'. Despite his antipathy towards African medicine, even Caltanisetta recognised *engariaria* as a useful medicine for curing the bladder.[24]

Mobile Medicines: Central African Healing Materials in the Atlantic World

When Governor Melo compiled a report on popular Angolan medicinals in the late eighteenth century, he demonstrated the mobility of these plant substances within West-Central Angola. *Kikongo* wood, which was by then used to cure acute fevers, erysipelas and skin lesions, was brought to Luanda from Benguela and Kilengues; *enkasa*, which had emetic 'virtues' and was used as an antidote against certain poisons, arrived in Luanda from the Kingdom of Kongo; *engariaria*, which was used for curing cramps and dysenteries, originated similarly in the Kingdom of Kongo; and *muriassangi* was found especially on the margins of Kwanza, near Massangano. The trade in these drugs was regional and systematic, and they could be bought in Luanda relatively easily, showing their continued popularity among the local population.[25]

The earliest hints that Central African medicinals enjoyed some popularity outside of Africa can be found in Cavazzi's account, which mentioned a plant called *pau da bata* being exported to Italy. Another Italian

[24] Carlo Toso, *L'anarchia congolese nel sec. XVII: La relazione inedita di Marcellino d'Atri* (Genoa: Bozzi, 1984), 69; P. Luca da Caltanissetta, 'Relatione della missione fatta nel Regno di Congo per il Padre Fra' Luca da Caltanissetta', in *Il Congo agli inizi del settecento nella relazione di P. Luca da Caltanissetta*, edited by Romain Rainero (Florence: La Nuova Italia, 1973), 151, 155, 163, 176, 193, 337. Theriac was a medical concoction used as an antidote and considered a universal panacea in the ancient and early modern world. Gilbert Watson, *Theriac and Mithridatium: A Study in Therapeutics* (London: Wellcome Historical Medical Library, 1966). Missionaries were not the only ones who feared poisoning, for it was sometimes suspected when military officials died suddenly in the interior. On the suspected use of poisons, see AHU, CU, Angola, Cx. 30, Doc. 2950, Carta do governador e capitão-general de Angola, Rodrigo César de Meneses, ao rei, 30 August 1734.
[25] 'De Dom Miguel Antonio de Mello acerca do Breu'.

source from the early eighteenth century refers to many vegetables from the mountains of Kongo, hinting that Capuchin networks would have made Kongolese *materia medica* available in Italy, a topic that would merit further study.[26] Early eighteenth-century pharmacopoeias give a clearer picture of the West-Central African drugs known in Portugal. In Lisbon, monastic pharmacies operated by Jesuits and Augustinians provided medicines to the city's ailing population. Augustinians, especially, were known for their texts on pharmacology, including the first continental pharmacopoeia written in vernacular Portuguese by Dom Caetano de Santo António, published in 1704.[27] The fourth edition of Dom Caetano's pharmacopeia, published in 1754 with the title *Pharmacopea lusitana augmentada*, includes only passing references to African medicinals. Canafistula and tamarind were mentioned among the medicinal plants imported from Angola, but these originated, were grown and enjoyed widespread popularity in South and South East Asia.[28] This clearly demonstrates that Angola was a part of global cross-cultural medical exchanges, not an isolated outpost in Africa. Similar to what was taking place in Brazil, plant-based drugs imported or transplanted by the Portuguese from India and Ceylon were spreading throughout West-Central Africa by the eighteenth century.[29]

The central figure in popularising medical knowledge from the tropics was the Portuguese doctor João Curvo Semedo, who published a set of books containing medical prescriptions based on medical prescriptions he called 'Curvian secrets'. Many of these treatments were made with ingredients from Africa, Asia and Brazil.[30] Curvo Semedo's work *Memorial de vários simplices* (Memorial of Various Simples) offers many examples of 'exotic' drugs exported from Angola. As evidenced in earlier works concerning Angola and Kongo, some of the Central African drugs were composed of animals. Hippopotami and elephant teeth, antelope claw, the vertebral bones of cobra and the teeth of wild boar (*engala*) were all mentioned among the drugs derived from animals. Among the drugs

[26] Cavazzi, *Istorica decrizione*, 142; Giuseppe Gazola, *Il mondo ingannato da falsi medici* (Venice: Marino Rossetti, 1716), 47.
[27] Walker, 'Acquisition and Circulation', 261–262.
[28] D. Caetano de Santo António, *Pharmacopea lusitana augmentada: methodo pratico de prearar os medicamentos na fórma galenica, e chimica* (Lisbon: Mosteiro de S. Vincente de Fóra, 4th ed., 1754), 26–27.
[29] On Asian medicinal plants in Brazil, see Walker, 'The Medicines Trade', 413.
[30] Furtado, 'Tropical Empiricism', 147; Benjamin Breen, 'The Flip Side of the Pharmacopoeia: Sub-Saharan African Medicines and Poisons in the Atlantic World', in *Drugs on the Page: Pharmacopoeias and Healing Knowledge in the Early Modern Atlantic World*, edited by Matthew James Crawford and Joseph M. Gabriel (Pittsburgh: University of Pittsburgh Press, 2019), 149–150, 158.

derived from plants, Semedo mentioned the root of *minhaminha*, which was used as an antidote to poison. Cadornega, writing around 1680, claimed that this had been 'recently' discovered in the *presídio* of Ambaca and was the finest antidote discovered until then. From Benguela, the Portuguese exported *kiseko* wood, which was used to cure headaches. Semedo also recognised one of the oldest botanical imports from West-Central Africa, namely *kikongo* wood, and claimed that it had the same effect as *kiseko*. Merolla, Curvo Semedo's contemporary, had also listed these three drugs in his book on West-Central Africa, and Cadornega's chronicle confirms that *kiseko*, along with *kikongo*, was a prevalent medicinal in Benguela.[31]

Some of Curvo Semedo's prescriptions including medicinal plants show clear continuities from the seventeenth century. Semedo, for example, recommended the *angariari* (or *engariaria*) fruit to provoke urine and to cure kidney stones and the bladder. Curvo Semedo seems to have been well aware of what had been written about local Angolan medicinals and probably had access to some of the manuscript materials. *Engariaria*, for instance, was described with the words Afonso Mendes had written in his treatise on Angolan medicinals around 1650. Another remedy also seems to come straight out of Mendes's manuscript. Semedo listed the root of a *mutututu* tree because of its great virtue in treating erysipelas and inflammation in the testicles, exactly as mentioned by Mendes. Some drugs listed by Mendes, however, were used differently by Curvo Semedo. The *mubango* tree, which Mendes included because of its usefulness in treating cold cramps and 'the air', was in Curvo Semedo's view used especially by pregnant women to alleviate childbirth pains. It was ground into powder and, when used like tobacco, made one sneeze. Curvo Semedo clearly had knowledgeable informants, as he knew that it came from Ambaca and Kasanje in the interior of Angola.[32]

Although the quantities of African medicinals imported into Portugal remains unknown, these pharmacopoeias, and especially Curvo Semedo's work, demonstrate that knowledge of West-Central African drugs was spreading in Portugal by the early eighteenth century. In Portugal, local doctors experimented with these ingredients and developed their own compounds, which they then offered to their customers. Here, one can see an antecedent to late nineteenth-century

---

[31] João Curvo Semedo, *Memorial de varios simplices que da India Oriental, da America e de outras partes vem ao nosso reyno* (Lisbon: Oficina de António Pedroso Galram, 1716), 11–12; Cadornega, *História geral*, III: 171, 381.
[32] Semedo, *Memorial de varios simplices*, 24, 29–30.

efforts by various pharmaceutical companies to bioprospect for plants in Africa and elsewhere in the tropics. It is clear that Portuguese doctors and pharmacists such as Curvo Semedo sought commercial advantages in developing these drugs, although they operated on a relatively small scale.

What about Central African natural products and medicines in Brazil? Since Brazil was the primary destination of West-Central Africans in the slave trade, and because of the well-studied interconnections of Angola and Brazil in the southern Atlantic, one would expect to find at least some celebrity drugs making the Middle Passage to the New World. After all, scholars have pointed out that Atlantic crossings of West African plants can be detected in *Candomblé* rituals, for example.[33] Another well-known example would be African oil palm, which held a central place in the development of Afro-Brazilian cultures and land-scapes. The historical trade in African palm oil between Bahia and several West and West-Central African societies helped construct a cultural economy for palm oil in Bahia, and it contributed to the social and ecological development of domestic palm oil production in and around Salvador.[34] Yet, the medical substances deemed most popular among Portuguese settlers in Angola – *kikongo, takula, engariaria* – seem not to have been systematically exported to Brazil. The meticulous surgeon Gomes Ferreira, who listed many plants that were commonly used in Minas Gerais in the early eighteenth century, noted that other plant medicines were arriving in Brazil from Angola. He listed a fruit called *tepe* or *pepe* as an essential ingredient in a remedy used to cure asthmatic defluxions (*defluxos asmáticos*). According to Gomes Ferreira, men who had business in Angola brought the *pepe* fruit and 'many other medicinal things' to Bahia. In the 1740s, surgeon João Cardoso de Miranda mentioned using Angolan salt in one of his medical concoctions. He called it *sal de Quissanga*, likely referring to salt from Kisama.[35]

[33] Robert A. Voeks, *Sacred Leaves of Candomblé: African Magic, Medicine, and Religion in Brazil* (Austin: University of Texas Press, 1997).

[34] Case Watkins, *An Afro-Brazilian Landscape: African Oil Palms and Socioecological Change in Bahia, Brazil* (unpublished Ph.D. dissertation, Louisiana State University, 2015), 118–176.

[35] Luis Gomes Ferreira, *Erário Mineral* (Lisbon: Officina de Miguel Rodrigues, 1735), I: 260, 333 and 471; II: 556–558 and 675–678; João Cardoso de Miranda, *Relaçaõ cirurgica, e médica, na qual se trata, e declara especialmente hum novo methodo para curar a infecçaõ escorbutica, ou mal de Loanda, e todos os seus productos, fazendo para isso manifestos dous especificos, e muy particulares remedios* (Lisbon: Officina de Miguel Rodrigues, 1747), 64. On earlier exports of *guandu* and guinea peas from Luanda to Brazil, see Cagle, *Assembling the Tropics*, 242. On Kisama's salt mines, see Beatrix Heintze, 'Historical Notes on the Kisama of Angola', *Journal of African History* 13 (1972): 407–418.

Another indication of the global movement of medicinals in the Portuguese Empire and in the Central African diaspora comes from the Inquisition case of Luzia Pinta, one of the most famous Central African healers in Minas Gerais during the eighteenth century. Sent to Lisbon in December 1741 for interrogation by the Inquisition, Luzia was described as a woman of around fifty years of age, tall and stout, with scarification marks close to her forehead and one on each cheek. She was an unmarried freed slave (*forra*) from Luanda, whose parents had been slaves. She had been baptised in Luanda in the Conceição parish. Luzia confessed to having used herbs and roots for healing purposes, but she denied the use of divinations and having a pact with the Devil. She identified the medicines she administered as the root of '*abatua*' (also known as *butua* in contemporary sources) and '*pau-santo*' and said that these made her patients vomit.[36]

A plant named *butua* was also found in West-Central Africa. It was identified by Cadornega as a plant imported from India. In the early nineteenth century, Angola's chief physician, José Maria Bomtempo, mentioned a few plants that were produced in Angola and Benguela. These were *abutua* (*Cissampellos Parreira*, L.) and *alcassús* (*Glycyrrhiza glabra*, L.). In the case of *abutua*, Bomtempo pointed to its potential economic value, writing that certain parts of West-Central Africa produced it in immense quantities. Finally, in the 1850s Welwitsch discussed a plant called *abutua* that he had found growing in the Golungo Alto, Cazengo and Dembos regions. Locals used its pounded roots as well as the leaves, branchlets, bark of the trunk and fruits as a decoction against diarrhoea, gonorrhoea and various other distempers, especially long-established syphilis. Its infallible efficacy was also recommended in cases of snakebites and as a sudorific in treating constipation.[37]

From Kongo to Lisbon: The *Enkasa* Tree

In 1731, Sergeant-Major Francisco de Buitrago sat down in Lisbon to write a book he called *Arvore da vida*. In English, the full title of the book

---

[36] Laura de Mello e Souza, *O diabo e a terra de Santa Cruz* (São Paulo: Companhia das Letras, 1986), 352–357; Mott, 'O calundu-angola'. The original documents are in ANTT, TSO/IL, Processo 252 (Processo de Luzia Pinta).

[37] Cadornega, *História geral*, III: 381; José Maria Bomtempo, *Compendios de Materia Medica* (Rio de Janeiro: Regia Officina Typografica, 1814), 27, 31; William Philip Hiern, *Catalogue of the African Plants Collected by Dr. Friedrich Welwitsch in 1853–61. Dicotyledons, Part I* (London: British Museum, 1896), 15–16.

manuscript ran *Tree of Life: The Discovered Treasure of a Tree, sister to the one from which the cross of our redemption was made; To free [oneself] from the evils of the Devil, for life and health of the bewitched or those vexed by the same Devil, and many other diseases; And many and singular remedies to many maladies all approved with many prodigious experiences, as is public and as can be seen from those treatises.* That Buitrago's manuscript was indeed intended for publication can be seen from the index that he compiled at the end of the book. However, it was never published; the book survives only in manuscript form in the Portuguese National Library. Religion and medicine were intrinsically inseparable in Buitrago's work, and he offered and dedicated the book to Our Lady of Conception. The book consisted of two treatises. The first treatise dealt with the virtues and prodigies of the bark of a tree that Buitrago called the tree of life. The second treatise was a compendium of 'many singulars' or natural remedies that Buitrago, a knight of the Order of Christ, had experimented with during more than twenty years of service in the colony of Angola.[38]

The tree of life was identified by Buitrago as the bark of the *enkasa* (spelled *emcassa* and *cassa* by Buitrago) tree. He argued that it was 'the most singular antidote in the whole world, not surpassed by anything; [it] is very singular and miraculous against *feitiços*'. It was used and esteemed among the Kongolese and many whites who had been to the Kingdom of Kongo. Buitrago claimed that it was sold in Lisbon. A friend of a friend who constantly received people from Kongo had ordered a great quantity of *enkasa* and sold it to others, declaring its great virtues, primarily against *feitiços* and poison. Buitrago referred several times to *enkasa* as the sister of the tree from which the cross of the crucified Christ had been made.[39] Given the proliferation of Christianity in the Kingdom of Kongo, this apparently reflected the Kongolese interpretation of *enkasa*. It seems to have been part of Kongolese folk Catholic mythology. In Kongo, people took suspected witches to the tree to see if they could escape from it or gave signs of being witches. Buitrago had given *enkasa* in Angola to a black who was about to die, after which the man had vomited 'various things' and been freed of his illness immediately. He

[38] Biblioteca Nacional de Portugal, Fundo Reservados 437, Códice 13114, Francisco de Buytrago, *Arvore da vida, Thezouro descuberto da Arvore irmaã daque se fez a cruz da nossa Redempção. Para livrar dos maleficios do Demonio, p.a vida e saude dos enfeitiçados ou vexados do mesmo Demonio, e outras m.tas enfermid.es E muitos e singulares remedios p.a muitos achaques aprovado tudo com muitas experiencias prodigiozas, como hé publico e se vera dos daq.les tractados.* Lisbon 1731, ff. 1r–5r. I use the modern spelling of Buitrago in the text rather than the spelling Buytrago that appears in the documentation.
[39] Buytrago, *Arvore da vida*, ff. 1r, 10v–11v.

had also tried it in Salvador, in Bahia, giving it to a slave who was soon freed of *feitiços*.[40]

The use of *enkasa* by the Kongolese to detect witches indicates its use in poison ordeals. Judicial ordeals were found in most Atlantic African societies, as John Thornton has shown. They commonly required giving the accused poison. If the accused vomited it up, they were held to be innocent; if not, then they either died of its effects or were held to be guilty. There were a variety of judicial ordeals in Central Africa, not all of them involving the use of poison. These included the plunging of hands in hot water or seizing hot irons. In these rituals, the innocent typically went unharmed. These ordeals had a remarkable continuity and geographical spread over the centuries. They have been interpreted not only as judicial procedures, but as a struggle between good and evil, against witchcraft itself. As such, they fit well in the larger context of healing and harming in Atlantic African medicine.[41]

Francisco de Buitrago's career in Angola is not well documented, but traces of it survive in official letters. In 1707, while serving as an adjutant in the infantry in Luanda, Buitrago was promoted to the post of Captain Engineer (*Capitam engenheiro*) because of his knowledge 'in the science of fortifications'.[42] After this, Buitrago disappeared from the documentary record until 1721, when he petitioned to be freed from service. In his letter, Buitrago documented that he had entered royal service in March 1692 and served for more than twenty years in Angola in various posts, including the posts of Captain-Major of the Ilha do Cazanga and Captain Engineer. In 1718, he had been allowed to leave Angola for Bahia in order to cure his ailments. However, this had not succeeded in Bahia and he had returned to Lisbon, where his treatment had continued.[43]

The first treatise of the manuscript documented in detail how Buitrago, after returning from Angola, used the bark of *enkasa* in Lisbon to exorcise people thought to have been bewitched. It was really an exorcist's manual and perhaps partly explains why the manuscript remained unpublished. In the early 1730s, the Inquisition of Lisbon

---

[40] Buytrago, *Arvore da vida*, ff. 6v–8r, 39v.

[41] John Thornton, *Africa and Africans in the Making of the Atlantic World, 1400–1800*, 2nd ed. (Cambridge: Cambridge University Press, 1998), 241. On poison ordeals and their historiographical interpretation in eastern Africa, see Langwick, *Bodies, Politics, and African Healing*, 42–46.

[42] AHU, CU, Angola Cx. 18, Doc. 2027, Consulta do Conselho Ultramarino ao rei D. João V sobre a nomeação de pessoas para o posto de engenheiro de Angola, 8 February 1707.

[43] AHU, CU, Angola Cx. 22, Doc. 2238, Consulta do Conselho Ultramarino ao rei, D. João V sobre o requerimento de Francisco de Buitrago, 11 January 1721.

accused several priests of performing illegal exorcisms.[44] Some of these priests were Buitrago's friends, as documented in his manuscript. More importantly, however, Buitrago's work shows how Western and West-Central African ideas of healing coalesced and were transferred from the colony of Angola and the Kingdom of Kongo to Lisbon.

Buitrago was not the only person to use *enkasa* in Portugal. A manuscript source from the municipal library of Porto reveals that *enkasa* was also used in the interior of Portugal in the eighteenth century. Noting Angola as the only source for this remedy, it repeats the same belief that the plant was related to the tree from which Christ's cross had been made. Noting the 'discovered and experimented' virtues of the tree, the manuscript states that it can be used for evacuating *feitiços* but also for expelling the Devil from a possessed person. It was also useful for deflux, flatus or flatulent pain, colic, ague, fevers and the bladder. The manuscript was dated 1753, suggesting that the remedy enjoyed popularity in Portugal and was constantly imported there for decades.[45]

Besides *enkasa*, Buitrago documented the names, uses and effects of fifty-four natural remedies (see Appendix A) that he had learned to use in Angola. He claimed that the variety and virtues of trees and herbs and other singulars in Angola and neighbouring provinces exceeded those found anywhere else in the world. In Buitrago's words, the people of Angola performed 'extraordinary and miraculous cures', but the Portuguese generally neglected and ignored them. Due to his many years of residence in the region, Buitrago had learned the virtues of many medicinals and the mode of using them. He stated that he had collected information 'at his own cost', hinting that monetary payments had been involved in obtaining knowledge from indigenous experts.[46]

---

[44] Márcia Moises Ribeiro, *Exorcistas e demônios: Demonologia e exorcismos no mundo luso-brasileiro* (Rio de Janeiro: Campus, 2003).

[45] I have been unable to consult the original source, which is partially transcribed in Eugénio dos Santos, 'O homem português perante a doença no século XVIII: Atitudes e receituário', *Revista da Faculdade de Letras: História*, II série, 1 (1984): 187–201. Richard Dennett's work attests to the continued importance of *enkasa* in early twentieth-century West-Central Africa. He observed its use in poison ordeals and in detecting witches in many locations. Among the Vili, the powdered bark was given to suspected witches and wizards as a test to prove their innocence or guilt. If the accused vomited the poison, they were deemed innocent. If the poison was retained, it either poisoned the witch or else acted as a strong purge, when the culprit was set upon and killed. Dennett was eager to find an *enkasa* tree, and as there were none in Luango, he took a walk of some 12 miles to find one. He described the *enkasa* tree he saw as measuring some 12 feet in circumference. There appeared upon its trunk a great oblong patch devoid of bark. Wanting to take a sample of the bark, he broke the blade of his knife, finding the tree much harder than he had imagined. R. E. Dennett, *At the Back of the Black Man's Mind or Notes on the Kingly Office in West Africa* (London: Frank Cass, 1906), 83, 127–129.

[46] Buytrago, *Arvore da vida*, ff. 5r–6r.

There were also ways of experimenting with new substances, as Pablo Gómez has shown for the early modern Caribbean. Sensual knowledge became a main avenue for ritual practitioners to identify, classify and control the natural world. Smelling not only alerted them to the 'virtues' of the herbs, but also helped them to feel and sense the immaterial world of spirits in very material ways and to cure illnesses that were caused by spells and poisons.[47] Buitrago's collection of plant medicines abounded with antidotes. Of the fifty-five medicinals, fourteen had use as an antidote (*contraveneno*). These were effective not only against snake and other animal bites, but also against poison, pointing to the prevalence of the harming register in everyday life. Some plants were useful for many purposes. For example, *engariaria*, which Buitrago had many times experimented with personally, was used not only as an antidote against the bites of poisonous animals, but to cure stone, carnosity, heat and internal sores. Some plants excited the senses by their smell. Buitrago mentioned that the *kiseko*, a white tree growing in Benguela, had a strong smell. He had used it personally and claimed that everybody uses it. The popularity of the tree was demonstrated by its being sold in pieces and as whole trees.[48]

Hybrid Moments

As discussed in Chapter 1, West-Central African healing specialists were experts in determining which spirits were plaguing the body and in appeasing ancestral spirits with feasts. They treated illness with natural medicines. Healers also had knowledge of a variety of antidotes in order to counteract the effects of poisonous plants. The selection of medicinal plants in Angola was extensive. The Europeans who wrote about local medicine in Angola in the seventeenth and eighteenth centuries listed over 120 different natural ingredients that could be used in different treatments. The great majority of medicine came from plants, with only twenty derived from animals and four from mineral sources.[49] The principal illnesses for which these remedies were used in healing practices were fevers, as was noted by early European visitors to the region.[50] Other common complaints included genital-urinary infections, venereal diseases and gastro-intestinal disorders. Other pharmaceutical uses of Central African medicine included the treatment of skin diseases and their use as antidotes.[51]

---

[47] Gómez, *The Experiential Caribbean*, 95–97, 103–114.
[48] Buytrago, *Arvore da vida*, 70v–73r, 74r–75r.   [49] Dias, 'Índice de drogas medicinais'.
[50] Pigafetta, *Relatione del reame di Congo*, 69.   [51] Dias, 'Índice de drogas medicinais'.

Portuguese settlers had quickly familiarised themselves with African medical practices. By the late sixteenth century, Duarte Lopes could report that, in the Kingdom of Kongo, natural medicine consisted of various herbs, trees and their bark, oils, waters and minerals. Fever was treated with a powder prepared from two trees that was mixed with palm oil and applied onto the body from head to toe. The cure for headaches was achieved by making cuts on the temple with small horns and then sucking through the horns so that they filled with blood. Cupping horns were used similarly on any ailing body part. Lopes saw how wounds were effectively disinfected with herbs. He concluded that people did not need doctors, surgeons and physicians or European medicine and mixtures, for they simply cured themselves with native plants.[52] Almost a century later, Cadornega observed that herbal remedies were often mixed with water in a pan and then people washed with this water. After repeating this a couple of times, the water was thrown onto a place where two roads crossed. The belief was that the first person who walked over the remains of the water took the disease away with him or her. People coming to a crossroads were careful to not walk over these remains and sought to bypass them as best they could.[53]

Some Portuguese openly believed in African healing practices, while others rejected them. This could cause conflict in therapeutic encounters. Lieutenant Pasqual Rodrigues de Queiroga was denounced in 1716 in Luanda for consulting African healers in order to heal his godfather, João de Moura da Silva, in Massangano. According to the testimonies, he had called a black diviner to his house, who had told him that the illness was caused by the *zumbi* of his children's wet nurse. According to the denunciations, the diviner used the *bolungo* ritual, which was used to locate witches. The diviner thus indicated that the wet nurse was behind Silva's illness. Queiroga had received a number of remedies from the diviner, but when he tried to persuade Silva to take them, the patient responded by chasing Queiroga out of the house. Besides believing in the advice of local healers, Queiroga was said to

---

[52] Pigafetta, *Relatione del reame di Congo*, 96.
[53] Cadornega, *História geral*, III: 258. The practice of taking herbal baths to alleviate or prevent illness was also reported in Minas Gerais, Brazil, in 1777. A healer named Roque Angola had an intimate relationship with his owner, a coloured woman named Brizida Maria de Araujo, who openly consented to and encouraged Roque's healing practice. Preparing the herbal bath was a hybrid practice, in which a crucifix was immersed in a caldron together with herbs. Roque and Brizida washed themselves with the water. After washing, they dressed in their best clothes and began a *calundu* ceremony. Brizida claimed that, in this ritual, the souls of the dead took possession of the living. According to witnesses, Roque was possessed by Brizida's deceased child. Kananoja, 'Infected by the Devil', 503–504.

wash himself only with water mixed with herbs that he conserved in a pot in his house. He was also rumoured to carry gazelle horns filled with poison as amulets.[54]

Medicines, then, did not signify only vegetable, mineral or animal substances, but were also used as medicinal charms and power objects. They were thought to have powers to transform and to do something, to change or protect the body.[55] Amulets and charms made of buffalo or gazelle horns were common in West-Central Africa. In the 1780s, Rafael de Castelo de Vide encountered numerous people in the Kingdom of Kongo who carried traditional talismans around their necks or wore clothing adorned with 'diabolic' symbols. When he tore these away, stamped on or burned them, people defended themselves by saying that they relied on their traditional ways because there were no priests to teach them.[56]

There is nothing curious or surprising about Portuguese men believing in African magical practices. After all, similar practices were used in Portugal at the same time. The idea that illness could be caused and cured by supernatural and physical means was common to Portuguese and African world views. José Pedro Paiva has shown that popular healers in Portugal, especially in the region of Minho in the north of the country, often engaged in spirit possession rituals. The contents of these rituals were more or less equal to the ones described in Angola. When it was thought that the spirit of a dead person was causing an illness, the healers moved violently and entered into a trance. In this state, the spirit that possessed them 'talked' and revealed the proceedings that were to be adopted to heal the illness. It was common that the spirit demanded a sacrifice from the patient. People usually offered bread, cheese and wine. Rather than seeing ritual offerings as a pagan practice, Paiva has pointed out that contacting the dead fitted perfectly into the Catholic model of asking for help from the souls of the dead in Mass and through prayers. The only doctrinal problem with spirit possession ceremonies was that, from an ecclesiastical point of view, it was not possible that the dead came to this world to talk to the living.[57]

---

[54] ANTT, TSO/IL, Caderno do Promotor 86, ff. 41–45v. See also Ferreira, *Cross-Cultural Exchange*, 186.

[55] Susan Reynolds Whyte, Sjaak van der Geest and Anita Hardon, *Social Lives of Medicines* (Cambridge: Cambridge University Press, 2002), 5–6.

[56] Academia das Ciências de Lisboa, Série Vermelha de Manuscritos, 396, *Viagem do Congolo, do Missionário Frei Rafael de Castello de Vide Hoje Bispo de S. Thomé*, 185–186, 190–191; Jan Vansina, personal communication, 13 November 2009.

[57] Paiva, *Bruxaria e superstição*, 106–107.

Therapeutic practices in Portugal were also based on local empirical knowledge of the virtues of certain herbs and plants. This ancestral knowledge was often transmitted orally and secretly from generation to generation. The application of natural medicine was normally spiced up with more or less orthodox Catholic prayers. Healers routinely requested the help of divine or saintly powers throughout the country. Cooking herbs and water and then giving the mixture to the patient to drink was a part of the healers' repertoire, as was applying concoctions of herbs to the parts of the body that were ailing.[58] In practical and symbolic terms, there was thus little that would have separated the Central African and Portuguese healing methods.

In early modern Catholic and Protestant thought, there was an important distinction between natural magic and diabolic magic. The suppression of popular magic in Europe, bolstered by the Reformations of the sixteenth century, has been seen as part of a campaign by the Church to Christianise the European peasantry.[59] By extending the medieval Christian idea of the diabolical pact, popular superstitions became systematically associated with demonic magic. However, Central African everyday practices such as folk healing were not always condemned as demonic magic, but they were interpreted as un-Christian superstitions. Capuchin missionaries and Portuguese settlers acknowledged that African healers cured people by offering them herbal medicine. They might condemn spirit possession rituals as diabolical, but they were also prone to condemning popular healers as charlatans and their rituals as deception.

In practical terms, much of the European medicine available in Angola must have been seen as ineffective and even counterproductive. Bloodletting rarely resulted in the recovery of the patient, but rather led to a deterioration in health. Bleeding by cupping was used by Africans as well, but it seems not to have been as severe. It is thus not surprising that medical knowledge in Angola was quick to become hybridised as the Portuguese learned the uses of local natural medicine from Central Africans. There was a great need for this knowledge among Europeans because the number of qualified doctors and the stock of European medicine in Angola were always low. Moreover, the consequences of humoural medicine must have led many people to conclude that the herbal remedies used by African healers inflicted less harm.

---

[58] Paiva, *Bruxaria e superstição*, 108–109.
[59] Jean Delumeau, *Sin and Fear: The Emergence of a Western Guilt Culture, 13th–18th Centuries* (New York: St. Martin's Press, 1990).

The hybrid nature of therapeutic practices in Angola is best revealed by correspondence concerning the hospital in Massangano. In 1702, the Capuchin missionary António Maria de Florença wrote to the king, complaining about the lack of medicine and the absence of a doctor and a surgeon in the Misericórdia hospital. His letter was brought to the attention of Angola's former governor, Luís César de Meneses, who commented on medical practices in Massangano. According to him, soldiers from the *presídios* of Muxima, Cambambe, Pedras and Ambaca came to be treated in Massangano. They were treated with '*remédios da terra*', or local natural medicine, by local specialists, who knew which herbs to use because of their long experience with various illnesses. Following the former governor's advice, the Overseas Council in Lisbon told Father António Maria that the soldiers in Massangano were best cured with local medicine, 'because experience shows that it is the best way to free them from danger than if they were cured with [European] medical arts'. Moreover, the council reminded the Capuchins that it would be impossible to send surgeons and doctors to Massangano voluntarily because of its reputation as a diseased place.[60] The Overseas Council thus gave its unwitting approval for the use of African medical practices in the interior of Angola.

Hybridity also worked the other way around. Local religious mixture was evident in Angola from the beginning. Catholic material culture definitely had an influence on Central African healing practices. Jesuits established a college in Luanda in 1593 to teach interpreters in the hope that they would then help them move Atlantic Creole Christianity closer to their ideal European model. They trained and sent 'chapel boys' to the interior to teach and prepare the way for them, as they had done with the sons of nobles in Kongo. Jesuits, eager to rid Angola of unacceptable indigenous religious practices, sought to identify and burn shrines dedicated to local deities. In the process, they began another practice that was to become commonplace in Angola. When baptising the *soba* of Songa in 1581, they replaced African 'idols' and religious instruments with Christian religious objects. Soon after this, the Mbundu began to appropriate Christian objects and install them in their shrines as objects of devotion.[61]

The hybrid practice of appropriating Catholic objects was noted by witnesses in inquisitorial inquiries led by the Jesuit Jorge Pereira in

[60] AHU, CU, Angola, Caixa 17, Doc. 1934, Consulta do Conselho Ultramarino ao rei sobre o parecer solicitado ao Luís César de Meneses, 21 May 1703. See also António Brásio, 'As Misericórdias de Angola', *Studia* 4 (1959): 144–146.
[61] Heywood and Thornton, *Central Africans, Atlantic Creoles*, 100–101.

Luanda between 1596 and 1598. They reported that in Kongo and Ndongo, Africans bought crucifixes, images of saints and even indulgences from New Christian merchants. One of these merchants had reportedly also sold 'false relics' or masks and dolls that he had called 'bones of saints' and 'children of God'. The cultural exchange really worked both ways, because Portuguese merchants also obtained African objects of religious value.[62] Heywood and Thornton have suggested that the Catholic Church spread in Angola not only in areas where regular priests travelled, but also outside of their jurisdiction, influenced by the secular clergy. One should also include Portuguese merchants as active agents in this process, because they were responsible for the adoption of Christian objects by Africans in many locations. As a result, as Heywood and Thornton have argued, 'a new Mbundu version of Atlantic Creole Christianity was taking shape' in Angola.[63]

Devotion to the saints was a fundamental part of Counter-Reformation religiosity. In the Kingdom of Kongo, this veneration took on a local meaning in the early eighteenth century with the religious movement of Dona Beatriz Kimpa Vita, who claimed to be possessed by Saint Anthony. The healing aspects of prophetic religious imagination were central to her emergence as a religious leader. As befits a saint, Dona Beatriz/Saint Anthony healed the sick and was said to be able cure infertility. She claimed that even women who had been sterile for a long time could have children if they devoted themselves exclusively to Saint Anthony. Dona Beatriz attracted an immediate following when she announced that she could heal the infertile. Women tied small ropes and threads onto Dona Beatriz's hand and feet as a sign of their faith, paralleling the practice of both Portuguese and Italian Christians who even today tie gifts of money and messages to the statue of Saint Anthony. But in Kongo it was also a common practice to wear chains or ropes on one's hands and feet on feast days. The Kongolese interpretation was that these cords made them slaves of the Madonna.[64]

In the Kingdom of Kongo, Dona Beatriz travelled extensively as Saint Anthony and claimed that she could heal the sick, especially the infertile. She found numerous followers among the common people, who accompanied her as she moved around. They sang the *Salve Antoniana* and proclaimed openly the tenets of her preaching. In order to further her

[62] José da Silva Horta, 'Africanos e portugueses na documentação inquisitorial, de Luanda a Mbanza Kongo (1596–1598)', in *Actas do Seminário Encontro de povos e culturas em Angola* (Lisbon: Comissão Nacional para as Comemorações dos Descobrimentos Portugueses, 1997), 307–312.

[63] Heywood and Thornton, *Central Africans, Atlantic Creoles*, 105.

[64] Thornton, *The Kongolese Saint Anthony*, 132–133.

goals, she commissioned her own missionaries from among her followers, calling them 'Little Anthonys' and sending them often in pairs to
preach throughout the kingdom. They told people that baptism served
no purpose in God's eyes and distributed little cast-metal statues of Saint
Anthony, called *Ntoni Malau*, that were intended to replace the cross and
other symbols of Christian worship.[65] Besides giving them a religious
reading, these objects can also be interpreted as medicinal charms. It
seems that belief in Saint Anthony remained constant in Kongo for many
years to come. In the middle of the eighteenth century, it was still
common that people carried statues of the saint carved out of wood
around their necks. At the same time, black soldiers who fought for the
Portuguese attributed all their victories to the same saint.[66]

The syncretic nature of Atlantic Creole Christianity was also observed
by Father Rosario dal Parco in Luanda. His report revealed that Catholic
priests sold relics to people who used Catholic objects as protective
amulets or medicinal charms.[67] Other documents confirm that the
market for Christian objects observed in the late sixteenth century was
still in place in the latter half of the eighteenth century. In 1767,
Portuguese soldiers confiscated a statue of Our Lady of Conception
among African 'idols' during one of their campaigns in the interior of
Angola, showing that Catholic images were ardently adopted and placed
among traditional objects of devotion.[68] Central Africans actively sought
to obtain these objects from churches, either by stealing them or by
persuading someone else to do so. In the 1750s, a slave named Luis
André obtained a chalice from a certain Pedro Oliveira de Pinto, who had
stolen a communion plate and a chalice from a chapel. As compensation,
Pedro received a bottle of *aguardente* for each. The chalice was later
seized from Luis André, who was sentenced to a year of penal servi-
tude.[69] A report by Bishop Alexandre in 1788 also pointed to the obvious
syncretism that had become a part of African religious practice in Angola.

---

[65] Thornton, *The Kongolese Saint Anthony*, 132–149.
[66] AHU, CU, Angola Cx. 37, Doc. 50, Oficio do Governador e Capitão General do Reino
de Angola (Marques de Lavradio) ao Conselho Ultramarino, 19 August 1750. In this
correspondence, it is claimed that the Kongolese called Saint Anthony the 'God
Saint Anthony'.
[67] P. Rosario dal Parco, 'Informations sur le royaume du Congo et d'Angola du P. Rosario
dal Parco, préfet des capucins en Angola et Congo, 1760', in Louis Jadin, 'Aperçu de la
situation du Congo et rite d'élection des rois en 1775, d'après le P. Cherubino da
Savona, missionnaire au Congo de 1759 à 1774', *Bulletin de l'Institut Historique Belge de
Rome* 35 (1963): 362.
[68] AHU, CU, Angola Cx. 51, Doc. 19, Carta do Governador Geral de Angola, 3 April
1767. In this case, the statue was sent to Brazil for restoration.
[69] AHU, CU, Angola Cx. 53, Doc. 37, Sentenças da Junta, 30 July 1769.

Chalices and other holy ornaments had disappeared from the majority of churches and were being used by Africans in their rituals. Holy images were placed in African homes alongside traditional statues, leading the bishop to state that images of Christ were adored side by side with those of 'the Devil'.[70]

Medical hybridity was not viewed favourably by Portuguese physicians. In a letter written in 1770, Governor Sousa Coutinho mentioned that, due to a conflict with Luanda's popular healers, or *curandeiros*, Chief Physician Damião Cosme had taken refuge in the governor's house.[71] Two decades later, Chief Physician José Pinto de Azeredo clearly condemned traditional popular healing practices in Angola:

> The black folk, even while living with whites and learning their customs, observing their religion, and speaking their language, never forget the heathen rites, mischief and superstitions. In their illness they do not want professors nor take pharmaceutical remedies; because they only have faith in their medicines that they call *milongos*, and these have to be administered by *feiticeiros* [sorcerers], or *curadores* [popular healers]. It is lamentable that many whites born in Angola, but even some Europeans, believe in the virtue of such remedies, and secretly subject themselves to similar doctors.[72]

Azeredo's comment shows that the feeble efforts, whether by the Inquisition or secular authorities, to rid the Portuguese colony of Angola of traditional therapeutic practices during the eighteenth century had not borne any fruit. Many white people found it more convenient to trust African popular healers than the surgeons and bleeders employed in the hospital of Luanda. In this way, people showed their distrust of the practice of phlebotomy that had dominated much of official medical thinking in Angola and elsewhere in the tropics. At the same time, however, the practice of making cuts in the skin and drawing blood in tiny quantities from sick people seems to have been an acceptable practice to both Africans and at least some Europeans.

Cross-cultural medical interaction persisted well into the nineteenth century. Omboni drew attention to the activities of African healers in Luanda and its hinterland, claiming that they lived alone in the woods, and, possessing practical knowledge of the effects of plants, also acted as doctors. People consulted them in groups and generally obeyed their suggestions. Medicinal preparations were sometimes made in secret

---

[70] AHU, CU, Angola Cx. 73, Doc. 28, Fr. Alexandre Bispo de Malaca, 20–24 June 1788.
[71] AHU, CU, Angola, Cx. 54, Doc. 53, Carta de D. Francisco Inocencio de Sousa Coutinho, July 11, 1770.
[72] José Pinto de Azeredo, *Ensaios sobre algumas enfermidades d'Angola* (Lisbon: Regia Officina Typografica, 1799), 53.

nocturnal meetings. According to Omboni, the 'ignorant' European soldiers of the forts and residents in the interior districts also consulted local folk healers secretly in cases of illness and scrupulously followed their advice.[73]

Collecting Information

The exact avenues of knowledge transmission from local Africans to Portuguese collectors remain obscure, as informants are usually not named in the sources. Information on the curative properties of plants certainly came directly from healers in the course of therapy. Information could also be bought, as Buitrago hinted in his manuscript when referring to the costs of collecting information on medicinal plants. Moreover, he claimed that the cures often circulated freely, as it was customary to 'make everything in the view of the sick, to free [the healers] from some bad suspicion'.[74]

As already mentioned, Afonso Mendes probably obtained his knowledge on plant medicines from African soldiers in Portuguese service and locals in the *presídios* of the interior. Portuguese settlers and traders who travelled in the Kingdom of Kongo or the hinterlands of Luanda and Benguela must have had experimental knowledge of local medicines. After all, they hardly had other options available. In this way, knowledge of herbal remedies must have accumulated over the decades and centuries, free to be used and shared with newcomers. Local African women, who had liaisons with Portuguese men in the port cities and in the interior, also facilitated access to sources of healing knowledge. In the case of João Pereira da Cunha, his partner Catarina Juliana directed him to a local African healer while they lived in Ambaca.

Central African mineral resources were as much a part of experimentation as plant medicines.[75] In December 1769, Governor Sousa

---

[73] 'Hanno loro sacerdoti che vivono solitari ne' boschi, ed avendo pratica conoscenza degli effetti di certe erbe fanno anche da medici .... I reggenti de' presidii e distretti portoghesi fomentano colla loro ignoranza quelle dannosissime superstizioni, perchè anch' essi in casi di malattia, nascostamente li consultano e ne seguono scrupolosamente i consigli.' Omboni, *Viaggi*, 93–94.

[74] Biblioteca Nacional de Portugal, Fundo Reservados 437, Códice 13114, Francisco de Buytrago, *Arvore da vida*, f. 5v. 'E pellas curas, q fazem he q se devulgão muitas couzas dellas, por ser costume entre o gentio fazer tudo a vista dos enfermos, p.ª os livrar de algua roim suspeita.'

[75] On persistent beliefs that mineral wealth could sustain the Angolan economy, see Governor Melo's report 'Acerca das riquezas desta Colónia, e da possibilidade ou impossibilidade de as aproveitar, 30 July 1799', *Arquivos de Angola*, First Series, 1:4 (1935): no page numbers.

Coutinho sent a sample of a green stone (*pedra verde*) to Lisbon. Its origin was a place called Serra de Bende, about eight or ten leagues from the *presídio* of Encoje in the lands belonging to a rebellious vassal of the King of Kongo. The locals called it the unguent stone (*pedra unguento*) because it healed all their sores and wounds. Missionaries, experimenters par excellence, used it to prepare paint, which they used in painting their churches. Besides giving a green dye, Sousa Coutinho assumed it contained copper. Fearing commercial competition by the French and English in Cabinda, he was unwilling to develop commerce in the product. Sousa Coutinho also wanted to hide the value of the green stone from locals and so had the stone brought to him secretly. Being certain that Angolan soils contained many similar treasures that should be brought under the spotlight of naturalists, Sousa Coutinho was, however, sceptical that locals were ambitious enough to develop a commerce in these products, commenting that locals always mixed their remedies with superstitious beliefs, believing that these made them virtuous.[76]

Sousa Coutinho's wishes to bring Central African minerals under closer scrutiny were fulfilled twenty years later, when Joaquim José da Silva sent samples of natural products to Lisbon. His shipment in November 1791 included minerals such as gypsum and marble, among many others.[77] In Portugal, however, these samples were either buried in the *Real Gabinete da Historia Natural in Ajuda* or looted by Napoleon's troops in 1808 and taken to Paris.[78]

By the late eighteenth century, the Portuguese in Angola had acquired a wealth of knowledge about natural medicine. Although this knowledge had been recorded in Capuchin writings, in Portuguese pharmacopoeias and in manuscript form, the late eighteenth-century officers and crown officials sent to Angola seem to have ignored these earlier writings completely and started their efforts at collection and systematisation from scratch. Joaquim José da Silva, a botanist sent to Angola, served in a double role as Secretary of Angola and as a scientific explorer. His three-year assignment became a lifetime residence, and he made field trips to Cabinda and the Rio Dande area (1783–1784), from Luanda to

---

[76] 'Sousa Coutinho para o Ex.mo Sr. Francisco Xavier de Mendonça Furtado com a remessa de hum caixote em que vai huma porção de Pedra Verde – Luanda, 4 December 1769', *Arquivos de Angola*, First Series, 1:1 (1933): no page numbers; AHU, CU, Angola, Cx. 54, Doc. 113, Ofício de Sousa Coutinho, 30 December 1770.

[77] 'Relação de productos Naturaes, que pela Secretaria de Estado da Repartição do Ultramar vão remetidos ao Real Gabinete – Luanda, 5 November 1791', *Arquivos de Angola*, First Series, 1:1 (1933): no page numbers.

[78] On French looting of natural history collections in Lisbon, see Filipa Lowndes Vicente, 'Travelling Objects: The Story of Two Natural History Collections in the Nineteenth Century', *Portuguese Studies* 19 (2003): 19–37.

Massangano (1784) and from Benguela into the interior of southern Angola (1785–1787). On his field trip to Cabinda, Joaquim José da Silva and his assistants were accompanied by Captain Álvaro de Carvalho e Matoso. Through his association and friendship with Silva, Matoso prepared a shipment of materia medica to Lisbon. The inventory list, published by Luiz de Pina in 1938 and in English translation by William Simon in 1976, provides a detailed account of several Angolan medicinal plants.[79] One is again struck by the inclusion of *kikongo* wood in Matoso's account. According to him, carbuncles, sores, cancers and all types of lesions that might suppurate were treated with 'a most singular remedy, much in use, and well tried, being the cure which is used instead of a harmful one'.[80]

Matoso's observation and detailed instructions for *kikongo*'s medicinal use show that the plant had enjoyed widespread popularity in West-Central Africa for over two centuries. Portuguese settlers had learned of its use from the local population and adopted it for curing their own infections. Matoso also listed other remedies that had already been mentioned in the preceding century. *Engariaria*, tusk of the wild boar and *engala* horn, *kiseko* and kola had all been tried by Mendes, Cadornega and the Capuchins and were listed in Portuguese pharmacopoeias. Writing of Angolan medicinal products, Matoso noted that these 'very often utilised' remedies had been tried many times 'with an indivisible effect' and had 'proven useful'.[81] The habitual use of local natural products by the Portuguese in Angola leaves no doubt that, in medical matters, Europeans learned from Africans rather than relied entirely on their own ways of treating diseases.

Portuguese attempts to collect information about Central African natural history were stepped up in the 1790s. Governor Almeida e Vasconcelos sent detailed instructions to captain-majors of the *presídios* to participate in sending samples to the *Real Gabinete*. Special care was to be taken when capturing, slaying and preserving animals. Military officers were also given guidance on how to dry and preserve plant specimens and remit minerals. Most importantly, collectors were asked to provide information on the provenance of specimens and their local uses. Finally, the instructions went beyond natural history and asked soldiers to collect 'with equal curiosity' arms, agricultural implements and indigenous idols and to provide observations on the religion, rites and laws of the locals.[82]

---

[79] Pina, 'Notas para a medicina'; Simon, 'A Luso-African Formulary', 112–114.
[80] Simon, 'A Luso-African Formulary', 113.
[81] Simon, 'A Luso-African Formulary', 112–113.
[82] 'Instruçõens Gerais aos Capitaens Mores, sobre a colheita, e remessa das Produçõens Naturais, que hão-de ser dirigidas ao Real Gabinete de Historia Natural, 17 October 1790', *Arquivos de Angola*, First Series, 1:4 (1935): no page numbers. It is unknown if

Although the captain-majors did not participate actively in providing knowledge on natural history, Joaquim José da Silva continued collecting and sending specimens. In February 1793, he sent a large collection containing several medicinals, including four pieces of the *kikongo* tree, *mututo* and *abutua* root and two pieces of *kiseko* wood. The shipment also included a piece of *takula* and information on using it as dye. According to Silva, a ball made by mixing *takula* powder and water, when sent from one chief to another, served as a declaration of war, and when fighting men painted their bodies with *takula* paint.[83]

The local markets were well developed and versatile products moved between the coast and the interior. Although the slave trade has been the main point of focus in narratives of Angolan history, Matoso's report points out that medicinal plants also moved along the trade routes. Kola nuts originating in the Kingdom of Kongo were imported to and sold in Luanda, where the inhabitants used them 'almost every day'. In exchange, Kongo traders received *nzimbu* shells that served as currency in their homelands.[84]

The mixing of European and African ingredients had also continued. For example, *engariaria* was mixed with brandy and gunpowder to make a concoction to cure diarrhoea and dysentery. Alcohol was an important ingredient in some medicines. Half a spoon of powder from the tusk of a wild boar given with sugar-cane brandy as well as three little balls of dark horse manure, well ground up, and half a pint of wine were regarded as 'excellent' remedies for pleurisies.[85]

---

these instructions ever led to any actions taken by captain-majors. If they did, the specimens and accompanying reports have not surfaced in the archives yet.

[83] 'Relação dos Productos Naturaes que pela Secretaria de Estado da Repartição do Ultramar, vão remetidos ao Real Gabinete da Ajuda, na Rela Fragata Minerva, em Cumprimento das Reaes Ordens de Sua Magestade, 18 February 1793', *Arquivos de Angola*, First Series, 1:4 (1935): no page numbers.

[84] Simon, 'A Luso-African Formulary', 113–114, *nzimbu* transcribed as 'Limbo' by Simon. According to Azeredo, *Ensaios*, 46, kola nuts were in constant use and chewed at all times with water, 'which makes it sweet and tasty ... it aids digestion and because of these benefits it has become such a luxury that companions offer pieces of it, which they call "legs", to one another as a courtesy, with the same gallantry with which we exchange snuff between us'. On the trade and use of the kola elsewhere in Atlantic Africa, see Paul E. Lovejoy, *Caravans of Kola: The Hausa Kola Trade 1700–1900* (Zaria: Ahmadu Bello University Press, 1980); Edmund Abaka, *Kola Is God's Gift: Agricultural Production, Export Initiatives and the Kola Industry of Asante and the Gold Coast c. 1820–1950* (Athens: Ohio University Press, 2005).

[85] Simon, 'A Luso-African Formulary', 112–113. On alcohol in West Central Africa, see José C. Curto, *Alcoól e Escravos: O comércio luso-brasileiro do alcoól em Mpinda, Luanda e Benguela durante o tráfico atlântico de escravos (c. 1480–1830) e o seu impacto nas sociedades da África Central Ocidental* (Lisbon: Editora Vulgata, 2002); Curto, *Enslaving Spirits*.

In the late eighteenth century, one can observe two conflicting tenden-
cies in the Portuguese attitudes towards African medicinals. On the one
hand, interest in botanical knowledge from different parts of the
Portuguese Empire was growing in Lisbon, resulting in scientific expeditions to Brazil, Angola and Mozambique. On the other hand, doctors
serving as chief physicians in Angola were clearly turning away from
using and experimenting with African plant-derived drugs, although they
might have recognised a few of these medicinals as useful in their practice. The primary intention of Portuguese physicians was to introduce
the newest Western medical thinking into Angola, including the
common usage of cinchona bark from Brazil in treating malaria (see
Chapter 5).[86]

Three centuries of European experimentation with indigenous
Angolan drugs was brought to a logical conclusion when, in 1798,
Governor Dom Miguel Antonio de Melo wrote about the positive experiences of the medical uses of *kikongo* wood, *enkasa* bark, *engariaria* fruit
and *muriassangi* root. The diseases for which the said drugs were used
had not changed over the centuries. Rather, the Portuguese had now
compiled more knowledge through experimentation. *Kikongo* was still
used to cure acute fevers, erysipelas and anthrax. Women used it with
palm oil as a cosmetic to adorn their faces and hair. For acute fevers, a
tablespoon of powder from the *kikongo* tree was dissolved in water,
showing that this medicine had a fixed dosage. Anthrax was cured by
covering skin lesions with *kikongo* powder and applying a poultice of
maize flour and palm oil to them. According to Melo, the continuous
experiences of curing anthrax with *kikongo* had demonstrated that, in
contrast to Portugal, the disease was not fatal in Angola.

Unaware of Buitrago's experiments with *enkasa* in Lisbon, Melo
thought that Europeans had not seen the tree before. It was known to
have emetic 'virtues' and was also used as an antidote against certain
poisons that abounded in the *sertão*. The first experiments with this
substance were always made with great caution, as it was well known
that large dosages were lethal. Melo was aware that blacks used it in their
judicial rituals and poison ordeals. *Engariaria* was another plant that had
a long history as a medicinal in Central Africa, but Melo was not familiar
with Capuchin writings about the plant. The plant resembled nutmeg

---

[86] Augusto D'Ésaguy, 'A abertura da Escola Médica de Luanda (duas obras inéditas do dr.
José Pinto de Azeredo)', *Imprensa Médica* 15:3 (1951): 31–37; Augusto D'Ésaguy, *Breve
notícia sobre a Escola Médica de Luanda (Documentos)* (Lisbon: Ed. Império, 1951); Jaime
Walter, *Um português carioca professor da primeira escola médica de Angola 1791 (as suas
lições de anatomia)* (Lisbon: Junta de Investigações do Ultramar, 1970).

and was used in curing cramps and bloody dysenteries. A teaspoon of *engariaria* powder was dissolved in water together with an equal amount of *kikongo* powder.[87]

Portuguese enthusiasm for West-Central African plant medicines can be compared with the scientific work of mapping the Congo River in the early nineteenth century by British explorers. By the time of Tuckey's expedition to the Congo in 1816, the epistemological effects of Linnaean systematisation were clearly discernible. The expedition's Norwegian botanist, Christen Smith, was more interested in amassing plants for physical examination than in their local names, uses and histories. He rarely recorded the vernacular names of plants in his journal and did not employ local assistants specialising in botany, although a Kongolese man named Ben served as his servant. When describing a plant Smith took for *Ximenia*, Smith noted that the locals called it *Gangi*. He also heard from Catholic priests 'long stories about its use in putrid fevers'. But that was the extent of Smith's interest. Unlike Portuguese amateur botanists before him, he did not compile a detailed list of local medicinal plants.[88]

When not hunting for new specimens on the land, Smith was confined to the ship on the river, making a focused effort to preserve and examine his valued plants, many of which undoubtedly were new to science. His activity can also be attributed to the constant haste that the expedition made in navigating up the River Congo. Whereas Buitrago spent years experimenting with *enkasa* in Angola and Lisbon, Smith only had time to scribble in his journal that 'Casa is a purgative legumen'. Later, people brought him its bark and leaves, telling him it was poisonous. Smith noted that the bitter *macasso* was a nut chewed by Kongolese elites, but he was not sure whether this was the kola nut. Smith's time on the river stands in great contrast not only to the efforts of Portuguese amateur botanists, but also to those of other Scandinavian botanists who were active in West Africa shortly before Tuckey's journey. Isert and Thonning on the Gold Coast as well as Afzelius in Sierra Leone were constantly interacting with local African informants or Europeans who had resided on the coast for a longer time (see Chapters 3 and 4). The nature of Tuckey's expedition made in-depth interaction with cultural

---

[87] 'De Dom Miguel Antonio de Mello acerca do Breu'.

[88] Christen Smith, 'Professor Smith's Journal', in *Narrative of an Expedition to Explore the River Zaire, Usually Called the Congo, in South Africa, in 1816, under the Direction of Captain J.H. Tuckey, R.N.* (London: John Murray, 1818), 261, 276. Smith's servant Ben 'left his native country when twelve years of age', and does not seem to have commanded specialised botanical knowledge.

go-betweens impossible, and Smith's imperatives lay in systematising his findings for botanical science.[89]

Conclusion

In West-Central Africa, the material world of medicine abounded with herbal, animal and mineral remedies. Experimenting with plant medicines and local curing methods was commonplace. From the early contacts onwards, the Portuguese constantly sought out local knowledge in their quest for health in a tropical environment. Exchanging medical knowledge formed the basis for cultural contacts, as local rulers requested European healing specialists and offered valued African medicinals as gifts to be sent to Portuguese kings. These exchanges were repeated over and over again in military regiments and households established by Portuguese men and African women. West-Central African medical knowledge and medicinals also spread throughout the Atlantic world, especially to Brazil and Portugal, by the eighteenth century. Further, religious connotations of healing were most prone to be cultivated cross-culturally, as the case of Saint Anthony of Padua's success in the Kingdom of Kongo attests.

Incorporating new medicinals into Luso-African pharmacopoeias was based, first and foremost, on experiment. The authority of healers, whether local *ngangas* or Portuguese men like Mendes and Buitrago, was based on public demonstrations of healing knowledge. Sensorial evaluation (taste, smell) of medical substances played a key role in their adoption. Expanding pharmacopoeias suggest that new plants and local specialties were added to lists of suitable remedies. With the 'discovery' of new ingredients in novel locations, news and knowledge of them travelled. Healers were mobile but so were the medicinals people used. Furthermore, Angola was a part of global exchanges. What had proven to work in India, moved with the Portuguese to West-Central Africa and Brazil.

[89] Smith, 'Professor Smith's Journal', 283, 286, 307, 328–329.

3 'Much Better Suited Than We Are, as Regards Their Health Care'
African Botanical Expertise and Medical Knowledge on the Gold Coast

Johannes Rask, a Danish clergyman who resided on the Gold Coast from 1708 to 1713, viewed West African bodies as relatively healthy and thought that people generally lived long. He wrote that locals did not come to be treated by Europeans unless they were absolutely sure that the treatment was 'effective' and only if they knew the surgeon or physician personally. He regarded the local healers he met on the Gold Coast as very skilful in treating external sores from a cut or having been pierced. People used palm oil in the treatment. Rask admitted thinking that

when picturing our apothecaries in Europe – filled with countless beakers, and glasses, boxes and bottles, from floor to ceiling; and thinking of the numerous saws, knives, stilettoes, scissors, forceps, awls with which our surgeons load their chests and cupboards – things of which the Negroes know nothing and have not even heard of them, yet they are much better suited than we are, as regards their health care.[1]

Rask did not make moral arguments about African healing knowledge, which to him implied the practice of herbalism. In contrast, many other early modern Europeans describing West Africa usually wrote about healing in the context of African religious practices, namely spirits or fetishes.[2] Modern anthropologists have similarly described African religious lives, witchcraft beliefs and magical world views, observing that illness and other misfortune resulted from witchcraft or other reasons having to do with the 'Other World' or occult powers.[3] African medical history and medical anthropology have challenged this view. Many

---

[1] Johannes Rask, *Two Views from Christiansborg Castle. Volume I. A Brief and Truthful Description of a Journey to and from Guinea,* translated by Selena Axelrod Winsnes (Accra: Sub-Saharan Publishers, 2008), 112 [145].

[2] E.g. Ludewig Ferdinand Rømer, *A Reliable Account of the Coast of Guinea (1760),* translated by Selena Axelrod Winsnes (Oxford: Oxford University Press, 2000), 83–98. See also Roberts, 'Medical Exchange on the Gold Coast'.

[3] On the Gold Coast especially, see M. J. Field, *Religion and Medicine of the Gã People* (London: Oxford University Press, 1937).

African societies, today as well as in the past, had several kinds of medical and religious experts. Some of these experts healed with what they regarded as spiritual powers, emanating either from local spirits or from the Christian God or saints, whereas other medical specialists are better described as herbalists.[4] Similar to what was observed earlier regarding Angola and Kongo, not all healing practised in Atlantic Africa should be regarded as spiritual or fetish worship; everyday illness – such as cold fever, coughing, chest pain and stomach ache – was treated with medicinal plants gathered from nature.[5] Summing it up, Danish merchant Ludvig Ferdinand Rømer wrote in the mid-eighteenth century that 'the sick person tries *first* to see if he can be helped with herbs or other [remedies] known to be effective in such an illness'.[6] African individuals and communities possessed botanical knowledge, and Europeans wanting to get rid of certain ailments did not necessarily need to visit a 'fetish man' in order to be cured.

By concentrating on the interaction between indigenous informants and European settlers, this chapter highlights African botanical expertise and medical knowledge on the Gold Coast. It invites the question: Were the Portuguese experiences of cross-cultural medical interaction in Angola and the Kingdom of Kongo exceptional? Just like in Angola and Kongo, local medical knowledge emerged as a viable healing alternative for European settlers, who were confined to West African coastal enclaves and could not always count upon a steady supply of imported European medicines. Cultural go-betweens,[7] many of them women, provided everyday healthcare and facilitated Europeans' access to local healers when necessary. Although the evidence is sparse, this can be detected in English, Dutch and Danish sources on the Gold Coast, which are examined in this chapter.

Early Medical Encounters

In their bid for global economic dominance in the early seventeenth century, Dutch traders seized upon major initiatives in Atlantic Africa.

---

[4] However, even a herbalist can believe that the plants used in the healing process 'work' because of the spiritual powers attached to them.

[5] Cf. Emmanuel Kwaku Akyeampong, 'Disease in West African History', in *Themes in West Africa's History*, edited by Emmanuel Kwaku Akyeampong (Athens: Ohio University Press, 2006), 194.

[6] Rømer, *A Reliable Account*, 90, italics added.

[7] On cultural brokers in the Atlantic world, see, e.g., Stephen Greenblatt, *Marvelous Possessions: The Wonder of the New World* (Oxford: Oxford University Press, 1991); Alida C. Metcalf, *Go-Betweens and the Colonization of Brazil: 1500–1600* (Austin: University of Texas Press, 2005); Toby Green, ed., *Brokers of Change: Atlantic Commerce and Cultures in Pre-colonial Western Africa* (Oxford: Oxford University Press, 2012).

In West-Central Africa, they followed the Portuguese traders in exploiting the supplies of *takula* on the Loango coast, especially at the port of Mayumbe.[8] *Takula* featured prominently among the trade items sought from West-Central Africa by the Dutch trader Pieter van den Broecke, who traded in Loango and Soyo in the early seventeenth century. There was an extensive regional market for *takula*, and van den Broecke traded it along the coast. On his second trip to Angola, van den Broecke bought 200 pieces of *takula* from a mulatto trader named Luís Mendes at Mayumbe to take to Kongo, where it was in great demand. Mendes worked for a contractor in Luanda, buying up 'all the redwood he could get'. During his second and third trip, van den Broecke brought 1,800 and 800 pieces of *takula*, respectively, to Amsterdam to test if dyers in Europe could use it. He noted that in Angola the Portuguese purchased *takula* in abundance and transported it along the entire coast, where it brought great profits.[9] *Takula* and *kikongo* continued to figure prominently for Dutch traders in the 1640s.[10] The Brazil Council of the Dutch West India Company (WIC) also expressed interest in *takula*, wanting to compare it with Brazilwood. Consequently, in 1641 the Dutch in Loango sent nine tonnes of Mayumbe redwood to Brazil for inspection.[11] Its use as a medicine seems to have continued on Dutch ships for at least several decades; in 1675, an 'Instruction for the Skippers in the Slave Trade' ordered each Dutch slave ship to have a supply of *takula* on board for distribution among the slaves.[12]

On the Gold Coast, shared conceptualisations of the human body are suggested by Wilhelm Johann Müller's seventeenth-century list of Akan vocabulary collected in Fetu. Müller listed fifty-five words related to parts of the human body. These included internal organs, such as liver, gall, heart, lungs, kidneys, spleen and bladder. Noticeably, in listing terms denoting persons of high and low status, Müller gave the local word for a doctor (*Ujodoru*). It is unclear whether it signified an

---

[8] 'Relação da costa de Angola e Congo pelo ex-Governador Fernão de Sousa, February 21, 1632', in Brásio, ed., *MMA*, 8: 124. On early Dutch activities on the Loango coast, see Mark Meuwese, *Brothers in Arms, Partners in Trade: Dutch-Indigenous Alliances in the Atlantic World, 1595–1674* (Leiden and Boston: Brill, 2012), 77–88.

[9] J. D. La Fleur, ed., *Pieter van den Broecke's Journal of Voyages to Cape Verde, Guinea and Angola 1605–1612* (London: The Hakluyt Society, 2000), 73, 80, 88, 93, 97, 102.

[10] 'Cornelis Hendrikz Ouman au Conseil de Recife'; 'Les XIX aux directeurs de Loanda'; 'Les XIX aux directeurs de la côte sud d'Afrique', in Louis Jadin, *L'Ancien Congo et l'Angola 1639–1655 d'apres les archives romaines, portugaises, néerlandaises et espagnoles* (Brussels and Rome: Institut Historique Belge de Rome, 1975), 1: 215, 470; 3: 764.

[11] Phyllis Martin, *The External Trade of the Loango Coast, 1576–1870: The Effects of Changing Commercial Relations on the Vili Kingdom of Loango* (Oxford: Clarendon Press, 1972), 57.

[12] A. M. G. Rutten, *Dutch Transatlantic Medicine Trade in the Eighteenth Century under the Cover of the West India Company* (Rotterdam: Erasmus Publishing, 2000), 99.

African herbalist or a European surgeon or physician. However, *Ujodoru* was clearly different from terms related to spiritual matters, which included several terms denoting soothsayers, sorcerers and fetish men.[13]

Despite mutual, occasionally intensive, interest in each other's healing methods, European and African medicine could coexist on the seventeenth-century Gold Coast with little seeming cultural transfer from one side to the other. The case in point concerns the preferred treatment for removing Guinea worms – an almost everyday occasion, if we trust Brun's and Hemmersam's accounts. Surgeon Samuel Brun advised his readers to pull the worms out gently, because if one grabbed them too hard they broke off and caused a terrible swelling. Goldsmith Michael Hemmersam, who contracted three cases of Guinea worm during his stay on the Gold Coast between 1639 and 1645, gave even more detailed advice, writing how it was best to pull out the worm little by little in the morning and evening. In his third case of Guinea worm, the worm broke off after only a quarter had been pulled out, causing a great swelling in his leg, which kept him in bed for four months; the leg finally had to be cut open to cure it. Hemmersam revealed that the locals had a different form of treatment. After they had pulled the worm out the length of a finger, they cut it off and smeared palm oil on it, tying the wound with a green leaf. The swelling that formed afterwards was cut open and the impure matter was let to run out. Then, the wound was washed with water strongly mixed with pepper and other herbs, so that it stung sharply. Afterwards, it was covered with a leaf and palm oil to relieve the pain.[14]

On the Gold Coast, early interaction with locals after the ousting of the Portuguese from Fort Elmina included a curious incident in May 1646, when a man named Doede, a representative of the Akan village of Elmina, arrived on behalf of all the captains and *caboseros* to visit General Jacob Adriaensz van der Wel in order to supply several beads to a local fetish man. The beads were to be used in a ritual to 'remedy the mortality' of the Dutch, who were dying in great numbers. In other words, local healing specialists were trying to help the Dutch overcome the constant threat of tropical illness. Van der Wel, outraged at this

[13] Wilhelm Johann Müller, 'Müller's List of Vocabulary', in *German Sources for West African History*, edited by Adam Jones (Wiesbaden: Franz Steiner, 1983), 269–328.
[14] Samuel Brun, 'Samuel Brun's Voyages of 1611–20', in *German Sources for West African History 1599–1669*, edited by Adam Jones (Wiesbaden: Franz Steiner), 91; Michael Hemmersam, 'Michael Hemmersam's Description of the Gold Coast, 1639–45', in *German Sources for West African History 1599–1669*, edited by Adam Jones (Wiesbaden: Franz Steiner, 1983), 121–122.

'godless' request, dismissed the fetish man's request.[15] This event shows how vulnerable the Dutch were in West Africa, but also the moral indignation caused by African religious healing. Would van der Wel have reacted similarly if locals had offered herbal remedies instead? Given the readiness of the locals to help the Dutch, one can surmise that such interactions had been common when the Portuguese occupied Elmina.

West-Central African attempts to acquire European medical knowledge, detailed in Chapter 2, were not unique. As had happened in Angola and the Kingdom of Kongo, so too the acquisition of medical knowledge occurred elsewhere in Atlantic Africa. Some West African rulers went as far as sending emissaries to Europe in order to acquire foreign medical secrets. In 1657, Ambassador Bans of the West African kingdom of Ardra landed in Cartagena de Indias. Sent by his ruler, Capoo, he was on his way to Madrid. While Bans's trip to the Spanish capital might have served political goals, obtaining medical knowledge was among the stated motives of the trip. Preoccupied with his own mortality and dynastic succession, King Capoo wished to learn from the Spanish sovereign and emulate his reputed longevity.[16]

Conversely, Europeans were no less interested in African medicines. In the second half of the seventeenth century, the English, for example, made more than twenty collections of plants in different parts of Atlantic Africa, especially in South and West Africa but also in Angola.[17] One of the most important contemporary organisers of these collections was James Petiver, a London-based pharmacist who corresponded with English officers, sea captains and settlers around the world. Petiver was in close contact with Hans Sloane,[18] and one of his letters to Sloane was published in the Royal Society's *Philosophical Transactions* in 1695. In the letter, Petiver described forty medicinal plants collected on the Gold Coast, mentioning the local name and uses of each plant. He compared the descriptions to other writings, such as Sloane's unpublished manuscript on Jamaica and Hendrik van Rheede's *Hortus Malabaricus*. This latter work attempted to demonstrate the global dispersal of plants

---

[15] Meuwese, *Brothers in Arms, Partners in Trade*, 305; Klas Ratelband, ed., *Vijf Dagregisters van Het Kasteel São Jorge da Mina (Elmina) aan de Goudkust (1645–1647)* ('S-Gravenhage: Martinus Nijhoff, 1953), 174.

[16] Gómez, *The Experiential Caribbean*, 16–18.

[17] These are catalogued in J. E. Dandy, ed., *The Sloane Herbarium: An Annotated List of the Horti Sicci Composing It; with Biographical Accounts of the Principal Contributors* (London: British Museum, 1958).

[18] On Sloane's work, see James Delbourgo, *Collecting the World: The Life and Curiosity of Hans Sloane* (London: Penguin, 2017).

beyond the Atlantic.[19] Sloane, whose work concerned Jamaica, undoubtedly pushed Petiver to this kind of universal thinking because it made
possible comparing the world's natural resources on a global scale.[20]

The forty plants described by Petiver in the *Philosophical Transactions*
had been collected by John Smyth, a clergyman in the service of the
Royal African Company at the Cape Coast Castle. Smyth also provided
the local names and information on the usefulness of these plants.
Smyth's information hints that the plants enjoyed widespread use among
Europeans on the Gold Coast; according to Smyth, each plant was
'good' for this or that disease. The diseases and ailments included itch,
smallpox, headache, toothache, buboes and bellyache. In addition,
Smyth had collected plants that were good for recovering strength,
improving a sick person's appetite, stopping the bleeding and killing
Guinea worms (*Dracunculus medinensis*).[21]

Smyth had local sources for this information. Information on two
plants had been provided by Mr. Edward Barter, who was a Eurafrican
educated in England. The Royal Africa Company had paid for his
schooling between 1690 and 1693, after which Barter returned to the
Gold Coast as a company employee.[22] Barter had told Petiver that juice
squeezed from a plant named *attrummaphoe* was good for making one
sneeze when snuffed up the nose. *Metacoe* was used on the Gold Coast
for making slow match.[23]

Petiver and his connections in Atlantic Africa and America[24] bring to
light several characteristics of knowledge production concerning Africa,
which differed considerably from relationships between Europeans and
Africans during twentieth-century colonialism. The plants collected by
Smyth were an indication that Europeans who settled in West Africa
could not afford to ignore African medical knowledge. On the contrary,

[19] James Petiver, 'A Catalogue of Some Guinea-Plants, with Their Native Names and Virtues; Sent to James Petiver, Apothecary, and Fellow of the Royal Society; with His Remarks on Them. Communicated in a Letter to Dr. Hans Sloane. Secret. Reg. Soc.', *Philosophical Transactions* 19 (1695): 679–684.
[20] Cf. Nicholas Canny, 'Atlantic History and Global History', in *Atlantic History: A Critical Appraisal*, edited by Jack P. Greene and Philip D. Morgan (Oxford: Oxford University Press, 2009), 328.
[21] Petiver, 'A Catalogue of Some Guinea-Plants'.
[22] Walter Rodney, 'The Guinea Coast', in *The Cambridge History of Africa*, Vol. 4, edited by Richard Gray (Cambridge: Cambridge University Press, 1975), 308. On Barter's later career as an influential trader, see William Bosman, *A New and Accurate Description of the Coast of Guinea. Divided into the Gold, the Slave, and the Ivory Coasts* (London: Ballantyne Press, 1907 [1705]), 51–52.
[23] Petiver, 'A Catalogue of Some Guinea-Plants', 681, 684.
[24] On Petiver's contacts in the Atlantic world, see Parrish, 'Diasporic African Sources', 289, 291.

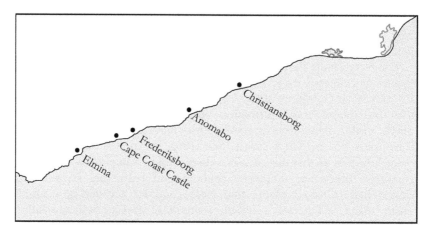

Figure 3.1 The Gold Coast.
Source: Map by Victor Wilson

Smyth conveys the message that African medical plants were acknowledged and used by Europeans in curing illness. Taking into account Smyth's social role as a priest in the Royal African Company's service, it is remarkable that he was not the least bit concerned by the indigenous religious context in which local medicinal plants would have been used on the Gold Coast. In other words, he separated the plants from their ritualised context, in which local healers provided their patients with medicines in spiritual settings.[25] What is remarkable about Smyth's collection and Petiver's description is that both gave credit to African medical knowledge and argued that African botanical riches could hold great significance for the whole of humanity – although in the end Petiver argued that African medical knowledge was not as well developed as European medicine because West Africans did not prepare compound medicines. At best, African medicines were simply ground up or dried and mixed with wine.[26]

Danes and the Dutch on the Gold Coast

Similar to the Portuguese in Angola, Dutch visitors to the Gold Coast described environmental and climatic patterns and constructed a

---

[25] Keeping in mind that the knowledge collected by Smyth was reported by Petiver, it is possible that it was not as easy to separate out natural history on the Gold Coast as it was in London.

[26] Petiver, 'A Catalogue of Some Guinea-Plants', 677–678.

medical geography of West Africa (see Chapter 7). Surgeon Samuel Brun accorded the fevers he encountered on the Gold Coast to the evil, intemperate air.[27] Dutch trader Pieter de Marees wrote about the local conceptualisation of seasons. On the Gold Coast, the months of April, May or June signalled the commencement of winter. It was a time of hot weather and profuse rains. Locals shunned the rain and considered it to be unhealthy for their bodies. De Marees noted that Europeans were badly affected during their voyages and when it rained much. Making a clear connection between climate and health, he pointed to the rains and miasma as a cause of great fevers. De Marees also claimed that West Africans found it no less unhealthy and avoided getting wet the best they could 'because of the unhealthiness of the body they experience from it'. If they did get wet, locals made a fire at night and lay down with their feet close to it as a preventative measure. Europeans interpreted this in a humoural framework. De Marees explained that it was done to draw downwards all humidity and evil humours acquired through the water, and Africans were right in doing so. Finally, they rubbed themselves with palm oil.[28]

Africa has often been described as a white man's grave before the rise of modern tropical medicine and the widespread use of quinine.[29] With certain reservations, this was the case. If one was able to survive in West Africa beyond the initial seasoning period, one had a fairly good chance of living for several years in European settlements.[30] A question worth thinking about is how European mortality compared to African mortality rates in precolonial Atlantic Africa. Quantitative sources are lacking to approximate an answer, but qualitative documentation shows that Africans suffered from sudden outbreaks of disease in the same way as Europeans. For example, the governor of Christiansborg Castle mentioned in October 1688 that an African named Ahinna Sarsaracoe 'is very ill and is afflicted with bloody diarrhea'.[31] Frequent smallpox epidemics raised mortality rates among Africans on the coast as well as on slave

[27] Brun, 'Samuel Brun's Voyages', 91.
[28] Pieter de Marees, *Description and Historical Account of the Gold Kingdom of Guinea*, translated from the Dutch and edited by Albert van Dantzig and Adam Jones (Oxford: Oxford University Press, 1987 [1602]), 110, 115; Marees's views on climate and humoural theory are also discussed in Elizabeth A. Sutton, *Early Modern Dutch Prints of Africa* (Farnham: Ashgate, 2012), 95–96.
[29] Curtin, '"The White Man's Grave"'.
[30] Harvey M. Feinberg, 'New Data on European Mortality in West Africa: The Dutch on the Gold Coast, 1719–1760', *Journal of African History* 15 (1974): 357–371; Holger Weiss, 'Tanskalaiset alusmaat Länsi-Afrikassa ylirajaisena yhteisönä', in *Pohjola, Atlantti, maailma: Vuorovaikutuksen historiaa 1600–1900-luvuilla*, edited by Kalle Kananoja and Lauri Tähtinen (Helsinki: Finnish Literature Society, 2018), 142–177.
[31] '23rd June 1688 – 7th April 1689: Daybook kept by Governor Fensman, Christiansborg', in Ole Justesen, ed., *Danish Sources for the History of Ghana*

ships.[32] West Africans were accustomed to inoculation against smallpox and had a role in bringing this specialised healing knowledge to North America. The practice was quite common on the coast, as noted by Isert in 1784.[33] However, smallpox did not spare African rulers. In April 1702, the King of Akwamu was rumoured to have contracted it.[34]

In the early seventeenth century, de Marees wrote that, based on their appearance, 'people seem to grow quite old here' despite being much subject to diseases.[35] A century later, Johannes Rask argued that, despite their poor diet, people lived longer because of their good humour and constant laughter.[36] Another Dane, Wulff Joseph Wulff, writing in 1836, emphasised the high incidence of disease. Commenting on the prevalence of malaria, or what the Danish termed 'climate fever', during the rainy season between March and August, Wulff claimed that 'mortality is far higher among Blacks than among the Whites'. He gave an environmental explanation for the prevalence of disease, explaining that it was caused by polluted air or miasma, as 'the rain drew the grass up to a height of tree meters, and since the sun heats it during the day, a terribly damp air rises from it, resulting in extreme humidity everywhere'.[37]

Early modern medicine in Atlantic Africa can best be described as fumbling. Major castles like the Dutch Elmina Castle and the English Cape Coast Castle had a hospital and a medicine shop. Elmina Castle also boasted a vegetable and herb garden, which provided fresh products to passing ships and a number of fresh medicinal herbs to the sick in the

---

1657–1754, 2 vols. (Copenhagen: Det Kongelige Danske Videnskabernes Selskab, 2005), I: 93.

[32] On the smallpox epidemic of 1700, see '27th July 1700: Governor Thrane, Christiansborg, to the Directors of the West India and Guinea Company, Copenhagen. General Letter', in Justesen, ed., *Danish Sources*, I: 118. At other times, letters mention high mortality rates on the Gold Coast without delving into the causes; e.g. '11th March 1719: Governor Rost et al., Christiansborg, to the Directors of the West India and Guinea Company, Copenhagen. General Letter', and '15th June 1719: Governor Rost, Christiansborg, to the Directors of the West India and Guinea Company, Copenhagen', in Justesen, ed., *Danish Sources*, I: 274, 276. On smallpox in the Atlantic, see Alden and Miller, 'Out of Africa'.

[33] Paul Erdmann Isert, *Letters on West Africa and the Slave Trade*, translated by Selena Axelrod Winsnes (Oxford: Oxford University Press, 1992), 219.

[34] '23rd December 1698 – 1st September 1703: Journal Kept at Christiansborg', in Justesen, ed., *Danish Sources*, I: 155.

[35] De Marees, *Description and Historical Account*, 179–180.

[36] Rask, *Two Views*, 111 [141]. On images of African labour, see Klas Rönnbäck, 'The Idle and the Industrious – European Ideas about the African Work Ethic in Precolonial West Africa', *History in Africa* 41 (2014): 117–145.

[37] Wulff Joseph Wulff, *A Danish Jew in West Africa: Biography and Letters 1836–1842*, translated by Selena Axelrod Winsnes (Legon-Accra: Sub-Saharan Publishers, 2013), 78.

hospital. While castle slaves or company blacks were also admitted to the Elmina hospital, sick domestic slaves were treated in their houses. Minor forts usually had smaller medicine cabinets with simple and compound medicines. Healthcare and drug supply were generally entrusted to surgeons. Treating tropical diseases was based on humoural medicine that relied on bloodletting and the use of strong purgatives. Contemporary views on these methods in West Africa are fragmentary. Willem Bosman, who resided on the Gold Coast for fourteen years, complained that Europeans only had spoiled medicines and unskilled doctors or barbers, who put many people at risk.[38] In the 1730s, English surgeon John Atkins described how the director-general of the Cape Coast Castle relied rather on the fetishes of his *mulatta* partner than on Atkins's advice.[39]

On slave ships, the care of the sick slaves and crewmembers was in the hands of ship surgeons, who had been trained to deal primarily with trauma cases, such as wounds, ulcers and amputations, and to apply bloodletting. The Dutch did not establish a training school for ship surgeons until 1769, a late stage considering that Dutch slave exports from West Africa fell drastically shortly thereafter.[40] In the same year, Dr David Henri Gallandat published a short book on ways to reduce slave mortality on the slave ships, *Noodige onderrichtingen voor de slaafhandelaren*. One of his first suggestions was that the slaves should always have enough fresh air. Since shipowners were rarely willing to invest in bellows, fire tools, wind wheels and ventilators, there was little alternative but to try to freshen the air by burning gunpowder, by lighting incense or juniper berries and by spraying vinegar and lemon juice. This was to be

[38] Bosman, *A New and Accurate Description*, 106. On Bosman's account, see also Albert van Dantzig, 'Willem Bosman's "New and Accurate Description of the Coast of Guinea": How Accurate Is It?', *History in Africa* 1 (1974): 101–108; Albert van Dantzig, 'English Bosman and Dutch Bosman: A Comparison of Texts', *History in Africa* 2 (1975): 185–216; Seth, *Difference and Disease*, passim.

[39] Atkins reminisced that he had first attended the Illness of one of her Children; and afterwards on the General himself, who on both occasions, I found, was so weak or so wise, as to give the preference of Fetishing to any Physical Directions of mine, wearing them on his Wrists and Neck. He was a Gentleman of good Sense, yet could not help yielding to the Silly Customs created by our Fears, and shews the Sway it bears in the Choice or Alteration of our Religion. (John Atkins, *A Voyage to Guinea, Brasil, and the West-Indies* [London: Ward and Chandler, 1737], 94–95). See also Norris Saakwa-Mante, 'Western Medicine and Racial Constitutions: Surgeon John Atkins' Theory of Polygenism and Sleepy Distemper in the 1730s', in *Race, Science, and Medicine, 1700–1960*, edited by Waltraud Ernst and Bernard Harris (London and New York: Routledge, 1999), 28–57; Seth, *Difference and Disease*, 196–207.

[40] Johannes Menne Postma, *The Dutch in the Atlantic Slave Trade 1600–1815* (Cambridge: Cambridge University Press, 1990), 244.

done while the slaves spent time on deck. Gallandat recommended that ship doctors speak to the slaves and reassure them that they would come to no harm and that the whites were not cannibals. It is doubtful whether the crew had much interest in easing the lot of the enslaved but certain that the multiplicity of African languages spoken in the slave quarters would have made communication very difficult.[41]

On the Gold Coast, the Dutch did not shy away from experimenting with local medicines. Some Europeans tapped local herbal knowledge to cure their ailments. The men working for the West India Company depended upon African women for companionship and marital relationships. More formal ties included marriages recognised in Dutch or Akan law. African women supplied their European partners not only with fresh fruits, but also with local medicine. Even though the Dutch maintained a hospital and imported medicines from the Netherlands, some Dutch men recognised the efficacy of African medicinals for certain ailments, such as malarial fevers. They experimented with the fermented sap of the oil of raffia palm against kidney stones, jequirity seed for ophthalmic purposes and kola nuts as stimulants. They also learned about coloquinte and strophantus as effective products. However, not everyone was satisfied. One officer complained in 1729 that during his illness, he had tried everything, even African medicines, but to no avail. Sometimes the use of local medical materials caused dismay among Dutch officials, as in 1750, when officer Van Doorst disapproved of officer de Sandra's use of medicines given to him by an African woman.[42]

The main products in the Dutch export trade were gold, ivory, slaves, grain, African sandalwood, palm oil, civet, kola nuts, melegueta pepper, redwood, salt, gum arabic and lime juice. Medicinal resins and gum resins obtained from African plants also included African kino (obtained from *Pterocarpus erinaceus*), African bdellium (from *Commiphora Africana*) and African myrrh (bisabol), which were used as wound dressings or plaster bases and internally for dysentery. Kino, described by Fothergill in 1757 as *gummi rubrum adstringens Gambiense*, was incorporated as an astringent in the London Pharmacopeia of 1787 and the Amsterdam Pharmacopeia of 1792. Around 1720, the value of pharmaceutical products amounted to 4 per cent of the total WIC trade from the Gold Coast. In some years, the export of kaolin (clay) was also

---

[41] Pieter C. Emmer, *The Dutch Slave Trade 1500–1850* (New York: Berghahn Books, 2006), 71–74.

[42] Harvey M. Feinberg, 'Africans and Europeans in West Africa: Elminans and Dutchmen on the Gold Coast during the Eighteenth Century', *Transactions of the American Philosophical Society* 79:7 (1989): 87–89, 96 n. 58; Meuwese, *Brothers in Arms*, 304; Rutten, *Dutch Transatlantic Medicine Trade*, 101.

mentioned. Clays were used locally as a healing material, and even today they are included in a number of pharmacopoeias and used to control diarrhoea.[43]

Melegueta pepper was an important product in the West African spice trade. In Europe, where it initially spread through the Medieval Saharan trade, melegueta was in great demand as a spice, commonly used in seasoning stews and as a medicine. Through the trans-Atlantic slave trade, it also became important to folk remedies in the Americas. More than a thousand species of pepper are known to grow in the tropical zone. In West Africa, peppers and herbal recipes spread regionally through networks of trade and migration. In addition to melegueta, the African export products included *Piper clusii* (Ashanti pepper) and *Piper guineense* (Guinea pepper), collected from Benin and traded in Elmina. *Piper cubeba*, or cubeb, was also cultivated in Benin and brought to Europe for the first time in 1485 by João Afonso d'Aveiro. Ashanti and Guinea pepper were used in traditional medicine as a carminative, vermifuge and diuretic and externally in ointments to treat rheumatism and headache. Early European references often situated melegueta pepper in contexts of romantic relationships, suggesting that it was used as an aphrodisiac.[44]

Other local products also found a medical application. Ivory, for example, was used as a medicine called *Ebur ustum*. Tamarind, common in the West African savannas, served to make water on ships drinkable, and it was also used as a laxative. West African elemi (from *Canarium Schweinfurthii*) was a common ingredient in wound ointments. Coloquinte apples were used as a purgative across Atlantic Africa.[45] Despite the great variety of potential natural medicines, no similar pharmacopoeias compiled by amateur botanists in Angola can be found on the Gold Coast in the seventeenth and early eighteenth centuries. This can be taken as an indication of different varieties of colonisation and settlement in West-Central Africa compared to West Africa. In Angola, the presence of Portuguese officers in the interior *presídios* forced Europeans to rely on local medicinal products and study them systematically, as was done by Afonso Mendes and Francisco de Buitrago. On the Gold Coast, the Dutch and Danish relied on their African partners to supply whatever local medicinals they were using but did not compose

---

[43] Rutten, *Dutch Transatlantic Medicine Trade*, 88–89. On medicinal clays in West Africa, see Bart E. van Dongen, Sharon E. Fraser and Timothy Insoll, 'The Composition and Origin of Ghana Medicine Clays', *Anthropology & Medicine* 18 (2011): 285–302.

[44] Rutten, *Dutch Transatlantic Medicine Trade*, 99; Osseo-Asare, *Bitter Roots*.

[45] Rutten, *Dutch Transatlantic Medicine Trade*, 90.

comparable inventories of local medicines before Isert's and Thonning's activities in the late eighteenth century (see the next section).[46]

Danish sources hint that European physicians and surgeons did not always enjoy great popularity, although this could be interpreted as a criticism of certain individual practitioners rather than as a criticism of the European medical system. In January 1683, Lykke, governor of Frederiksborg Castle, wrote that no one was willing to be treated by the barber-surgeon Nicolay Fensman. Lykke himself had decided to seek treatment at the Cape Coast Castle after Fensman almost crippled him. Similarly, in 1745 Governor Billsen trusted the surgeon in Dutch service more than the Swede who worked for the Danes.[47] At other times, as in 1710 and 1752, Christiansborg had no medical personnel.[48] A doctor was needed, however, not only to treat the Danish soldiers and African castle slaves but also to examine the enslaved Africans who were sold to the Atlantic slave traders. Governor Herrn commented in 1722 that his expertise was not sufficient for examining the health of slaves, and therefore he had hired a doctor from a slave ship to serve at the Danish castle.[49] The same happened in 1752, when a ship captain 'traded' one of the surgeons in his service to a mulatto soldier with the Danes.[50]

Besides the lack of doctors, Europeans struggled with maintaining the pharmacies at their forts and castles. The Dutch were perhaps much better organised in supplying medicines regularly to West Africa than the Portuguese to West-Central Africa, but even they complained about the continuous shortage of drugs. Each year, an order list was sent to Amsterdam. When medicines did not arrive, Dutch officers sometimes bought medicine cabinets from passing ships, and many high-ranking officers had a private medicine chest. Antimony compounds, unpopular

[46] On Danish efforts, see C. D. Adams, 'Activities of Danish Botanish Botanists in Guinea 1783–1850', *Transactions of the Historical Society of Ghana* 3 (1957): 30–46.
[47] '13th January 1683: Governor Lykke, Frederiksborg, to the Directors of the West India and Guinea Company, Copenhagen', in Justesen, ed., *Danish Sources*, I: 77; '1st June 1748: Declaration by Friderich Pedersen Svane, Copenhagen', in Justesen, ed., *Danish Sources*, II: 746.
[48] '14th April 1710: Governor Lygaard, Christiansborg, to the Directors of the West India and Guinea Company, Copenhagen', in Justesen, ed., *Danish Sources*, I: 229; '9th April 1752: Governor Hachsen et al., Christiansborg, to the Directors of the West India and Guinea Company, Copenhagen, General Letter', in Justesen, ed., *Danish Sources*, II: 852.
[49] '10th February 1722: Governor Herrn, Christiansborg, to the Directors of the West India and Guinea Company, Copenhagen, General Letter', in Justesen, ed., *Danish Sources*, I: 287.
[50] '9th April 1752: Governor Hachsen et al., Christiansborg, to the Directors of the West India and Guinea Company, Copenhagen, General Letter', Justesen, ed., *Danish Sources*, II: 852.

by the early eighteenth century because of their toxicity, were increasingly used on the Gold Coast for the treatment of threadworm disease. Popular syphilis remedies, such as guaiac, sassafras, sarsaparilla and smilax china, were also imported regularly, and New World medical crops infiltrated the material culture of West African herbalists fairly easily. The use of kaolin (bolus) and theriac against flux and dysentery was also common. The use of cinchona bark to treat malaria began on the Gold Coast in the early eighteenth century. With the high costs of transporting medicine from Europe and a fair chance of their contamination, directors in Amsterdam at least twice (in 1644 and 1684) gave instructions to collect native drug plants as a replacement for European medicines.[51]

As primarily a commercial enterprise, the WIC was not interested in studying the medicinal uses of native plants. Some directors-general in Elmina took initiatives to send African plant drugs and aromatic herbs to Amsterdam. In 1719, Butler shipped a small sample of 'aromatic beans in pods' to be considered as a possible economic asset. A few years later he thought he had found coloquinte apples, which in Holland would be valuable, but no indication of a substantial export of these products has been found. Four decades later, Director-General J. P. T. Huydecoper pointed to the 'infinitely large number of curative herbs, unknown to Europeans, which Negroes use to cure internal and external disease … and that would certainly yield a good branch of commerce if only a botanist were present'. This did not raise excitement in Amsterdam. The export of pepper species, especially melegueta, formed an exception.[52]

With regard to medical supplies, the Danes were struggling as late as 1843, when Governor Carstensen reported on the complete disarray of the state of affairs at the pharmacy. He complained that remedies arriving on the Gold Coast were closed by corks, opened for use irregularly and put back temporarily with the cork loosely attached. Indispensable remedies lost their power within a few weeks. Very few objects in the pharmacy were labelled. According to the inventory lists, everything should have been there, but almost everything was useless, and Carstensen found himself asking: 'Have the mixtures, the remedies which have been given to those unhappy patients, been collected from this rotten store

---

[51] Rutten, *Dutch Transatlantic Medicine Trade*, 92–97; Roberts, 'Medical Exchange on the Gold Coast', 494–497.

[52] Rutten, *Dutch Transatlantic Medicine Trade*, 98. On Dutch botanical knowledge of West Africa in the early nineteenth century, see M. J. Reynhout, *Redevoering behelzende Kruid- en Geschiedkundige Waarnemingen omtrent de Goudkust* (unknown publisher, 1824).

room.' The problem, therefore, lay in carelessness. Carstensen referred to the house pharmacies kept by Europeans at their homes and argued that by appropriate means, even European medicine could be preserved in West Africa. Finally, he recommended that necessary remedies should be ordered from England.[53]

Dutch and Danish sources describe cross-cultural medical exchanges on the Gold Coast and show that local elites had a sympathetic attitude towards European medical practices, although there is little evidence of African popular healers' eagerness to adopt foreign remedies.[54] Europeans supplied the Ashanti with medicines, such as tincture of rhubarb and tincture of cinnamon. Even if Europeans occasionally expressed doubts about their doctors, this did not hinder Africans from seeking treatment at European forts. In April 1701, the Danes reported that Addo, ruler of Akwamu, was seeking treatment for the 'French disease', or syphilis, at Accra from a Dutch 'master'. He stayed for a month at the Dutch fort.[55] It is unclear whether Addo really suffered from syphilis, an American disease that had arrived to Africa with the Europeans,[56] or whether he had contracted yaws, a treponemal disease endemic to Africa. This raises the question of whether Africans thought of syphilis as a white man's disease, which would lead to a hypothesis that Africans thought that Europeans had a potent treatment for it. West Africans had learned the use of sarsaparilla[57] as a treatment for syphilis from the Portuguese and the Dutch. It was bought from slave ships and was in common use.[58]

---

[53] Edward Carstensen, *Closing the Books: Governor Edward Carstensen on Danish Guinea 1842–50*, translated from the Danish by Tove Storsveen (Accra: Sub-Saharan Publishers, 2010), 39–40.

[54] Cf. Roberts, 'Medical Exchange on the Gold Coast'.

[55] '23rd December – 1st September 1703: Journal kept at Christiansborg', in Justesen, ed., *Danish Sources*, I: 143–144.

[56] However, one of the contemporary names for syphilis, the 'French disease', shows that early modern Europeans were confused about the origins of the disease. Sheldon Watts, *Epidemics and History: Disease, Power and Imperialism* (New Haven, CT and London: Yale University Press, 1997), 122–134; Jon Arrizabalaga, John Henderson and Roger French, *The Great Pox: The French Disease in Renaissance Europe* (New Haven, CT and London: Yale University Press, 1997), 24–25.

[57] Sarsaparilla (*Smilacaceae*) was a medicinal plant originally from tropical America, which was dried and brought to Europe, where it was mixed with rum to form a compound medicine.

[58] Rask, *Two Views*, 112 [144]; de Marees, *Description and Historical Account*, 173. Rømer mentioned in a 1745 letter that venereal disease was treated with mercury on the Gold Coast. '28th February 1745: L. F. Rømer, Cape Coast Castle, to the Directors of the West India and Guinea Company, Copenhagen', in Justesen, ed., *Danish Sources*, II: 649. Rømer, *A Reliable Account*, 178, also mentioned the steam cabinet as a standard treatment for syphilis at the time.

Venereal disease seems to have been fairly common on the Gold Coast, and women were often deemed the cause of disease. Bosman wrote at length about 'all our Venereal Ware-houses and their contain'd Stores', and John Atkins laid the cause of venereal disease at the feet of 'common women'.[59] Rømer implied that African traders sometimes consciously infected Europeans. Rømer claimed that John Currantee of Anomabo often entertained Europeans in his house and invited them to pass a night with a woman, sometimes bringing in infected women. When he later heard that Europeans had become ill or were lying in a steam cabinet (standard treatment for syphilis at the time), Currantee was allegedly tremendously pleased by it.[60]

Even if Africans occasionally relied on the care provided by European doctors, it appears that this practice was limited to rulers, elites and company employees in European service.[61] European barbers asked for large payments for their services.[62] In 1750, a ruler named Tette Krii asked for the governor of Christiansborg to send a small quantity of the same medicine that had been given to a servant of a certain slave trader. Tette Krii wanted to treat a relative who had a great hole in his foot.[63] According to Rømer, bloodletting was the most suspicious European method in African eyes. He advised slave ship surgeons to administer bloodletting only in emergency, and even in those cases that it be done so that neither other slaves nor the patient being treated saw the operation. Rømer argued that 'Blacks do not understand that this is done for their benefit, and they think we are going to kill them.'[64]

Johannes Rask was not alone in appreciating local medical knowledge. Hans Christian Monrad wrote in the early nineteenth century that Europeans sometimes placed themselves in the hands of the local blacks when suffering from malaria.[65] He had personally gone to an African healer when suffering from yellow fever and urged Europeans to take heed of local knowledge:

Normally the Negro doctor concerns himself with the cure of only one illness; he keeps his medicines secret. However, the cure would be worth the trouble of

[59] Seth, *Difference and Disease*, 185–186.   [60] Rømer, *A Reliable Account*, 178.

[61] For example, the mulatto employees in Dutch service used the hospital maintained by the West India Company and relied on European medicines and techniques. Feinberg, 'Africans and Europeans in West Africa', 91.

[62] Bosman, *A New and Accurate Description*, 110.

[63] 'November 1750: Johan Suurman, Keta, to Governor Platfues, Christiansborg', in Justesen, ed., *Danish Sources*, II: 798.

[64] Rømer, *A Reliable Account*, 199.

[65] H. C. Monrad, *A Description of the Guinea Coast and Its Inhabitants*, translated by Selena Axelrod Winsnes. (Accra: Sub-Saharan Publishers, 2009), 204.

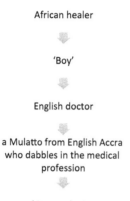

African healer

'Boy'

English doctor

a Mulatto from English Accra
who dabbles in the medical
profession

his own doctor

Figure 3.2 Wulff's experience of medical pluralism on the Gold Coast

buying the secret from them. Especially does their cure of yellow fever merit the attention of the West Indian doctors. They say that there grow no herbs for death [*sic*], but it is entirely possible that the healing herb could grow alongside the illness, or, more correctly, at the place where the illness originated.

The above-mentioned Negro to whom I addressed myself cured me both simply and rapidly. Three times a day, morning, midday and evening, he had my entire body washed in water in which a number of both nicely scented and bitter herbs had been soaking for a long time. In addition, I had to drink three handfuls, each time, of the same water in which I was being bathed. After having taken this cure for 3 to 4 days I felt to a surprising degree, much better, and in a short time I was quite recovered. My doctor called upon his fetish very frequently, and forbade me to eat palm oil or legumes during the cure, which, he told me very seriously, his fetish had forbidden.[66]

Monrad, a theologian who served as a chaplain on the Gold Coast, did not see a problem in an African healer's medico-religious treatment. Similarly, Wulff Joseph Wulff also wrote in detail about his encounter with a local healer and a variety of other practitioners (Figure 3.2). Contracting an illness that he self-diagnosed as jaundice and climate fever on a trip to a Danish plantation, Wulff first took recourse to a local healer who bathed him several times a day. The cure continued for three weeks. Wulff claimed that, at one point, the healer almost beat him to death, so he asked to be treated by bathing only. He also received a strong laxative from the healer, but it was of no help and only led to a worse attack of illness.[67]

---

[66] Monrad, *A Description of the Guinea Coast*, 206.
[67] Wulff, *A Danish Jew in West Africa*, 174.

Continuing to rely on his local assistants, Wulff reported receiving some tamarind water from one of his 'Boys',[68] after which he felt immediate relief and thanked the Boy, next after God, for saving his life. The black healer did not offer any more medicine but continued to administer baths to Wulff thrice daily, 'each time first with green soap, then with limes, and finally with scented green leaves'. Because of a worsening rash, however, Wulff dismissed the healer. He next turned to an English doctor serving on a Navy ship. After an examination, Wulff was given a large dose of quinine powder and Spanish fly, made of dried beetles (*Cantharides vesicatoria*). Furthering cross-cultural medical exchanges, the English doctor arranged for 'a Mulatto from English Accra who dabbles in the medical profession' to look after Wulff and see to it that he took his powders. Wulff also received opium pills and, finally, several good laxatives, after which he came down with extreme diarrhoea. Despite such treatment, the rash and other symptoms – headache, vomiting gall and diarrhoea – continued. The Mulatto doctor continued seeing to Wulff, administering footbaths, shaving off his moustache and hair, and placing plasters of Spanish fly on his temples and sides and mustard plaster on his legs. He was also bled once during the illness, presumably by the Mulatto doctor, who took 'two teacups full'. Wulff reported that his veins were always quite red in appearance during the illness, but when they turned blue again, the Mulatto doctor, who was now clearly in charge of Wulff's treatment, declared that the illness was over. Even after recovering some strength, Wulff wrote that he was 'covered from head to foot with yellow, suppurating boils, [my] legs covered with holes and sores, and both hands are covered with scabs'. Yet, the local opinion was that this was a definite sign that the climate illness was really and properly over.[69]

Writing to his parents a few months later, Wulff continued to complain about his illness. By now, he was convinced that the best thing to do was to be his own doctor: 'The wisest thing I have done, I am convinced, is that I have dismissed both the white as well as the black doctors.' Calling them scoundrels, Wulff claimed that they knew no more about malaria than he did, but continued to make experiments upon experiments on

---

[68] In fact, the two 'Boys' employed by Wulff likely had an intimate knowledge of local botanical knowledge. Asang was the son of a 'fetish man' and Astée was a fetish man in Labadi. At one point, Wulff reported observing the Yam Custom at Labadi, where Astée presided, 'totally possessed by his fetish'. Wulff never commented upon what these Africans gained by being in his service, and one can only surmise at their motives, which might have included information gathering and protection seeking. Wulff, *A Danish Jew*, 91, 161–162.

[69] Wulff, *A Danish Jew*, 174–179.

everyone who wished to make use of them. He ordered the medicines he wanted from the pharmacy in Christiansborg to treat himself. After he became completely swollen from head to toe, Wulff took laxatives regularly, washed two or three times a day in cold water and kept a careful diet. He went for a good walk every afternoon and walked the balcony of his house at five o'clock in the morning.[70]

Cross-cultural medical interaction was remarkably common on the Gold Coast. Gender played an important role in it. As elsewhere in Atlantic Africa, the European settler population was predominantly male, which led to informal relationships between white men and black or coloured women.[71] Elias Svane, a chaplain in Danish service, wrote a long letter on the relationships between local women and Danish men. According to Svane, it was much better for Danes to buy slave women than to marry free Africans because slaves were easier to convert to Christianity. All fetishes were to be confiscated from the slaves and they had to be kept away from African religious ceremonies. According to Svane, however, it would have been best to send only married men with their spouses to the Gold Coast.[72]

Although the role of women is rarely remarked upon in the documentation, they had a central role in running households and treating diseases. Writing in 1836, Wulff remarked that all the whites lived with local women, 'and one has the advantage thereby that they take very good care [of the man] when he is ill'. According to Wulff, newcomers to the coast should follow local customs and habits if they wanted 'to avoid a dose of an extremely unpleasant medicine'.[73]

European men had to admit that they were powerless over certain maladies and let themselves be healed by African women. Rømer's advice to slave ship captains describes the situation clearly. Although it was given to ship captains sailing the Atlantic, there is no doubt that a similar practice, dictated by centuries of experience, was maintained on the coast:

Should the slaves fall victim to the [endemic] illnesses of the land, such as worms, etc., a couple of the female slaves can be allowed to take over, after we have

---

[70] Wulff, *A Danish Jew*, 182–183.
[71] Brooks, *Eurafricans in Western Africa*; Kananoja, 'Healers, Idolaters and Good Christians'; Candido, *An African Slaving Port*; Pernille Ipsen, *Daughters of the Trade: Atlantic Slavers and Interracial Marriage on the Gold Coast* (Philadelphia: University of Pennsylvania Press, 2015).
[72] '15th March 1724: Elias Svane, Christiansborg, to the Directors of the West India and Guinea Company, Copenhagen', in Justesen, ed., *Danish Sources*, I: 302.
[73] Wulff, *A Danish Jew*, 86.

supplied them with *mallaget* and *piment*, palm oil, and citrons, from which they can prepare [African] medicines, and the sick will feel well afterward.[74]

Isert and Thonning: Practising Locally, Thinking Globally

Two Danes who lived on the Gold Coast amassed significant botanical collections and familiarised themselves with the medicinal flora of the region. Surgeon Paul Erdmann Isert was in the Danish service between 1783 and 1786. Peter Thonning, who had similarly received medical training, served on the Danish Gold Coast from 1799 to 1803. Isert and Thonning, as well as a few other Danes, collected approximately 2,000 specimens for Martin Vahl, a professor of botany in Copenhagen. Over 600 species are represented in the collection. But in addition to the specimens, Danes provided information on the locations where the plants were found, their local names as well as their uses.[75]

Isert published his letters on the Danish Gold Coast originally in German. In *Reise nach Guinea und den Caribäischen Inseln in Columbia*, he did not focus on local healing practices per se, although he described Ga culture extensively. Isert, however, provided information on how Europeans treated certain tropical diseases. In his own practice, Isert applied bloodletting and purgatives as well as compound medicines. Like his Portuguese contemporaries in Angola, he utilised quina bark from South America (see Chapter 5).[76]

Although Isert's letters did not provide detailed descriptions of natural environments – perhaps regarding them as uninteresting to readers – he clearly saw that the natural history of the Gold Coast should be studied and placed in a global context. In January 1785, Isert was in Ouidah and wrote a letter to Sir Joseph Banks, head of the Royal Society. Banks sponsored natural historical expeditions to different parts of the world, and the collected specimens were taken to London, where they made up a significant part of collections in the Kew Gardens. When writing to Banks, Isert mentioned that, in a short time, he had collected a large number of specimens, but being so far from Christiansborg he could not send them to Banks. Instead of a large collection, Isert sent thirteen

---

[74] Rømer, *A Reliable Account*, 199.
[75] According to F. N. Hepper, *The West African Herbaria of Isert & Thonning: A Taxonomic Revision and an Index to the IDC Microfiche* (Kew: Bentham-Moxon Trust & Royal Botanic Gardens, 1976), 11–12, the collections in Copenhagen also included samples sent from the Gold Coast by Julius Philip Benjamin von Rohr, Ole Haasland Smith and Lars Mortensen.
[76] Isert, *Letters on West Africa*, 203–204.

plants and asked Banks to sponsor his 'natural philosophical' research in West Africa. He wanted an annual compensation of 400–500 pounds because travelling and buying specimens from locals was expensive. In his letter, Isert referred to his collecting activities in passing. Besides his own expeditions, he bought specimens from locals, who also provided him with information on the uses of plants.[77] Without local knowledge, plant collections would have been considerably smaller and their description would have been limited to the physical attributes of plants.

Isert's and Thonning's descriptions of plants varied in their breadth and scope. The simplest descriptions gave a very general location of where the plant grew and when it was in flower. For example, *Agingeli* (*Uvaria ovata*) was reported to grow 'here and there not rare; flowers in May and June'. *Calotropis procera* grew in 'sandy places at La and Prampram. Flowers in March and April.'[78] The most detailed descriptions provided information on medical, economic and dietary uses among the locals. The description of *Cassia occidentalis* is a perfect example:

Is used by the natives in different ways, e.g. the bark of the root is scraped off, boiled with pytto (native beer) and is drunk in cases of dysentery. The same bark is finely macerated along with a few grains-of-paradise [Aframomum] and with aid of lemon juice is made into an ointment with which ringworm is coated over. The leaves are used to induce the opening of bowels and to soothe pains in the abdomen and are boiled for this purpose with pytto. The bark of the root has a bitter slightly astringent taste, it is said to be recommended as a good substitute for china-bark [cinchona]. The leaves have a stupefying odour, which much resembles opium.[79]

Isert and Thonning did not name their informants, but one can easily see that they relied on local sources of knowledge and cultural go-betweens. Thonning listed the local names of 163 different plants, which indicates that he either collected and observed them together with locals, or, like Isert, bought specimens and the knowledge connected to them. When exploring West African natural environments, Thonning was never alone. In his notes, he alluded to constantly being accompanied by a personal servant, an African or a Eurafrican residing in the Danish castle, an interpreter, a person met by accident in the woods or another European who had resided longer on the coast. These local experts showed him things, answered his queries, told him the local names of plants and provided their own interpretation of what was transpiring.[80]

[77] Isert, *Letters on West Africa*, 290–292.   [78] Hepper, *The West African Herbaria*, 26–27.
[79] Hepper, *The West African Herbaria*, 34.   [80] Hopkins, 'Danish Natural History', 384.

Because a large part of Thonning's collection was destroyed, informants have long since vanished from the documentation, if they were ever
noted there as individuals in the first place. However, the natural historian gave credit to his African assistants four decades after returning to
Europe:

My journeys were concerned precisely with the investigation of their country,
woods, plants, products, their history, constitution, religion, customs, etc.; this
the negroes understood very well, and were always very obliging with answers to
my questions, and brought me unbidden items that they thought might be of
interest to me, and it was clearly their desire that I should discover something that
might make their country interesting to the whites. The negroes never laid
hindrances in the way of my travels, but welcomed my arrival and received me
with glad cries and hospitality.[81]

Conclusion

In the early modern period, natural historical collections outside of
Europe were made in collaboration with indigenous assistants and
informants. African, American and Asian sources of knowledge often
have a silent presence in sources written by Europeans. In their published
work and even their private journals, natural historians rarely provided
information on the identities of informants. Yet it is clear that locals
always acted as cultural brokers for outsiders. It is also evident that
settlers and scientists trusted and appreciated local knowledge. This
appreciation was not relayed when they returned to Europe, although
without locals, natural historical collections could not have been made.
In Atlantic Africa, go-betweens were numerous and included black
Africans, Eurafricans and Europeans who had resided on the coast for
a longer time. The role of women in transmitting medical knowledge was
significant. Ultimately, this shows how reliant early modern Europeans
were on their African partners. In other words, Africans governed over
space and knowledge.

On the Gold Coast, Europeans to a large extent relied on African
healing knowledge. This was not something only the Portuguese commonly did. Medical exchanges and healing in the context of cross-
cultural interaction was, in reality, a two-way process, one which affected
Africans as well. Perhaps they did not benefit to the same extent from
European medicines, but they were interested in and open to trying new

---

[81] Cited and translated in Hopkins, 'Danish Natural History', 397.

practices. Similarly, Europeans who settled in West Africa experimented with local medicinals and sought to tap the sources of indigenous healing knowledge by consulting with their African companions and slaves and by seeking access to specialist herbalists and healers. In the end, some of them accumulated knowledge that allowed them to act as their own doctors with a mixed bag of medicines.

4 Remedies on the Spot
Science, Agricultural Development and Botanical Knowledge in Sierra Leone ca. 1800

> The diseases to which the Europeans are subject from the climate on the coast, may be reckoned among the greatest inconveniences to establishments of white people in that part of the world ... Nevertheless there are remedies on the spot well known among the negroes, which effectually cure the diseases that cannot be escaped.[1]

After visiting Senegal in the 1780s, Swedish abolitionist Carl Bernhard Wadström published his work *Observations on the Slave Trade*. Describing the West African coast, he included a short passage on 'the Diseases', as was often customary in early modern European accounts of Africa. Wadström noted the challenges posed by the disease environment and the high mortality rates impacting European colonisation efforts, but he also acknowledged another fact well known to Europeans living in Atlantic Africa, namely that Africans had remedies for many of the illnesses that foreigners suffered from.[2]

Carl Bernhard Wadström was a staunch supporter of Swedenborgian ideals and egalitarianism, and ideologically he had much in common with his countrymen, the botanist Adam Afzelius, Anders Sparrman and the Nordenskiöld brothers. The teachings of the Swedish seer Emanuel Swedenborg (1688–1772) centred on the vision that the 'human form divine' was to be found in the interior of Africa. At the core of these ideas were the claims that the African was in no way inferior to the white person and that Africa was ripe for useful cultivation and legitimate trade. Afzelius, along with the Swedes August Nordenskiöld, Daniel Padenheim and Jakob Strand, ended up in Sierra Leone in the 1790s to seek this utopia.[3]

---

[1] Carl Bernhard Wadström, *Observations on the Slave Trade and a Description of Some Part of the Coast of Guinea* (London: James Phillips, 1789), 50–51.

[2] Wadström did not return to this topic in his *Essay on Colonization*, though it also included a substantial section on health and disease. Carl Bernhard Wadström, *An Essay on Colonization*, 2 vols. (London: Darton and Harvey, 1794), I: 42–48.

[3] Deirdre Coleman, *Romantic Colonization and British Antislavery* (Cambridge: Cambridge University Press, 2005), 64. For an early important study on Swedenborgianism in

Carl Bernhard Wadström was the leading Swedenborgian author of this group. Deirdre Coleman has characterised his thinking on colonisation as anti-imperial and anti-commercial. Although not completely immune from contemporary excitement about the commercial potential of Africa, his thinking lacked the ambition for engaging in intensive plantation-scale colonisation. Instead, it relied on a utopian vision of a classless and egalitarian rural community in the African interior.[4] Wadström travelled to Senegal in 1787 and 1788, accompanied by the naturalist Anders Sparrman, and he published *Observations on the Slave Trade* in 1789. His travels left him excited with the agricultural abundance of the Upper Guinea coast. Wadström found that 'millet, rice, potatoes, pulse, and many other excellent vegetables are cultivated on the coast with very little trouble, and in a profusion perfectly astonishing to an European'. He wrote about the 'abundance of the most wholesome and delicious fruit', and he observed the potential for sugar-cane and tobacco cultivation. Wadström and Sparrman also listed several species of cotton and different kinds of indigo and gum as other valuable crops that thrived in Atlantic West Africa. Finally, Wadström also took note of 'a great variety of the most valuable and beautiful woods', bringing back samples of fourteen species barely known to European botanists.[5]

This chapter examines Africans as providers of plants and local medical knowledge in Sierra Leone by focusing on the documentation produced by Adam Afzelius and Thomas Winterbottom, an English physician. It shows that, in Sierra Leone, the indigenous knowledge collected by Europeans was completely provided by Africans. Two local men, Peter and Duffa, clearly stand out among African informants. They provided more than half of the plants studied by Afzelius, and a typical entry in the botanist's journal usually began thus: 'Peter and Duffa brought...' Yet, the journal remains silent on who Peter and Duffa really were. Typical of scientific voyagers, Afzelius and Winterbottom rarely discussed the identities of their assistants and informants. Although they

Sweden, see Robert Sundelin, *Svedenborgianismens historia i Sverige under förra århundradet* (Uppsala: W. Schultz, 1886).

[4] Coleman, *Romantic Colonization*, 71–72.

[5] Wadström, *Observations on the Slave Trade*, 42–44. The same subject was also dealt with in Wadström, *An Essay on Colonization*, 31–38. On Wadström's trip to Africa and his ideas on colonization, see Klas Rönnbäck, 'Enlightenment, Scientific Exploration and Abolitionism: Anders Sparrman's and Carl Bernhard Wadström's Colonial Encounters in Senegal, 1787–1788 and the British Abolitionist Movement', *Slavery & Abolition* 34:3 (2013): 425–445; Jonas Ahlskog, 'The Political Economy of Colonisation: Carl Bernhard Wadström's Case for Abolition and Civilisation', *Sjuttonhundratal* 7 (2010): 145–167. For a critical biography of Wadström, see Philip K. Nelson, *Carl Bernhard Wadström: Mannen bakom myten* (Norrköping: Föreningen Gamla Norrköping, 1998).

accepted and valued African botanical and medical knowledge, their informants remain almost anonymous and completely faceless. Yet, the African contribution was integral to early modern natural history and provided the basis for the scientific studies conducted by Afzelius and his students.[6]

Portuguese Precedents on the Upper Guinea Coast

Portuguese explorers initiated cross-cultural medical encounters in West Africa in the fifteenth century. Definitions of medicine at this time and in the following centuries were open and expansive. On the Upper Guinea Coast, forms of medical knowledge shifted and circulated between littoral areas and their hinterland. Changing patterns of trade, migration and settlement associated with Mandé influence impacted changing notions of illness and therapy. Similar to West-Central Africa, early travellers and missionaries made a distinction between biophysical and spiritual healing. The boundaries between body and mind were fluid, and so were the affinities between Christian, Islamic and 'animist' knowledge. Europeans referred to local herbal remedies with respectful interest and appropriated their curative properties, whereas African shrines were dismissed as idol worship. However, as Philip Havik has shown, West African herbal and spiritual healers were consulted by both local people and foreigners because of their perceived therapeutic powers.[7]

For Jesuits on the Upper Guinea Coast, spiritual assistance was as good a remedy as a material cure. Commenting on the worst illness he had ever experienced, Jesuit Father Barreira wrote that confidence in God served as a medicine that had enabled him to recover his health and rid himself of a swelling of abnormal size, which had brought about high fever and a lack of appetite. Speaking the holy name of Jesus and making the sign of the cross was also taught to African converts as a type of holy medicine or protective remedy against the Devil.[8]

Besides relying on spiritual cures, Jesuits and other Portuguese travellers quickly familiarised themselves with local healing materials. Jesuits, who were themselves actively involved in the art of healing, complained

---

[6] On African or black informants in the Americas, see Schiebinger, *Secret Cures of Slaves*.

[7] Philip Havik, 'Hybridising Medicine: Illness, Healing and the Dynamics of Reciprocal Exchange on the Upper Guinea Coast (West Africa)', *Medical History* 60 (2016): 181–205.

[8] Doc. 31, 'Barreira's Annual Report for 1608–1609, Chapter 8, p. 1', and Doc. 45, 'Father Sebastião Gomes, Letter from Santiago, October 1613, p. 15', in A. Teixeira da Mota and P. E. H. Hair, *Jesuit Documents on the Guinea of Cape Verde and the Cape Verde Islands, 1585–1617 in English Translation* (Liverpool: Dept. of History, University of Liverpool, 1989).

that European traders often sought assistance from African healers.[9] Due to their common use in daily life, kola nuts were one of the most common medicinals used in medical encounters in Sierra Leone. André Alvares d'Almada compared their use to the popularity of betel leaves in India. According to him, West Africans believed that kola nuts served as a medicine for the liver and the bladder, and the Portuguese employed them for the same purpose, though not as often as the locals. Blacks also chewed kola nuts and rubbed their forehead with kola paste if they had a headache.[10]

Almada's reference to kola as a medicine for the liver and the bladder points to the fact that Europeans in West Africa shared with locals certain ideas about the functioning of human bodies. A question worth considering is, to what extent had doctrines of humoural medicine spread to Islamic West Africa? Although the evidence is sketchy, this facet of cross-cultural medical encounters certainly cannot be ruled out. In the Guinea Bissau region, itinerant Islamised healers of Manding extraction not only converted Africans but also produced amulets and talismans, disseminating healing methods based on the powers of these charms. One of the most remarkable healers in Bañun in the early 1600s was an individual from Malacca, whose presence demonstrates the global connections between West Africa and East Asia. Wearing a long white *bubú*, as worn by Muslim clerics, and a number of talismans around his neck and on his forehead, this Muslim healer from South East Asia scorned Christians and accompanied locals in their religious activities. Local dignitaries sought him out for his Oriental healing skills, which he combined with African practices. Eventually imprisoned on the Cape Verdean island of Santiago, he fled to Angola, where he might well have continued his medical practice.[11]

Ethnomedical Research in Sierra Leone

Sierra Leone emerged in the late eighteenth century as a settlement for Africans based in England. After the first settlement failed, the Sierra Leone Company, incorporated in 1791, took over. The main part of the population consisted of former slaves from North America, who had left the United States for the British colonies of Nova Scotia and New

---

[9] Havik, 'Hybridising Medicine', 189.

[10] André Alvares d'Almada, *Brief Treatise on the Rivers of Guinea* (Liverpool: Dept. of History, University of Liverpool, 1984), 56.

[11] Havik, 'Hybridising Medicine', 189, 198–199. Elsewhere in West Africa, Islamic medicine took the form of prayers and secret incantations; see, e.g., Abdalla, 'Diffusion of Islamic Medicine into Hausaland'.

Brunswick. Over a thousand Nova Scotians arrived in Freetown in 1792 and soon settled down to life in a pioneer community. The Sierra Leone Company governed the colony and hoped to make profits from trade.[12] Among the Company's staff in Sierra Leone was Adam Afzelius, a Swedish botanist, whose main task was to collect plants for his sponsor, Sir Joseph Banks, president of the Royal Society in London. In Sierra Leone, Afzelius was joined by Thomas Winterbottom, a physician, who showed great interest in West African medical practices.[13]

Afzelius and Winterbottom conversed with numerous locals and settlers in Sierra Leone. They were equally interested in local and pan-African knowledge and did not disdain women as informants. A significant part of Winterbottom's work concentrated on women's diseases in Sierra Leone, and Afzelius's journal points out that women contributed significantly to the information published by the physician. All this makes Freetown an important scene of scientific research in West Africa and the Black Atlantic world. The work of Afzelius and Winterbottom, and of Henry Smeathman before them,[14] throws into question the image of Africa as a scientific backwater despised by European colonists of the nineteenth and twentieth centuries. These two men firmly believed that blacks in Sierra Leone could provide important information that could be of use for the whole of humanity and that the diversity of Upper Guinean flora could offer opportunities for scientific discoveries. As has already been demonstrated, Afzelius and Winterbottom were not alone in their conviction that much could be learned from blacks in the early modern Atlantic world; similar ideas – including the view that women possessed much important medical knowledge – could be found in other parts of Atlantic Africa as well.

Adam Afzelius was a disciple of Linnaeus, who first travelled to Sierra Leone in 1792. Because of ailing health, he travelled back to England in August 1793 but returned to Freetown in 1794, staying there until 1796. Sir Joseph Banks, whom he had befriended after travelling from Uppsala to London in 1789, sponsored his botanical work. Banks was one of the

---

[12] Stephen J. Braidwood, *Black Poor and White Philanthropists: London's Blacks and the Foundation of the Sierra Leone Settlement, 1786–1791* (Liverpool: Liverpool University Press, 1994); James St. G. Walker, *The Black Loyalists: The Search for a Promised Land in Nova Scotia and Sierra Leone 1783–1870* (Toronto: University of Toronto Press, 1992).

[13] The most comprehensive biography on Afzelius and his activities in Sierra Leone is a work in Swedish by Sten Lindroth, 'Adam Afzelius. En linnean i England och Sierra Leone', *Lychnos* (1944–1945): 1–54. A shorter English version appeared in Sten Lindroth, 'Adam Afzelius: A Swedish Botanist in Sierra Leone', *Sierra Leone Studies*, New Series, 4 (1955): 194–207.

[14] Deirdre Coleman, *Henry Smeathman, the Flycatcher: Natural History, Slavery, and Empire in the Late Eighteenth Century* (Liverpool: Liverpool University Press, 2018).

masterminds behind the African Association. Banks, in his capacity as an informal advisor on the Royal Botanic Gardens, dispatched and sponsored several collectors around the world to send him specimens, and Afzelius was part of this global network. In practice, Banks and the Sierra Leone Company outfitted and paid for his work on the natural history of Freetown and its environs. Banks and Afzelius were united by more than a passion for science. They were both ardent abolitionists and interested in making comprehensive emancipation a reality by introducing social improvements and promoting useful knowledge.[15]

In 1788, Wadström had obtained free land lots in the new Sierra Leone colony for himself and eleven others of his sect, including Adam Afzelius, August Nordenskiöld and Jakob Strand, all of whom later sailed to the colony. Their objective was to locate the New Jerusalem in the interior of West Africa.[16] The utopian Swedenborgian ideals fit well with the English colonisation schemes that took shape in the 1780s. Idealists began to campaign for the abolition of the slave trade not only because such an action was deemed morally just, but also because it was seen as the best way to foster legitimate commerce in Africa. Commentators began to encourage the development of African agriculture, and men like Afzelius were perfectly suited to study the local conditions and riches of the West African natural world. After all, the potential for commerce with Africa had scarcely been tapped, as the sporadic fits of enthusiasm by the Royal African Company demonstrate. In the early eighteenth century, the company had sought to promote export trades in cotton, indigo, pepper and medicines, but these projects were doomed by the inability of the British to establish authority on the coast.[17]

These ideas, however, had continued to circulate and had taken root in 1771, when Henry Smeathman was sent out to the Grain Coast to study its flora and fauna. Smeathman clearly recognised the prospects for agricultural development and returned to England in 1780 with elaborate plans to colonise Sierra Leone.[18] Granville Sharp and others took up Smeathman's ideas, envisioning the settlement of Sierra Leone as a

---

[15] Eric Herschtal, *The Science of Antislavery: Scientists, Abolitionism, and the Myth of Slavery's Backwardness* (unpublished Ph.D. thesis, Columbia University, 2017), 216–227.

[16] Coleman, *Romantic Colonization*, 78–79.

[17] Christopher Leslie Brown, 'Empire without America: British Plans for Africa in the Era of the American Revolution', in *Abolitionism and Imperialism in Britain, Africa, and the Atlantic*, edited by Derek R. Peterson (Athens: Ohio University Press, 2010), 86–87, 93–94.

[18] On Smeathman's voyage to Sierra Leone, see Starr Douglas and Felix Driver, 'Imagining the Tropical Colony: Henry Smeathman and the Termites of Sierra Leone', in *Tropical Visions in an Age of Empire*, edited by Felix Driver and Luciana Martins (Chicago: University of Chicago Press, 2005), 91–112; Starr Douglas, 'The

beachhead for civilisation and as a way to commodify production. These ideas finally led to the establishment of the Sierra Leone Company in 1791. In a sense, Adam Afzelius and Thomas Winterbottom took up Smeathman's work and started to further explore the botanical riches of the colony.

Winterbottom, like many botanists in this period, was a practising physician. In the beginning of his two-volume work on Sierra Leone, he lamented the difficulties he had experienced in obtaining knowledge from the locals there. According to him, it was partly due to the unwillingness of local healing experts to 'disclose the secrets of their medical art'. Language formed another barrier, which was only 'imperfectly remedied by the assistance of an interpreter'.[19] Despite these challenges in obtaining information, Winterbottom's work on local medical knowledge in Sierra Leone is remarkably rich. How was it possible if everything related to healing was secret? Although Winterbottom did not name his informants in his published work, it can be inferred that he was a close observer of local healing practices and was in close contact with African specialists, interacting with and interviewing them constantly. For example, when discussing venereal disease, he claimed that 'African physicians boast that they are able to cure this disease in all its forms, and in every stage, for which purpose they employ a variety of remedies, chiefly sudorifics or violent purgatives'.[20]

Winterbottom's work was further enriched by his correspondence with Afzelius, who provided the Linnaean names of medicinals. Afzelius's journal demonstrates that the two were already working closely together in Freetown. Winterbottom provided medicinal plants to Afzelius on several occasions, along with information on their local names and uses.[21] The two also ventured out together to observe local ritual practices in the vicinity of Freetown. In his journal, Afzelius recorded minutely how he and Winterbottom, along with Mr Witchell and Mr Gray, went out to see a poison ordeal. Invited by Jimmy Queen, a Temne ruler on the west side of White Man's Bay, the four men ventured out to his village in June 1795. The excursion gave Afzelius an opportunity to observe the local flora, but he also described the poison ordeal in great

Making of Scientific Knowledge in an Age of Slavery: Henry Smeathman, Sierra Leone and Natural History', *Journal of Colonialism and Colonial History* 9 (2008).

[19] Thomas Winterbottom, *An Account of the Native Africans in the Neighbourhood of Sierra Leone; to Which Is Added an Account of the Present State of Medicine among Them*, 2 vols. (London: Hatchard & Poultry, 1803), II: 2.

[20] Winterbottom, *An Account of the Native Africans*, II: 32.

[21] Adam Afzelius, *Sierra Leone Journal 1795–1796*, edited by Peter Kup (Uppsala: Almqvist & Wiksells, 1967), 29r, 34v–35r, 38r, 121r, 127v, 157r, 163v, 164v, 168r, 191v, 210v.

detail. In the trial, a Bullam man accused of killing another Bullam man was forced to eat a piece of kola nut and drink red water, an infusion of the bark of *Erythropleum guineense*, on an empty stomach. In the ritual, the accused was deemed innocent if he threw up all the kola nut he had eaten, as happened on this occasion.[22] The resemblance to West-Central African poison ordeals is striking.

Afzelius's journal provides an intimate view on the workings of a colonial botanist in Sierra Leone. The living conditions were quite modest. In May 1795, Afzelius resided in Freetown in a wooden house, made of boards and shingle and thatched with grass. The house was flimsily constructed, and it shook when a person walked on the floor.[23] Only rarely does he mention venturing out to collect plants, and even then, he seems to have done so mainly in the public gardens of Freetown, occasionally accompanied by a Temne-speaking informant.[24] It was far more common for him to rely on local Africans or Europeans to bring him specimens and inform him on the uses of different plants. Some Africans, aware of Afzelius's work, brought him plants in exchange for small sums of money. For example, on 26 May 1795, he 'bought of Natives a branch of a tree full with small berries, which they called *Manennika* ... I bought also an Agaricus of a vermilion colour or rather a little more red, so that he may be called roseus. The Native name of it was *Maninko*.'[25]

The difficulties in obtaining information from Africans were sometimes underlined by clear attempts to lead Europeans astray. On one occasion, Afzelius recorded how he had '[b]ought of Little Andrew a Lycoperdon', which the seller claimed was an edible mushroom. However, passers-by unanimously informed Afzelius that it was poisonous, and Little Andrew was forced to confess that he had tried to deceive the botanist to induce Afzelius to buy all the mushrooms he had brought with him.[26] However, at other times practical questions were resolved in simple conversation, as the following example recorded by Afzelius demonstrates:

Some weeks ago we were one morning at breakfast conversing, whether it was possible to make butter in Sierra Leone or not, when Mamadoosamboo solved the question by informing us that they made plenty of butter in the Foulahs

[22] Afzelius, *Sierra Leone Journal*, 67r–97v. It was apparently not uncommon for Europeans to observe this public ceremony. Afzelius (244v–251v) described it again in February 1796, and in his book, John Matthews, *A Voyage to the River Sierra-Leone, on the Coast of Africa* (London: B. White, 1788), 125–127, also explained it briefly.
[23] Afzelius, *Sierra Leone Journal*, 33r.   [24] Afzelius, *Sierra Leone Journal*, 29r, 31r.
[25] Afzelius, *Sierra Leone Journal*, 39r.   [26] Afzelius, *Sierra Leone Journal*, 38r–38v.

country. But as it was to[o] hot in daytime, they used to be employed about it in
nighttime.[27]

Visiting African rulers and dignitaries also shared information with
Europeans in Freetown. In June 1795, a Bullom ruler named Pa Jack
from north of the Sierra Leone River and a Temne ruler named Prince
George told Afzelius in a casual conversation the local names of the
Inktree, 'both saying that the people knew the tree, but did never make
any use of it'. Afzelius's relationship with Pa Jack was a long-standing
one, as a journal entry from January 1796 reveals: 'Pa Jack came over
from the other side in the evening and supped with us – We then
conversed with him about several plants and got by him informed ...'[28]
Besides visiting Africans, commercial agents from the Sierra Leone
Company also acted as informants. For example, an agent named
Trien brought a specimen of spice bark to Winterbottom from the
Sherbro.[29] Afzelius's presence in Freetown seems to have led to random
and chance encounters with informants, who brought him specimens on
one or two occasions in exchange for small financial compensation. In
the beginning of January 1796, a man named Amarah is mentioned twice
in Afzelius's journal. He provided Afzelius and Winterbottom with a
great deal of information on a total of nineteen plants, including their
vernacular names and medicinal and other uses.[30]

Winterbottom's stay in Sierra Leone did not concentrate solely on
collecting information, but also experimenting with it. On 12 January
1796, Afzelius reported that Winterbottom had given him a plant, which
the Kru called *Sassara Winghee* and which was used in curing sore legs.
About a month later, Winterbottom told Afzelius that he had healed the
toes of two Africans by using *Sassara Winghee* and *Apel*, washing the sores
with a decoction of the former and strewing a powder of the dried and
uppermost leaves of the latter on the toes afterwards.[31]

In modern terms, Afzelius and Winterbottom could be characterised
as ethnomedical researchers, who observed, collected, interviewed, compared and even experimented.[32] Their knowledge of local flora and its

[27] Afzelius, *Sierra Leone Journal*, 48v.

[28] Afzelius, *Sierra Leone Journal*, 56r–56v, 157v, 161r.

[29] Afzelius, *Sierra Leone Journal*, 99v.

[30] Afzelius, *Sierra Leone Journal*, 123v, 125r–127v.

[31] Afzelius, *Sierra Leone Journal*, 299v.

[32] An example of comparing African and European medical knowledge comes from
Winterbottom, *An Account of the Native Africans*, II: 10–11, who observed that, in
Sierra Leone, locals paid no regard to the phases of the moon when collecting
medicines for use. However, a local belief upon the coast was that people can only die
at high or low tide. Winterbottom noted that the tide's influence had been credited also

medical uses was greatly enhanced by their interaction with local informants, whose expertise formed the basis of scientific research. This was an
intellectual order, one which turned the colonial order on its head. In this
picture, Africans emerge as the true masters of their domain, which they
undoubtedly were. Without them, the scientific achievements of a
European botanist and a physician would have been considerably less
comprehensive and extensive. Yet, even in his private writings, Afzelius
hardly gave any information on his most reliable and hardworking
informants.

'Peter and Duffa Brought Following Plants'

Of Afzelius's informants and assistants, two men, Peter and Duffa,
clearly stand out. Both are indexed as servants by Peter Kup, the modern
editor of Afzelius's journal. The journal itself gives no information about
the two men, despite their central role in collecting plants for Afzelius.
Neither does it contain information on how the relationship between
Afzelius, Peter and Duffa was formed. Peter is simply first mentioned by
Afzelius on Wednesday, 20 May 1795: 'Peter brought me a great deal of
forest Plants and among them was also Haemanthus Multiflorus, which
had begun to flower not long time ago.'[33] On the following day, Afzelius
recorded that 'Peter brought again many plants, partly the same as
yesterday.'[34] Then, on 1 June, 'Peter brought me today a collection of
fine plants.'[35] But Peter did not only bring plants for Afzelius to study –
he also brought information on their local uses, as the following examples
demonstrate:

Gardenia crinite he called Coúta, or in English written Coútèe, the leaves of
which rubbed between the fingers smell as Anthoxantum odoratum, and in this
state the Natives use to rub their forehead with them to take away headach [sic].[36]

Peter informed me about the name and use of some native plants viz:

1. Banisteria Leona Cav. is called Matácky, and the seeds or rather the wole [sic]
   fruit of it bruised and rubbed in the hair kills lice, and is for that purpose used
   by the natives.[37]

Peter probably assisted Afzelius throughout the autumn of 1795, but this
cannot be confirmed because his journal ends abruptly on 4 August

in European medicine, namely in the work of Willem Piso, but already having root in the
writings of Aristotle.
[33] Afzelius, *Sierra Leone Journal*, 31v–32r.   [34] Afzelius, *Sierra Leone Journal*, 32r.
[35] Afzelius, *Sierra Leone Journal*, 47v.   [36] Afzelius, *Sierra Leone Journal*, 49r.
[37] Afzelius, *Sierra Leone Journal*, 102r–102v.

1795 and only recommences on 1 January 1796. Afzelius's other loyal assistant, Duffa, might have entered his service during this five-month break in the journal. He is first mentioned on 7 January. The two are first mentioned working as a pair on 11 January, and after this date they mostly brought plants together, bringing their largest collection of thirty-seven specimens on 25 February.[38]

Afzelius paid Peter and Duffa as well as his other assistants a fixed sum for each specimen. On one occasion, he distributed rum to his helpers in order to motivate them to collect everything they could find. In this way, he managed to collect not only a great number of plant specimens, but also a great number of living animals, including birds, beasts of prey, snakes and an alligator. He also collected insects that he described in a publication after returning to Sweden.[39]

Peter's and Duffa's contributions to Afzelius's plant collection were enormous. Working mostly together, but also separately, they provided more than 50 per cent of the plants Afzelius collected in Freetown, and given the five-month gap in documentation, this proportion might have been considerably higher. The number of specimens they brought numbered over 300, and most of them were collected during January and February of 1796. Peter and Duffa were both Temne speakers and often provided Temne names for the plants they brought. However, it is hard to infer their level of knowledge about the local uses of these plants. Especially towards the end of his collaboration with the two, Afzelius rarely recorded information on how the plants were used. This might have reflected the fact that many specimens brought by Peter and Duffa were duplicates of plants Afzelius already had in his collection and had described earlier. It might also signify that Peter and Duffa first brought plants that were most interesting to them and those that were valued locally, later starting to bring random plants that locals usually ignored.

Race, Gender and Pan-African Knowledge in Sierra Leone

European images of Africa and Africans were manifold. While much has been written about the literary construction of racial hierarchies in European thought concerning Africans, it should also be acknowledged that the portrayal of African 'otherness' cannot be generalised to concern all European sources on Africa in the precolonial period. John Fage has argued that early modern Europeans 'generally thought of African

---

[38] Afzelius, *Sierra Leone Journal*, 135v, 150r, 301v–304r.
[39] Lindroth, 'Adam Afzelius: En linnean', 41.

societies as different from their own but not as innately inferior ... Europeans were beginning to assume that they were superior to other peoples, but even so it was until the second half of the nineteenth century that practical evidence of this became apparent in the field of tropical Africa.'[40]

Scholars concerned with European portrayals of Africans as inferior would be well advised to look more closely at what was actually happening in Africa between whites and blacks in the early modern period. The medical practices described by Afzelius and Winterbottom bring to the fore a more complex and nuanced picture of racial hierarchies and intellectual order in late eighteenth-century West Africa. According to Winterbottom, Europeans in Sierra Leone frequented African healers. Just like the locals, they could travel to distant villages 'in order to take medicines from some one who has acquired celebrity for the cure of a particular disorder; this is frequently some old woman, to whom even Europeans will often trust themselves in preference to their own countryman'.[41]

In Sierra Leone, African women were important carriers of indigenous medico-botanical knowledge. This was duly noted by Lieutenant John Matthews in the 1780s, when he wrote that in Sierra Leone, 'the office of physician ... is carried on by old women, and the cures they perform are truly astonishing; particularly in external wounds, by the use of simples, which their woods and fields afford in abundance'.[42] During his travels in the 1770s, Henry Smeathman married the daughter of a local ruler. The arrangement helped him to negotiate a framework of local connections, or in other words, a network, which enabled him to travel and collect specimens throughout the coastal regions of Sierra Leone.[43]

The medical interaction between Africans and Europeans, as described by Afzelius and Winterbottom, turned the racial and gender-based intellectual hierarchies on their head. While living in Freetown, the two men freely took advantage of African women's medical expertise. In January 1795, they had a chance to interview Miss Betsy Heard, whom

[40] J. D. Fage, *A Guide to Original Sources for Precolonial Western Africa Published in European Languages: For the Most Part in Book Form* (Madison: African Studies Program, University of Wisconsin – Madison, 1994), vii.
[41] Winterbottom, *An Account of the Native Africans*, II: 11.
[42] Matthews, *A Voyage*, 136. It is questionable whether Sierra Leone was the only part of the coast where women specialised in popular healing. Surgeon Atkins described in the 1730s how the director-general of the Cape Coast Castle relied more on the fetishes of his coloured mistress than Atkins's advice. Atkins, *A Voyage to Guinea*, 94–95.
[43] Douglas, 'The Making of Scientific Knowledge'.

they had long waited to see.[44] Betsy Heard was a mixed-race slave trader, who as a young woman had visited England, and who now lived among the Mandinga people. Afzelius described the meeting in his journal:

> She breakfasted with us and as soon as this was done, she, the Doctor [Winterbottom], I and a [sic] old respectable woman, Namoona-moodu's Sister, went so far as to the next brook on the different roads, and collected a number of plants, which we brought home in the Doctor's room and there Miss Herd [sic] shewing her skill and knowledge of Africa's Medical Plants and at the same time her politeness to us in telling us without reserve the medical uses of the following plants.[45]

Miss Heard was one of the most knowledgeable and efficient informants that Afzelius and Winterbottom encountered. During the course of a single day, she revealed the secrets of thirty-five plants. What makes this encounter remarkable is that Miss Heard not only gave the names of plants but also provided detailed instructions on their medical properties. By comparison, on their most efficient day Peter and Duffa, working as a pair, brought about the same number of plants but did not have much to say on their local uses. Miss Heard was a native Susu speaker, for this was the language in which she named the plants. In contrast to male inform-ants, she was especially knowledgeable about healing ailments typical to women and children.[46] This made her all the more valuable to Winterbottom, who used this information to compose chapters on their diseases.[47]

Like many other earlier European collectors and botanists in Africa and the Black Atlantic world, Afzelius and Winterbottom recognised the central role of women in guarding medical knowledge and practising healing in their everyday lives. Yet, neither Betsy Heard nor other African informants found a place in publications regarding scientific discoveries. Their role was downplayed and silenced, perhaps because eighteenth-century European men were reluctant to show their intellectual debt to black women – or any women, as European women were still excluded from academic life, too. In his private journal, Afzelius could reveal his

---

[44] Afzelius, *Sierra Leone Journal*, 149r–149v, 194r–200v. On 11 January, Afzelius recorded that 'Calamina or Miss Herd [sic] had passed by some days ago from Bance Island without calling here, to the great disappointment of the Doctor, who had expected much information from her on the African diseases.' On Betsy Heard as a slave trade in Sierra Leone, see Bruce L. Mouser, 'Women Slavers of Guinea-Conakry', in *Women and Slavery in Africa*, edited by Claire C. Robertson and Martin Klein (Madison: University of Wisconsin Press, 1983), 320–339.
[45] Afzelius, *Sierra Leone Journal*, 194r–194v.
[46] Afzelius, *Sierra Leone Journal*, 194r–200v.
[47] Winterbottom, *An Account of the Native Africans*, II, chs. 12 and 13.

admiration for Betsy Heard, but in Winterbottom's published account this anticipated and fruitful meeting went without mention.

The botanical and medical knowledge collected by Afzelius and Winterbottom was not confined to Sierra Leone and the Upper Guinea Coast but extended to other parts of the Black Atlantic world as well. In Winterbottom's case, the textual references to medical knowledge in other parts of Africa and on the other side of the Atlantic Ocean were evident in occasional footnotes referring to the works of travellers and physicians. Yet, one can assume that he and Afzelius also learned a great deal from ship captains and crews who passed by Sierra Leone on their slaving voyages and from Africans of different origins, who for one reason or another had ended up in Sierra Leone. A specific example is provided by Afzelius, who wrote in August 1795, regarding the Guinea worm, that it 'not only attacks the feet, as has hitherto been believed, but also other and higher parts of the body as legs, knees, thighs etc., as we have been informed by people from the Gold Coast, where this worm is common'.[48]

The Nova Scotian settlers of Sierra Leone were an important source of pan-African knowledge. One settler named Mrs Logan showed Afzelius how she made soap out of banana stems and leaves, collecting as many as she could and putting them out to dry near her house. Then, she tore the dried stems and leaves into smaller strips and burnt them to ashes used for the soap.[49] It is important to note that Sierra Leone emerged as a space where pan-African knowledge converged. First, it forcibly moved across the Atlantic from different regions of Africa to the New World, while practical botanical knowledge then returned to Africa in the late eighteenth century. Revolutions in the Atlantic world also instigated return movements of blacks from the Americas to Africa, which meant that bodies of knowledge were concentrated in places like Sierra Leone.

One of Afzelius's most remarkable informants was a man named Cyrus Williams, who either himself or whose parents were from West-Central Africa. Afzelius did not disclose Williams's background in detail, but as Williams gave him the names of plants in a Bantu language, Afzelius recorded them as 'Angol', or Angola. Judging by his English name of Cyrus Williams, he had been a slave in an English colony in the New World, but the fact that he was able to give Bantu names to plants suggests that he had been born in Africa and had intimate knowledge of West-Central African flora. His information points to the wide distribution of certain plants along the Atlantic coast of Africa, and even more

---

[48] Afzelius, *Sierra Leone Journal*, 121v.   [49] Afzelius, *Sierra Leone Journal*, 36r.

remarkably, to the similar uses of certain plants in Angola and Sierra Leone. For example, Afzelius recorded that '*Sengasaing* Angol. is the same as Congiare and Pongia the bark of which the Angola people use to dye yellow with as well as our neighbours'.[50]

Besides Africans who crisscrossed the ocean, slave ship captains and crews actively participated in circulating medical knowledge. Winterbottom's work includes several references to information he culled from publications regarding disease in the West Indies, but he and Afzelius also interviewed ship captains. In March 1796, the two joined a trading expedition to the Los Islands off Conakry in present-day Guinea. In Domingee, captains Mighee and Carr joined them for dinner. Afzelius related that the former had first served as a surgeon on a slave ship and had now advanced to the position of captain. Mighee and Winterbottom had a long conversation about different diseases and the methods for curing them. African healing methods were certainly used on slave ships to combat some diseases. Regarding flux and how to cure it, Mighee related that

he had seen [it] on all parts of the coast but more amongst them that lives [*sic*] on Yams than Rica – Amongst other things they use for it is Guava bark as an astringent, which they sell parceled up and dried at a Portuguese Island to the Leeward. On the Gold Coast the natives only use clystin.[51]

Historians of science and medicine in the Atlantic world have highlighted the contributions of Amerindians and enslaved Africans in shaping knowledge about natural history in the Americas. Bodily and botanical knowledge arrived from Africa to the Americas and left an indelible mark on healing systems and medical cultures. However, hybrid healing knowledge continued to circulate back and forth in the Atlantic world. With returned Africans, and through the experience of slave ship captains, it shaped and informed medical knowledge in Atlantic West Africa.

With the amount of medical knowledge that Afzelius and Winterbottom collected, Sierra Leone could perhaps have achieved medical self-sufficiency if it had seriously been tried. But the nineteenth century brought to West Africa Europeans who were much more confident in the scientific progress that was contesting old doctrines in medicine. They were also much more arrogant in shunning and discounting African healing knowledge. Especially in Sierra Leone, this change in attitude was fairly sudden. The nineteenth century brought with it the

---

[50] Afzelius, *Sierra Leone Journal*, 170r–171v.
[51] Afzelius, *Sierra Leone Journal*, 37v (part two).

rise of the witch doctor discourse to Atlantic Africa, and this drastically changed the nature of medical interaction.

Conclusion

Whereas early modern scientists still relied on African expertise, the imperial explorers of the second half of the nineteenth century more often had a negative view of African knowledge. Classifying and taming nature by scientific methods was typical of colonial knowledge production, which underlined European superiority compared to 'pagan darkness'.[52] This change in European attitudes is best described by the Swiss botanist Hans Schinz, who travelled in South-West Africa between 1884 and 1887. Schinz remarked that he had to collect everything by himself.[53] However, the experiences of medical interaction between Europeans and Africans in precolonial Africa shows that a more open attitude towards local knowledge was, and is, possible.[54]

The question that must be posed regarding the examined sources concerns their representativeness. Afzelius and Winterbottom, both ardent abolitionists, certainly regarded African botanical and medical knowledge as rich, useful and valuable. Certainly, they were less excited about the ritual healing practices than about the actual materia medica. But were their views exceptional in precolonial Atlantic Africa or in the wider Black Atlantic world? This is certainly not the case. The use of both African medicinal plants as well as participation in local religious rituals is well documented among the Portuguese settlers in West and West-Central Africa. However, neither were the Portuguese exceptional in this regard. The French, the Danish and the English in West Africa, along with the Dutch in West and South Africa, were all similarly interested in precolonial African medical knowledge for at least three reasons. First, the constant shortage of European medicines, physicians and surgeons in precolonial Africa drove Europeans to experiment and frequent local medical specialists. African women taken as partners by

[52] Johannes Fabian, *Out of Our Minds: Reason and Madness in the Exploration of Central Africa* (Berkeley: University of California Press, 2000); Leila Koivunen, *Visualizing Africa in Nineteenth-Century British Travel Accounts* (London: Routledge, 2009).

[53] Gitte Beckmann, ed., *'Man muss eben alles sammeln': Der Zürcher Botaniker und Forschungsreisende Hans Schinz und seine ethnographische Sammlung Südwestafrika* (Zürich: Neue Zürcher Zeitung and Völkerkundemuseum der Universität Zürich, 2012).

[54] See, e.g., Stacey A. Langwick, 'Healers and Scientists: The Epistemological Politics of Research about Medicinal Plants in Tanzania', in *Evidence, Ethos and Experiment: The Anthropology and History of Medical Research in Africa*, edited by P. Wenzel Geissler and Catherine Molyneux (New York: Berghahn Books, 2011), 263–295.

Europeans played an important role in caring for the sickly men and in providing access to local healers. Second, curiosity, sometimes driven by economic interest, played a role for some Europeans. After all, African medicinals, like materia medica from other parts of the world, could be marketed in Europe as 'exotic'. Third, by the late eighteenth century there was definite scientific interest driven by Linne's taxonomic work. In Africa, Linne's students Afzelius, Sparrman and Thunberg are perhaps the best-known examples of botanists documenting local flora, but the Portuguese were similarly organising scientific expeditions in the late eighteenth century, displaying an interest in developing the market for African medicinals in Europe. Isert's and Thonning's activities on the Gold Coast as well as Winterbottom's and Afzelius's work in Sierra Leone fit into this larger context of scientific research.

5   Healers, Hospitals and Medicines
European Medical Practice in Angola

In 1743, Angola's chief physician, Eusébio Catela de Lemos, complained about the activities of unlicensed popular healers in Luanda. He alleged that their corrupt and false medicines put the ill at risk and had already caused deaths or injuries. At the centre of these accusations stood an Englishman named Henry Masterman (Port. Henrique Mestre man), who had first arrived in Lisbon twelve years earlier. There, he had first been employed as the servant of a druggist (*droquista*) and then worked in a pharmacy (*bótica*). A turn of events, or 'some accidents', had forced Masterman to move to Pernambuco, where he continued to work as a pharmacist/druggist and was baptised as a Catholic. Because of his unpopularity in Brazil, Masterman moved to Angola, where he got married and continued to practise not only as a pharmacist but also as a doctor and surgeon in medicine. When Luanda's physician and surgeon tried to examine his knowledge of medical theories, Masterman replied that he did not know how to argue medically, he only knew how to prepare prescriptions and cure ailments on a practical level. Chief Physician Lemos argued that Masterman should not be allowed to practise medicine or surgery and sought to arrest and punish him.[1]

To defend his right to practise medicine, Masterman had collected testimonials from several people he had allegedly cured. For example, José Miranda de Vasconcelos certified that for many years Masterman had engaged in surgery, medicine and pharmaceutical work, with general acceptance of and applause for his successful cures.[2] However, Lemos replied by arguing that it was well known in Luanda that the signatories

---

[1] AHU, CU, Angola, Cx. 36, Doc. 3445, Carta do governador e capitão-general de Angola, João Jacques de Magalhães, ao rei, 16 November 1743. Masterman was probably present in Luanda by 1740; a letter from that year refers to a Catholic foreigner trained as a druggist (in São Paulo instead of Pernambuco). See AHU, CU, Angola, Cx. 34, Doc. 3283, Consulta do Conselho Ultramarino ao rei D. João V sobre a carta do governador e capitão-general de Angola, João Jacques de Magalhães, 12 October 1740.

[2] AHU, CU, Angola, Cx. Cx. 36, Doc. 3403, Requerimento do cidadão inglês Henrique Martiman, morador na cidade de Luanda, ao rei, earlier than 21 January 1743.

had never admitted Masterman into their homes to treat them. The Englishman was not the only unofficial white healer in Luanda, claimed Lemos, but he did not name any others. One of them, however, can be identified as the pharmacist Pedro Marques Pereira, who similarly collected testimonials from Luandans to prove his ability to practise the medical arts. A Capuchin writing on his behalf testified that Pereira had great experience in curing diverse infirmities.[3] The only way to control these practitioners, the chief physician argued, was to have them officially examined and licensed if they proved capable. Evaluating these accusations in Lisbon, Doctor Cipriano Pinheiro Pestana pointed out that they should be directed to the chief physician of Portugal. Lemos, who resided with the governor in Luanda, did not have authority to punish anyone suspected of heterodox medical practice.[4]

Masterman was one of the European practitioners to try his luck in the colony of Angola. Never a popular destination among Portuguese physicians and surgeons, and far from Lisbon's central authority, the doors were wide open for different kinds of European practitioners to establish themselves in Angola. As this chapter shows, African healers were not the only ones whose practice could come under the scrutiny of ecclesiastical or secular authorities. The legitimacy of white healers was similarly discussed from time to time. Medical pluralism reflected mostly local African practices and values, but global influences were also present in the form of the charitable brotherhoods, which ran hospitals in Luanda, Benguela and Massangano. They are also evident in the arrival of quina bark from Brazil as early as the 1720s and patent medicine from Portugal soon thereafter.

Physicians, Surgeons and Barbers

Early modern healthcare in Europe was characterised by medical pluralism. The therapeutic landscape in southern Europe included different forms of healing. David Gentilcore's model of medical pluralism includes three concentric and permeable rings, which labels three types of healers and sources of healing as well as etiological categories, namely medical, ecclesiastical and popular. The medical category refers to learned or university medicine, and it includes healing provided by

---

[3] AHU, CU, Angola, Cx. 36, Doc. 3421, Consulta do Conselho Ultramarino ao rei sobre requerimento do boticário e familiar do Santo Ofício, capitão Pedro Marques Pereira, 24 April 1743.

[4] AHU, CU, Angola, Cx. 36, Doc. 3445, Carta do governador e capitão-general de Angola, João Jacques de Magalhães, ao rei, 16 November 1743.

physicians, surgeons, barbers and pharmacists at hospitals or privately. Admittedly, university medicine is a misleading term as surgeons and barbers gained practical training via apprenticeships instead of academic training. Yet, surgeons and barbers often carried out treatment on the orders of the physician, so grouping them together makes sense. Ecclesiastical healing included not only the spiritual services – prayers, blessings, exorcisms – offered by priests, but also the perceived healing power of shrines, saints and living saints. Living saints and lay exorcists functioned both within ecclesiastical and popular idioms of healing, whereas charlatans rightly belong to the popular and medical spheres. The role of midwives, in turn, overlapped with all three categories. Gentilcore's model allows for historical change, and the circles are continually shifting in relation to one another, as are the places of individual healers and sources of healing.[5]

Gentilcore's model fittingly describes the multicultural colony of Angola, where a pluralism of healers prevailed. Factors such as availability, cost, reputation, suitability of the healer to the disease and its underlying causation as well as the past experiences of the sick themselves, affected the reactions and solutions of individuals in seeking a cure. Most treatment was undoubtedly carried out in the home, and in this regard Portuguese settlers were assisted by their local African partners and slaves. The number of European physicians and surgeons was limited, and therefore it is not surprising that many Portuguese turned to local sources of healing knowledge and materials (discussed in detail in Chapters 1 and 2).

Little is known about the earliest Portuguese physicians and surgeons serving in Angola. Only one seventeenth-century physician, Aleixo de Abreu, published a book documenting his experiences with tropical diseases in West-Central Africa. The presence of surgeons is documented sporadically. Sometimes new governors nominated to Angola chose their medical staff personally. In 1624, when Fernão de Sousa did not find a sufficiently qualified doctor to follow him to Africa, he took surgeon Marcos de Sequeira with him. Sequeira's role was to provide medical care on the journey from Lisbon to Luanda and to continue with similar duties in Angola. Another surgeon, António Martins Manso, received the same order to cure sick and wounded soldiers on the sea on his way to serve as the chief surgeon in Luanda.[6] Surgeons were primarily attached to military units and followed them on their

---

[5] Gentilcore, *Healers and Healing*, 3.
[6] AHU, CU, Angola, Cx. 2, Doc. 142, Requerimento do nomeado para governador de Angola, Fernão de Sousa, ao rei, preceding 19 January 1624; AHU, CU, Angola, Cx. 11,

campaigns to the interior. They were especially needed during the war against the Dutch, when the governor requested that a doctor and medicines be sent to Angola.[7]

In the aftermath of ousting the Dutch from Angola, nominating medical officers was part of the reorganisation of the colony. Luanda received a chief physician and a pharmacist, whereas a chief surgeon was assigned to Benguela. Antonio Lopes de Oliveira's nomination as Angola's chief physician was justified by the argument that Angola was a very sickly country where the inhabitants perished from the 'absence of necessities'. Before his nomination, the chief physician of Portugal orally examined this Coimbra-educated doctor. Other specialists included the pharmacist Manoel Pereira, who moved to Luanda from Lisbon, where he had his shop and where 'all the people tried out his science'. Benguela's chief surgeon, Bernardo Pinto, had in turn served with the troops that had restored Angola to Portugal, and he continued to serve in the infantry in Benguela. Around the same time, Father João da Piedade, who had earlier served in the city of Tangier, was nominated as the general administrator of the military hospital in Luanda. His responsibilities included taking care of the treatment of the sick. Piedade, a Third Order Franciscan, petitioned personally for the nomination to this post. In deliberating his nomination, officials referred to another priest who had a similar responsibility in the province of Alentejo, demonstrating the active role taken by clergy in running medical establishments in Portugal and its overseas territories.[8]

For a long time, chief physicians served as the personal doctor of the governor and other high-ranking officials. Newly nominated governors sometimes sought the nomination of doctors that they knew personally. This was the case with Rodrigo de Miranda Henriques, nominated as

Doc. 1302, Consulta do Conselho Ultramarino ao príncipe regente D. Pedro sobre o requerimento do cirurgião, António Martins Manso, 2 May 1673.

[7] AHU, CU, Angola, Cx. 4, Doc. 382, Consulta do Conselho Ultramarino ao rei sobre carta do governador de Angola, 10 February 1646.

[8] 'Do Bot.ro Manoel Pereira, 11 March 1648', 'Do fizico mor L.do An.to Lopez de Oliveira, 26 May 1649', 'Do Surgião mor do Reino de Benguella Bernardo P.to', 16 December 1649', 'Do P.e M.tre frei João da Fonsequa, 20 May 1650', all in *Arquivos de Angola*, First Series, 1:2 (1933): no page numbers; AHU, CU, Angola, Cx. 4, Doc. 441, Consulta do Conselho Ultramarino ao rei sobre requerimento do medico licenciado pela Universidade de Coimbra, António Lopes de Oliveira, solicitando o título de fisico-mor do reino de Angola, 6 May 1649; AHU, CU, Angola, Cx. 4, Doc. 439, Consulta do Conselho Ultramarino ao rei sobre requerimento do religioso da Ordem Terceira de São Francisco, frei João da Piedade, solicitando o ofício de administrador geral do hospital de Angola, 5 May 1649; AHU, CU, Angola, Cx. 4, Doc. 467, Consulta do Conselho Ultramarino, ao rei, sobre o requerimento do religioso da Terceira Ordem de São Francisco, padre frei João da Piedade, 23 November 1650.

governor in 1651, who petitioned for the nomination of *licenciado* Jordão Correa, an experienced doctor who had studied at Coimbra and practised medicine for many years in different villages. He was accompanied by the pharmacist Miguel Correa, who ran his own shop in Lisbon before embarking to Luanda.[9]

There are few indications of the salaries received by medical staff in Angola. In 1666, a royal provision defined the salary of the chief physician as 70$000 *reis*, while the surgeon received 30$000 *reis*. These sums were to be paid by the Santa Casa de Misericórdia (see below in the 'Administering Hospitals' section).[10] Around the same time, the governor gave an order to forward 100 *cruzados* to surgeon Daniel Serra, who treated soldiers outside of Luanda, in 1666.[11] Yet, surgeons' earnings were modest. Surgeon António Alvares requested that the king fund his voyage to Angola in the company of Governor Luís César de Meneses in 1697 because he was poor.[12] By the 1730s, however, the annual compensation due to the chief physician had risen to 150$000 *reis*. The chief surgeon's salary was also discussed around the same time. It was suggested that it should be in the order of 10$000 reis per month, or 120 $000 reis annually, signifying a fourfold increase.[13]

The training and expertise of European practitioners stationed in Angola varied. The University of Coimbra was the centre of medical learning in Portugal during the early modern period, but generally speaking, many Portuguese doctors received their training elsewhere. Salamanca was the most common Iberian destination, but many students also found their way to France and Italy. The Netherlands, in turn,

---

[9] AHU, CU, Angola, Cx. 4, Doc. 482, Consulta do Conselho Ultramarino, ao rei, sobre o requerimento do governador do reino de Angola, Rodrigo de Miranda Henriques, 5 June 1651; AHU, CU, Angola, Cx. 5, Doc. 493, Consulta do Conselho Ultramarino, ao rei, sobre o requerimento do boticário, Miguel Correia, solicitando o cargo de boticário do hospital e presídios de Angola, 10 July 1651. *Conselho Ultramarino* had no news of the recently nominated chief physician, Antonio Lopes de Oliveira, but noted that the physician might have passed away given the climate of Angola.

[10] AHU, CU, Angola, Cx. 9, Doc. 1057, Provisão (cópia) do rei estipulando o ordenado dos governadores de Angola, 4 April 1666.

[11] AHU, CU, Angola, Cx. 9, Doc. 1031, Portaria do governador de Angola, André Vidal de Negreiros ao provedor da Fazenda Real, capitão Tomás Figueira Bultão, 18 January 1666. A *cruzado* was worth $400 *reis*.

[12] AHU, CU, Angola, Cx. 16, Doc. 1837, Consulta do Conselho Ultramarino ao rei sobre requerimento do cirurgião António Alvares, 11 February 1697.

[13] The rise in the chief physician's salary is documented in AHU, CU, Angola, Cx. 34, Doc. 3253, Relação dos rendimentos da Fazenda Real de Angola no ano de 1739, undated; the chief surgeon's salary is discussed in AHU, CU, Angola, Cx. 34, Doc. 3283, Consulta do Conselho Ultramarino ao rei D. João V sobre a carta do governador e capitão-general de Angola, João Jacques de Magalhães, 12 October 1740.

became the favoured destination for Portuguese Jews and New Christians, whose admission to the University of Coimbra was prohibited altogether in 1671.[14] Some of the doctors and surgeons sent to Angola were recent university graduates with very little experience, while others had very little formal training but a wealth of experience. Some had a combination of both. For example, Manuel Francisco Preto, who petitioned for nomination as the surgeon-major of Angola in 1639, had a university degree and seven years of practical experience working on seafaring vessels and in Brazil. He had been involved with the military activities in the conflict between the Dutch and the Portuguese in Paraíba and Pernambuco, and he was eager to serve as a military surgeon in Angola, expecting an excessive workload in a diseased country.[15] João Baptista Monteiro, who petitioned for nomination as a military surgeon in 1700, referred to his experience as a naval doctor, having embarked to Brazil several times.[16] In 1732, one pharmacist who had acquired experience working at the Royal Hospital in Lisbon requested that he be nominated as chief surgeon of Angola. Although he had taken lessons in surgery, he had not yet received a formal recognition of his skills. The Overseas Council recommended nomination only if he first passed the formal examination for a surgeon. One council member, however, disapproved and argued that only men born in Angola (*naturais da terra*) should be nominated as surgeons in Angola, as they had acquired direct experience with diseases in that country. At least some Portuguese, then, thought that local experience in the tropics counted more than formal training in the metropole.[17]

Surgeon-Major Francisco Tavares de Ataíde made an exceptional petition in 1674, asking to be nominated as chief physician in addition to his position as chief surgeon. Ataíde had already served five years in Angola. He boasted of 'curing the whole infantry of the maladies that pertained to his art of surgery, as well as to those of medicine'. Invoking

---

[14] Mário Sérgio Farelo, 'On Portuguese Medical Students and Masters Travelling Abroad: An Overview from the Early Modern Period to the Enlightenment', in *Centres of Medical Excellence? Medical Travel and Education in Europe, 1500–1700*, edited by Ole Peter Grell, Andrew Cunningham and Jon Arrizabalaga (Farnham: Ashgate, 2010), 132–142.

[15] AHU, CU, Angola, Cx. 3, Doc. 302, Consulta do Conselho da Fazenda ao rei sobre o licenciado Manuel Francisco Preto que pediu o cargo de cirurgião-mor do reino de Angola, 4 March 1639.

[16] AHU, CU, Angola, Cx. 16, Doc. 1893, Requerimento do cirurgião João Baptista Monteiro, ao rei solicitando provimento no lugar de cirurgião-mor da Infantaria da cidade de Luanda, que se encontrava vago, 15 December 1700.

[17] AHU, CU, Angola, Cx. 29, Doc. 2827, Consulta do Conselho Ultramarino ao rei D. João V sobre o requerimento do boticário aprovado António Inocêncio Pita, 12 August 1732.

his great experience, Ataíde argued that he could serve as chief physician since there were no qualified doctors in Angola. The Overseas Council asked for the opinion of Portugal's physician-major, who examined Ataíde's claims and recommended his nomination for the position of Angola's *físico-mor*.[18]

The array of formally nominated doctors and practitioners of medicine with university or apprentice training opens up the question of whether any Portuguese popular healers offered their services in Angola besides Masterman, mentioned at the beginning of this chapter. Indications are rare, but one potential clue can be found from 1715, when King João V granted a licence for Angola's chief physician, Manuel de Andrade de Goes, to return to Portugal. The licence was granted on condition that Jorge Ferrer de Espinosa was still alive in Luanda. Espinosa had been practising healing in Angola for several years. However, the wording of the king's letter leaves the exact nature of Espinosa's practice open, for it stated that he healed with medicine – *estar curando de Medicina*. Espinosa's practice thus seems to have been closer to university medicine than that of a folk healer. King João made the point that Angola was not to be left without a doctor, for the residents were bound to suffer if there was no one to assist them with their illnesses.[19]

There are likewise some clues regarding the transmission of medical knowledge from Portuguese doctors to Africans. The classes on medicine offered by Chief Physician José Pinto de Azeredo in the late eighteenth century have often been cited as the first example of medical training in Angola, but there might have been earlier precedents, and at least there were plans to train medical personnel in Luanda as early as the beginning of the eighteenth century.[20] Manuel de Andrade de Goes was granted permission to practise medicine in Angola, both to cure soldiers and also to teach medicine to all residents who wanted to learn. He resided in Luanda for over a decade.[21]

---

[18] AHU, CU, Angola, Cx. 11, Doc. 1364, Consulta do Conselho Ultramarino ao príncipe regente D. Pedro sobre o requerimento do cirurgião-mor de Angola, Francisco Tavares de Ataíde, 22 November 1674.

[19] 'Provisão autorizando o regresso à Metrópole do Fisico Mor Manuel de Andrade de Goes, desde que não houvesse falecido o curandeiro Jorge Ferrer de Espinosa, 24 May 1715', *Arquivos de Angola*, First Series, 11:9 (1936): 147–148.

[20] Walter, *Um português carioca*; d'Esaguy, *A abertura da escola*.

[21] AHU, CU, Angola, Cx. 17, Doc. 1944, Informação do que fora concedido e exigido ao médico, Manuel de Andrada e Góis, em resultado do requerimento analisado pelo Conselho Ultramarino, com resolução a 9 de Junho de 1703, no qual se comprometia a ir servir como médico em Angola, after 9 June 1703.

As the Inquisition cases discussed in Chapter 2 make clear, Africans were trained as barbers in Luanda, where they appear in the documentation as assistants to the Portuguese surgeons but also as independent practitioners. They were also present in the Kingdom of Kongo in the second half of the seventeenth century, as documented by Capuchin Father Dionigi de Carli, who was bled by a black barber in the Duke of Bamba's service. He had been trained in Luanda and, according to Carli, was very good at his practice.[22] It serves as evidence that the Kongolese elites, at least, continued to make use of European knowledge, although such encounters are rarely documented in European sources. There are indications, however, that the presence of barbers had a very long continuity in West-Central Africa and elsewhere in the Lusophone Black Atlantic well into the eighteenth and nineteenth centuries. Sometimes when there were no physicians present in Luanda, the city's population had to rely on the barber-surgeons serving on ships.[23] In Brazil and Angola, *barbeiros* were not only barbers but also bloodletters who performed minor surgeries. In Brazil, where many African slaves and freedmen practised as *barbeiros*, the profession existed until at least the end of the nineteenth century.[24]

Perhaps the best evidence of the presence of barbers in Angola is provided by the census counts of the late eighteenth century, which demonstrate that barbers were present in Luanda and most of the Portuguese establishments in the interior (see Tables 5.1 and 5.2). Noticeably, the population counts, which listed people by phenotype or colour – using the categories white, black and mulatto – show that almost all barbers in the interior as well as on the coast were black. Only in 1803 did a single mulatto barber appear in Encoge. Some settlements had an elevated number of black barbers. For example, the district of Icolo and Bengo had three black barbers in 1797, and Massangano had five in both 1797 and 1798. Benguela, which had two surgeons and one pharmacist (all white), had as many as sixteen black barbers. But their

---

[22] Dionigi de Carli, *Viaggio del P Dionigi de'Carli da Piacenza, e del P. Michel Angelo de' Guatini, da Reggio Capuccini* (Reggio: Prospero Vedrotti, 1671), 109.

[23] AHU, CU, Angola, Cx. 50, Doc. 4694, Oficio do governador e capitão-general de Angola Francisco Inocêncio de Sousa Coutinho ao secretário de estado da Marinha e Ultramar Francisco Xavier de Mendonça Furtado, 4 April 1766.

[24] Mariza de Carvalho Soares, 'African Barbeiros in Brazilian Slave Ports', in *The Black Urban Atlantic in the Age of the Slave Trade*, edited by Jorge Cañizares-Esguerra, Matt D. Childs and James Sidbury (Philadelphia: University of Pennsylvania Press, 2013), 207–230; Tania Salgado Pimenta, 'Barbeiros-sangradores e curandeiros no Brasil (1808–28)', *História, Ciências, Saúde – Manguinhos* 2 (1998): 349–372; Mariana P. Candido, 'Different Slave Journeys: Enslaved African Seamen on Board of Portuguese Ships, c. 1760–1820s', *Slavery & Abolition* 31 (2010): 404.

Table 5.1 *Black* **barbeiros** *in the colonies of Angola and Benguela,*
1797–1798 and 1803[1]

	1797	1798	1803
Icolo and Bengo	3	n/a	n/a
Dande	1	n/a	n/a
Benguela	16	13	n/a
Massangano	5	5	4
Encoge	2	5	6 (+1 mulatto)
Cambambe	1	1	4
Muxima	1	2	5
Pungo Andongo	5	5	3
Ambaca	0	1	9
Caconda	0	n/a	0
Novo Redondo	3	3	n/a
Golungo	n/a	n/a	12
Total	37	35	43 (+1 mulatto)

[1] AHU, CU, Angola, Cx. 91, Doc. 41, Mappas statísticas, 15 April 1799; AHU, CU, Angola, Cx. 109, Doc. 37, Mappas statísticas, 17 March 1804.

Table 5.2 **Barbeiros** *in Luanda, 1799 and 1802–1803*[1]

	Masters	Officials	Apprentices	Total
1799	7	29	11	47
1802	8	14	6	28
1803	4	15	13	32

[1] AHU, Cx. 94, Doc. 1, Mappas statísticas, 1 January 1800; AHU, Cx. 105, Doc. 44, Mappas statísticas, n.d.; AHU, CU, Angola, Cx. 109, Doc. 49, Mappas statísticas, 10 April 1804.

number was most elevated in Luanda, where several masters trained barber apprentices. Although the short time span does not make it possible to draw definitive conclusions, the number of black barbers seems to have remained quite stable.

Barbeiros remained popular in Luanda and elsewhere in Angola into at least the second half of the nineteenth century. Joachim John Monteiro, a resident in Angola in the 1860s, wrote that one encountered barbers' shops in several places. He described the Mbundu *barbeiros* as very skilful in the use of the lancet. One of his local assistants in Cambambe was a 'capital hand at bleeding', and on an occasion Monteiro 'took some pains to sharpen it [his knife] properly on a hone'. Being accustomed to operating with a blunt instrument, the barber nearly killed the first man he operated upon. However, he thanked Monteiro afterwards, believing that 'no blood-letter would be able to compete with him'.[25]

The presence of barbers also demonstrates that Atlantic Africa was not merely sending people, plants, disease and knowledge to the West Indies in what Londa Schiebinger has termed the Atlantic world medical complex. Schiebinger has pointed out that only a trickle of medical knowledge returned from the West Indian 'center of calculation' along the African slave trade nexus and that 'West Indian knowledge may well have transshipped to Africa via Europe'.[26] This, however, leaves out the fact that medical knowledge was circulating directly from Europe to Africa and being selectively adopted in local communities. Medical knowledge was a part of the cultural creolisation taking place in West-Central Africa. This means that Atlantic creoles who had appropriated European medical knowledge in places like Luanda, Benguela and the Kingdom of Kongo were arriving in the Americas with an understanding, and sometimes practical experience of, European medicine. This is evident especially in Brazil, where black barbers had a substantial presence in the medical market of Rio de Janeiro well into the nineteenth century.[27]

Miraculous Cures, Medical Ignorance and Colonial Scandals: The Case of Chief Physician Aboim

The 1720s were a turbulent time in Angola's history, as the ports of Luanda and Benguela were rocked by a series of scandals. One of these scandals concerned the nomination of Father João Teixeira de Carvalho as school master of the cathedral in Luanda. Carvalho's activities between Benguela, Luanda and Rio de Janeiro and his career advancement had long been contested by authorities in Angola, including the governor, who threw various accusations at him, including that of practising Judaism. Yet, he also had strong protectors, including the Bishop of Luanda and Colonel Antonio da Fonseca Coutinho, who belonged to one of the richest families in Luanda. According to Selma Pantoja, these scandals reflected internal power struggles in the colony of Angola, where the slave trade was on the rise in this period.[28]

---

[25] Joachim John Monteiro, *Angola and the River Congo*, 2 vols. (London: Macmillan, 1875), 2: 262–263, cited in Soares, 'African Barbeiros', 213–214.
[26] Schiebinger, *Secret Cures of Slaves*, 153.
[27] On Atlantic creoles, see Heywood and Thornton, *Central Africans, Atlantic Creoles*.
[28] Selma Pantoja, 'Personagens entre mares atlânticos: Visões de Luanda setecentista', *Revista de História Comparada* 7 (2013): 136–148.

Father Carvalho's 'scandalous' behaviour came to light in 1719, when he was arrested for publicly dealing with foreign slave traders in Benguela, which was strictly forbidden. The next year, he was connected with the case of captain Antônio de Freitas Galvão (see Chapter 1), who was accused of heterodox religious practices, namely publicly adoring a goat and sacrificing a calf in Benguela. When Father Carvalho, 'a prejudicial cleric', intervened in the case, the Overseas Council recommended its delegation to the Inquisition. In 1726, Carvalho was accused of stabbing his concubine, Mariana Fernandes, who was rumoured to be in a relationship with a man named André Ferreira Gil. He was also accused of ordering his slaves to attack another man for having a relationship with the same woman. However, the bishop intervened in the case on Father Carvalho's behalf, which caused an uproar in Luanda.[29]

These were not the only strange happenings in Luanda and Benguela around this time. The most obscure case concerns Angola's chief physician, Tomé Guerreiro Camacho e Aboim, who, much like Father Carvalho, had been at the centre of controversy in Luanda for several years. He arrived in Luanda in 1717 accompanying the newly appointed governor, Henrique de Figueiredo e Alarcão. The chief physician came under scrutiny in 1720 when the governor reported that most people who were treated by him perished. In other words, Aboim was accused of lacking experience and expertise in treating tropical diseases. Instead of seeking treatment from him, many sick allegedly relied on surgeons 'who barely knew how to bleed', pharmacists and even the nurses employed at the hospital. They all boasted a better record of curing the sick. The many diseases that ravaged Luanda almost annually and Aboim's complete lack of skill, wrote the governor, had led the municipal council to request a new doctor from Rio de Janeiro. The settlers in Luanda were even prepared to pay the new doctor's compensation – amounting to a *conto de reis* (1:000$000) – from their own pockets.[30]

The citizens of Luanda turned to Rio de Janeiro because it was said that the ports of Brazil had enough sufficiently qualified doctors. The new doctor from Rio was a Naples-born Spaniard named Felipe Cortes

---

[29] AHU, CU, Angola, Cx. 22, Doc. 2258, Consulta do Conselho Ultramarino ao rei D. João V sobre a carta do ouvidor-geral de Angola, Francisco de Santa Bárbara e Moura, de 13 de Dezembro de 1720, 16 September 1721; AHU, CU, Angola, Cx. 25, Doc. 2488, Carta do ouvidor-geral de Angola, Francisco Pereira, ao rei sobre o Bispo daquele reino, proteger o clérigo João Teixeira de Carvalho, 28 March 1726.

[30] AHU, CU, Angola, Cx. 22, Doc. 2222, Carta do governador Henrique de Figueiredo, ao rei, 18 August 1720. Aboim's appointment date is from AHU, CU, Angola, Cx. 24, Doc. 2413, Requerimento do físico-mor de Angola e cavaleiro fidalgo de Sua Majestade, Tomé Guerreiro Camacho Aboim, ao rei solicitando aumento do soldo, earlier than 12 July 1725.

Velasco, who also practised surgery. Although 180 people had agreed to contribute to his salary, some Luandans expressed doubt about his credentials. The paper trail showed, however, that Dom Felipe's right to practise medicine had been ascertained six years earlier by the kingdom of Portugal's chief physician, João Bernardes de Morais, and further, that Rio's governor believed in its authenticity. Therefore, the majority saw no impediment to hiring him. After Velasco's arrival, the municipal council noted that ecclesiastics, who had opposed the hiring of a new physician and refused to contribute to his salary, were the first ones to use his services. Moreover, it was claimed that the whole city found Aboim's practice repugnant.[31]

The controversy surrounding the recruitment and hiring of a new physician is understandable. Prior to 1720, physicians and surgeons had been nominated by the king to serve in Angola and had usually accompanied a new governor's entourage. By agreeing to compensate the doctor's fee personally, Luandans took the matter into their own hands, bypassing customary practice and imperial bureaucracy. However, this was not the end of the story. Camacho e Aboim wrote a lengthy letter to the king in self-defence of his actions. Much like with Father João Teixeira de Carvalho, the chief physician had powerful enemies in Luanda's colonial hierarchy, including Governor Henrique de Figueiredo e Alarcão. According to Aboim's complaint, the governor had thrice ordered soldiers to kill him, but they had always failed. On the third occasion, he had been beaten through the streets of Luanda before being thrown into prison. The governor had then ordered that charges be brought against him. Aboim claimed that the governor had machinated a smear campaign against him, which included requesting a new physician from Rio de Janeiro. In his view, he had been successful in his practice and had many years of experience in treating tropical diseases in the Central African climate.[32]

In his letter, the chief physician brought up several abuses directed at him by the governor and his cronies. According to him, the *ouvidor geral* Francisco de Santa Bárbara e Moura and the governor's accomplices in Luanda's municipal council had invented the inflammatory accusations that Aboim killed all his patients. In the governor's name, Moura had personally inspected the medicines used in the hospital and claimed that Aboim gave poison to his patients, including quina (*china china*, or

---

[31] AHU, CU, Angola, Cx. 22, Doc. 2259, Despacho do Conselho Ultramarino, 17 September 1721.
[32] AHU, CU, Angola, Cx. 22, Doc. 2267, Requerimento do físico-mor de Angola, Tomé Guerreiro Camacho e Aboim, undated.

cinchona bark) and sheep's trotter. As such, the cinchona bark, as a new material and the healing technology connected to it, could have led to protests among patients, but this was never implied in the documentation. Instead, critics emphasised Aboim's character as the root problem. Therefore, one is not surprised to find out that he was also accused of being a drunkard.

The governor's goal was clearly to intimidate people to avoid seeking treatment from him. When this failed, because Aboim had the clergy's support, the governor tried to banish him from the city, but this effort failed as well since the municipal council did not approve of it. Finally, he was thrown into the public jail of Luanda. During his imprisonment, the governor ordered the surgeons and pharmacists to treat the city's inhabitants. If they refused, they were also threatened with prison. Aboim also claimed that a 'heretic' (i.e. Protestant) surgeon was hired from a foreign ship during this time. This was of little avail because more than a hundred people, including Capuchin Father Arcanjo, allegedly died while Aboim was in prison. Further, he claimed that the new doctor brought from Rio, Felipe Cortes Velasco, was a mere soldier and had never been a surgeon, being recognised as a 'comedian' after only a short while. Aboim, who claimed that Velasco refused to be examined by him, effectively turned the accusations around and argued that it was the Spaniard who killed people by malpractice. However, as shown in Chapter 7, surgeon Velasco wrote medical statements well grounded in humoural theory to at least two officers petitioning to leave Angola for health reasons, so he seems to have had at least some competence.

The confusion about Aboim continued after Alarcão had been replaced as governor in 1722. The interim governor, José Carvalho da Costa, complained that the chief physician had been responsible for Alarcão's death. Referring to Aboim's 'great ignorance, malevolence, and loathing', Costa claimed that few people went to Aboim for treatment. Allegedly, people rose from the sick bed only to be put into the grave, and therefore, Costa repeated the earlier requests that a new chief physician be sent to Angola.[33]

Despite these protests, Aboim continued to practise medicine in Luanda after his release from prison. In a personal testimony given after eight years in Luanda, he requested that the king raise his annual compensation and assist in his living costs, which had increased since his arrival in Angola. Aboim claimed that he worked excessively in Luanda's hospital and had personally fallen ill several times. Besides treating

[33] AHU, CU, Angola, Cx. 25, Doc. 2546, Carta do governador e capitão-general de Angola, Paulo Caetano de Albuquerque, ao rei, 3 April 1727.

soldiers, he referred to treating free and enslaved blacks, orphans and widows as well as the rich and the poor. Aboim also wrote that he needed four blacks to assist him in his work, but he was having constant problems with runaway and sick slaves, having already lost fifteen of them. Apparently, this was no idle bragging, for the officials of the municipal council and the Misericórdia brotherhood confirmed Aboim's diligence in treating his patients, pointing out his heroic commitment when malignant fevers and contagious diseases raged in Luanda in 1718 and 1720. Moreover, Aboim served the priests and slaves in Luanda's convents without remuneration. Two priests eulogised his work by claiming that, of the more than 500 patients treated in the hospital in one year, only 30 died, attributing many miraculous cures to the chief physician and his prodigious medicines.[34]

The governors of Luanda controlled the flow of information from Angola to Lisbon, thereby greatly contributing to what we can know about this case. Aboim was able to get an occasional letter out of the colony, probably by using his ecclesiastical contacts. The case took another twist when Aboim was denounced to the bishop, who used his inquisitorial powers to imprison him. The bishop eventually banished him to Cambambe. The actual timing and contents of the denunciation are unknown, but in two letters from April 1727 Governor Albuquerque referred to Aboim's imprisonment by the Inquisition, pointing out that Luanda had been without a physician for years. He also continued to accuse Aboim of medical abuse, which had led to numerous deaths. Apparently, Aboim's duties at the hospital were delegated to military surgeons, especially Surgeon-Major António Henriques, who became Albuquerque's trusted man in providing healthcare to ailing soldiers and settlers.[35]

In 1727, Aboim was able to send a complaint about his treatment to Lisbon. He complained that he had again suffered an attack on his life. The attack was performed by four Benguela blacks, who presumably had been following the orders of Antonio da Fonseca Coutinho. When the chief physician went to complain to Governor Albuquerque, the

---

[34] AHU, CU, Angola, Cx. 24, Doc. 2413, Requerimento do físico-mor de Angola e cavaleiro fidalgo de Sua Majestade, Tomé Guerreiro Camacho Aboim, ao rei, earlier than 12 July 1725.

[35] AHU, CU, Angola, Cx. 25, Doc. 2546, Carta do governador e capitão-general de Angola, Paulo Caetano de Albuquerque, ao rei, 3 April 1727; AHU, CU, Angola, Cx. 25, Doc. 2547, Carta do [governador e capitão-general de Angola], Paulo Caetano de Albuquerque, ao rei, 3 April 1727; AHU, CU, Angola, Cx. 27, Doc. 2683, Requerimento do cirurgião-mor António Henriques, ao rei, 14 February 1730.

governor had replied that worse treatment awaited him in Évora, hinting that Aboim would have to go through an Inquisition trial and an *auto-da-fé*. According to Aboim, his enemies went to denounce him to the bishop with allegations of witchcraft and blasphemy, of having a pact with the devil and of certainly being a Jew. Antonio da Fonseca Coutinho was presumably behind these machinations.[36] Finally, Aboim was sent to Recife but was not allowed to travel to Portugal. In 1730, he once again petitioned the king and tried to get a permission to return to Lisbon.[37]

How then can the enmity between the governors and the chief physician be explained? The case fits quite well with other descriptions of deep divisions in Luanda's colonial hierarchy and seems to have been a personal or factional issue.[38] Yet, it should be asked if it also had a medical dimension. One can see a potential conflict brewing in accusations of medical abuse, but the documentation shows that many people held the chief physician in high regard. The unfamiliarity with new medicines, such as cinchona, offered by Aboim to his patients might be one source of conflict, but, given the proclivity of settlers in Angola to experiment with local natural medicines, it is doubtful. In the end, one must believe the weight of evidence in favour of Aboim. Instead of Aboim, Governor Henrique de Figueiredo e Alarcão was responsible for the death of Luandans who did not receive treatment when Aboim was hindered from doing his job.[39]

Administering Hospitals

African healers' compounds were not the only choice for people residing in Luanda, Benguela and the *presídios* of the interior. The Portuguese

---

[36] AHU, CU, Angola, Cx. 26, Doc. 2575, Consulta do Conselho Ultramarino ao rei D. João V sobre o requerimento do físico-mor de Angola, Tomé Guerreiro Camacho e Aboim, 31 January 1728.

[37] AHU, CU, Angola, Cx. 29, Doc. 2801, Parecer do Conselho Ultramarino sobre o requerimento do ex-físico-mor de Angola, Tomé Guerreiro Camacho de Aboim, 29 April 1732. Aboim's correspondence with the Inquisition can be found in ANTT, TSO, Caderno 7 de Ordens do Conselho Geral.

[38] Cf. Pantoja, 'Personagens entre mares atlânticos', passim.

[39] It is noteworthy that one of the officers sent to kill Camacho e Aboim in the early stages of the conflict was João Pereira da Cunha, who was himself imprisoned by the Inquisition two decades later. According to one of Aboim's letters, Cunha had been sent to Angola because of *malefícios* performed in Portugal. Cunha had murdered a man in Porto, but Aboim's use of the word *malefícios* gives the murder a supernatural connotation. Further, when Cunha wrote in his own defence in the 1740s, he referred to the case of Aboim as an example of how officers in Luanda used the Inquisition to get rid of their competitors and enemies. AHU, CU, Angola, Cx. 22, Doc. 2267, Requerimento do físico-mor de Angola, Tomé Guerreiro Camacho e Aboim, preso em Luanda, ao rei, undated; ANTT, TSO/IL, Processo 9691, Processo de João Pereira da Cunha, f. 24v. On Cunha's case, see Kananoja, 'Healers, Idolaters and Good Christians'.

established hospitals from the early seventeenth century onwards. The brotherhood of the Santa Casa da Misericórdia (Holy House of Mercy) was one of the most significant providers of healthcare in the Portuguese colonial world, including Angola. Essentially a lay organisation, the first branch of the Santa Casa was established in 1498 in Lisbon. Its establishment was based on the older model of charitable assistance in Europe. The first printed *Compromisso*, or statutes, of the Misericórdia (1516) contained nineteen chapters. It defined the seven spiritual and seven corporal works of charity to be practised by all brothers. In addition to ransoming captives and visiting prisoners, the members were expected to cure the sick, bury the dead and offer clothes, food, drink and shelter to the poor.[40]

With the onset of Portuguese overseas expansion, Misericórdias spread globally and had an important role in the construction of empire.[41] In the east, the Misericórdias of Goa, Macao and Japan administered hospitals, admitting large numbers of Portuguese needing medical aid. In Brazil, Misericórdias were established in many towns in the colonial period. Their importance was widely recognised by ecclesiastical and lay authorities. Branches of the brotherhood were often entirely responsible for running hospitals and providing medical treatment to ailing patients. For example, in Bahia the Misericórdia was the sole administrator of the hospital, and all expenses were covered by the brotherhood. Insufficient funds and an absence of official financial support, however, made the running of hospitals challenging.[42]

The overseas Misericórdias were intimately linked to secular and religious power structures.[43] Angola became a part of the global reach of Misericórdias, when Paulo Dias de Novais founded the first confraternity in Luanda soon after his arrival there in 1575. It only enjoyed modest success in the initial decades, but it gained a new lease on life during the governorship of Bishop D. Frei Simão Mascarenhas (1623–1624). The hospital of the Misericórdia served the population in treating 'diseases of the land', and it perhaps enjoyed some success in momentarily decreasing mortality rates. D. Francisco do Soveral, who served as the Bishop of Angola from 1627 to 1642, became known as a great benefactor of the brotherhood. During his time, four infirmaries were constructed for the

---

[40] On the background and establishment of Portuguese Misericórdias, see A. J. R. Russell-Wood, *Fidalgos and Philanthropists: The Santa Casa da Misericórdia of Bahia, 1550–1755* (London: Macmillan, 1968), 1–23.

[41] Laurinda Abreu, 'O papel das Misericórdias dos "lugares de além-mar" na formação do Império português', *História, Ciências, Saúde – Manguinhos* 8 (2001): 595–597.

[42] Russell-Wood, *Fidalgos and Philanthropists*, 24–41.

[43] Abreu, 'O papel das Misericórdias', 592.

hospital, each serving patients with different diseases. In order to take care of the spiritual obligations of the Misericórdia, an altar was placed at the centre of the four wards. According to Cadornega, more than 400 people were annually treated in the hospital, and in some years the number rose to more than 600, if the rains were extremely abundant during the rainy season. The hospital staff included a doctor and a surgeon as well as nurses and slaves to assist in treating the sick. The hospital also employed a white barber and a black barber as his substitute.[44]

In the 1660s, an open conflict emerged between the Houses of Mercy in Luanda and Massangano. When officers in Massangano established their own Misericórdia, the brotherhood in Luanda complained that this was against regulations, as the officers in Massangano did not have royal permission to set up a lay brotherhood. Moreover, they argued that the alms collected in Massangano should have been directed towards the upkeep of the House of Mercy in Luanda. Finally, the low number of soldiers in Massangano – forty according to the complaint – was a poor justification for the maintenance of a hospital in Massangano, as they could easily have been cured in Luanda. The Luanda brotherhood used economic arguments as the main reason why another Misericórdia should not be established in Angola. However, the officers in Massangano responded that the Luanda brotherhood was only seeking to serve its own interests, not those of Massangano's population. They pointed out that Massangano constantly received a large number of soldiers that needed treatment. The distance of forty leagues to Luanda's hospital was too much to be covered by ailing patients. There were also numerous widows and orphans in Massangano who needed to be looked after. Pleading from a position of modesty and obedience, the new brotherhood asked the king to grant it a licence to carry out its pious and caring functions.[45]

This exchange continued for some months, with the Luanda brotherhood taking an active stance in defending its interests. The brethren pointed out that a major part of the resources needed for maintaining the hospital in Luanda came from the alms collected in Angola. While the brotherhood received 200$000 *reis* from the crown, it used between 7,000 and 8,000 *cruzados* annually to run a clinic for infantrymen.

[44] Brásio, 'As Misericórdias de Angola', 107–112; Cadornega, *História geral*, III: 21–22.

[45] AHU, CU, Angola, Cx. 7, Doc. 772, Carta do ex-governador de Angola João Fernandes Vieira, ao rei, 9 April 1661; AHU, CU, Angola, Cx. 7, Doc. 779, Representação dos moradores da vila da Vitória de Massangano, ao rei, 12 July 1661. See also Russell-Wood, *Fidalgos and Philanthropists*, 36–37.

Therefore, the Misericórdia in Massangano emerged as its direct rival for scarce resources. The town council of Luanda joined the chorus of criticisms directed against Massangano's 'poorly disciplined residents', who, they argued, were about to establish a lay brotherhood at their own initiative. However, it turned out that the officials of the new brotherhood had been granted permission by the *cabido* of Kongo to establish a hospital in Massangano. Governor André Vidal de Negreiros, who participated in the deliberations, argued that, while the residents of Massangano could have their hospital, they should not be allowed to run a Misericórdia in the interior of Angola.[46]

Officials in Lisbon condemned the actions of the brothers in Massangano, turning to medical arguments to prove their point. One official who had served in Angola argued that the limited population of Massangano, composed mainly of resident Portuguese and Africans, was not as heavily subjected to diseases as the military units in Luanda, and even when they were attacked by illness, they had better remedies for taking care of themselves. However, the soldiers and seamen in the capital could only turn to the Misericórdia to receive treatment. With the opinion so strongly opposed to the establishment of the new brotherhood, the king resolved to shut down the Holy House of Mercy in Massangano.[47]

However, a little over a decade later the residents of Massangano were more resolute than ever to reinstitute the brotherhood. Referring to their heroic defence of Portuguese possessions in Angola during the Dutch occupation, the brotherhood requested that the king grant a licence to the Misericórdia of Massangano, which had already begun building a new hospital in the village. This time, the Overseas Council was in favour of letting the Massangano residents have their way, and in August 1675 the Misericórdia received official approval.[48] Governor Meneses's letter of 1703 confirms the existence of the hospital in Massangano. He wrote that Massangano 'always' had had a hospital where the soldiers

---

[46] AHU, CU, Angola, Cx. 7, Doc. 782, Carta da Casa da Misericórdia da cidade de São Paulo da Assunção do reino de Angola, ao rei, 14 August 1661; AHU, CU, Angola, Cx. 7, Doc. 783, Carta dos oficiais da Câmara de São Paulo da Assunção do reino de Angola, ao rei, 14 August 1661; AHU, CU, Angola, Cx. 7, Doc. 784, Carta do governador do reino de Angola André Vidal de Negreiros, ao rei, 18 August 1661.

[47] AHU, CU, Angola, Cx. 7, Doc. 815, Carta de Bento Teixeira de Saldanha, ao secretário do Conselho Ultramarino Marcos Rodrigues Tinoco, 9 December 1662; AHU, CU, Angola, Cx. 7, Doc. 819, Carta do provedor e irmãos da Santa Casa da Misericórdia de São Paulo da Assunção do reino de Angola, ao rei, 3 February 1663.

[48] AHU, CU, Angola, Caixa 12, Doc. 1383, Consulta do Conselho Ultramarino ao príncipe regente D. Pedro sobre o requerimento dos moradores da vila da Vitória de Massangano, 29 July 1775.

from the *presídios* of Muxima, Cambambe, Pedras and Ambaca came for treatment. In the same breath, however, he admitted that it was impossible to get medical personnel to work there unless one could banish someone suitable to the interior.[49]

The Misericórdia of Massangano was not the only problem for the hospital in Luanda. The brotherhood of Luanda struggled with financial administration throughout its existence, and there were constant complaints that the hospital could not function because of a lack of staff and medicines. The costs of treating the sick and helping the poor far surpassed the resources of the brotherhood. Several schemes were devised to amass capital. In the 1660s, the Misericórdia sought royal permission to collect 2,000 *zimbos* monthly from each household on the island of Corimba. Permission to collect such a tribute had been given by the governor in 1658, but islanders did not want to pay because the order had not received royal confirmation. In petitioning for this right, the brotherhood of Luanda referred to a similar royal mercy given to Bahia's Misericórdia. In its deliberations, the Overseas Council heard the testimony of Bento Teixeira de Saldanha, who pointed out that the *muxiloandas* of the island were poor and useful as fishermen and sailors. Efforts to collect *zimbos*, however, would be limited and often not yield 2,000 pieces per month. The Overseas Council therefore recommended that the Misericórdia be given only the right to collect contributions of fruit, eggs and chickens given freely as donations.[50]

In 1693, the secretary of the Misericórdia was granted the right to approve and open the testaments of patients treated in the hospital, with the hopes that, in their last hour, people would give generously to the brotherhood.[51] At the same time, the Misericórdia had to claim compensation for the amount it was owed by the state to buy clothing for the sick. The king ordered that 200$000 *reis* be paid to the brotherhood or else all slave ships would be stopped from leaving Luanda.[52] However, this did

---

[49] AHU, CU, Angola, Caixa 17, Doc. 1934, Consulta do Conselho Ultramarino ao rei sobre o parecer solicitado ao Luís César de Meneses, 21 May 1703.

[50] AHU, CU, Angola, Cx. 7, Doc. 924, Consulta do Conselho Ultramarino, ao rei D. Afonso VI, sobre o requerimento do provedor e irmãos da Santa Casa da Misericórdia da cidade de São Paulo da Assunção, 23 August 1664.

[51] AHU, CU, Angola, Cx. 14, Doc. 1764, Consulta do Conselho Ultramarino ao rei D. Pedro II sobre requerimento do provedor e irmãos da Mesa da Casa da Santa Misericórdia da cidade de São Paulo de Assunção de Luanda, 25 February 1693.

[52] AHU, CU, Angola, Cx. 14, Doc. 1768, Consulta do Conselho Ultramarino ao rei D. Pedro II sobre decreto real de 3 de Março de 1693 determinando que o governador de Angola, Gonçalo da Costa Meneses, proibisse a saída de qualquer navio carregado de escravos de Angola até que o contratador de Angola, Diogo da Fonseca Henriques passasse as letras para o pagamento da quantia que o dito

not lead to the much anticipated financial prosperity. Therefore, in 1695 the Misericórdia of Luanda was granted a licence to sell 500 slaves annually. The argument in favour of the decision referred to the large expenses of visiting the prisoners and hiring a doctor, surgeon and barber as well as other servants. The high prices of medicines and provisions for the sick wards were also quoted in the Misericórdia's favour. This decision, however, later led to accusations that the brotherhood drove the prices down by selling its quota of slaves too cheaply.[53]

According to António Brásio, the hospital of the Misericórdia was always primarily a military hospital. Yet, by the mid-eighteenth century even soldiers began to avoid being treated in the hospital, arguing that there were never enough medicines and that patients died of hunger. These complaints led the governor, Count of Lavradio, to seek reforms in the financial administration of the brotherhood in 1750. Despite the attempt to provide more funds to the Misericórdia, it continued to decline in the second half of the century.[54]

There is very little information on the Misericórdia besides the administrative documentation. However, personal testimonies were provided in the early eighteenth century, when a number of men were asked about the reputation of Angola's surgeon-major, Matias Carvalho de Sousa. He had requested membership in the Order of Christ, and the testimonies were part of the process. Carvalho de Sousa had been born on the island of São Miguel in the Azores and had served in Angola for sixteen years (1701–1717). He had worked in the Misericórdia hospital in Luanda, often treating soldiers free of charge because of the meagre resources at his disposal. He had also cured the sick persons living in poverty in Luanda. The men who testified on Carvalho de Sousa's behalf confirmed his devotion to his patients. He was praised for his zealous and careful work as well as his generosity in often giving medicines free of charge.[55]

Despite being the only facility for soldiers needing medical attention, there are indications that the officers serving in Luanda's military forces did not always have to go to the hospital in order to receive treatment. In the 1720s, Angola's chief physicians were ordered to treat officers in their

contratador devia ao Hospital de Todos os Santos da cidade de Luanda relativa a ordinária destinada à compra de roupas para os enfermos, 5 March 1693.
[53] AHU, CU, Angola, Cx. 15, Doc. 1818, Consulta do Conselho Ultramarino ao rei sobre carta do provedor e irmãos da Misericórdia da cidade de São Paulo de Assunção do reino de Angola, 29 January 1695. See also Brásio, 'As Misericórdias de Angola', 113–119.
[54] Brásio, 'As Misericórdias de Angola', 121–126.
[55] AHU, CU, Angola, Cx. 21, Doc. 2186, Requerimento do cirurgião-mor de Angola, Matias de Carvalho de Sousa, ao rei solicitando o hábito de Cristo, before 19 July 1719.

homes. The governor sought to put this order into effect, but it is not clear the extent to which it was followed in this or other periods. Compensation due to the physician seems to have been a central issue, for Chief Physician Aboim, who was at the helm in the 1720s, would have liked to charge a fee for home visits.[56]

The hospital also became a site of Luanda's constant scandals in the 1720s, when the board of the Misericórdia complained that prisoners who were brought from the jail for treatment were watched over by armed guards in the hospital wards. Moreover, the board was concerned that many people who came to the hospital for treatment were arrested and sent to the *presídios* in the interior. The Misericórdia also complained that government officials embezzled funds meant for pious works. In his response, Governor Albuquerque denied all these accusations, claiming that prisoners received treatment in the jail and that the brotherhood had received its funds as agreed for several years. In the governor's view, these falsehoods were machinated and circulated by dishonest men. Yet, in light of the constant bickering between competing factions in the city around this time, the complaints by the Misericórdia board likely contained some truth as far as the treatment of prisoners went, but the brotherhood's bookkeeping demonstrated that the local government had complied with its upkeep quite satisfactorily.[57]

In Benguela, official healthcare developed in small steps. In 1674, Francisco de Távora, the governor of Angola, took the initiative in constructing a hospital in Benguela in addition to a fort and a church. The hospital was intended primarily as a military hospital to heal soldiers, who died in 'infinite' numbers. Its maintenance was covered by the tithes collected in Benguela, and Távora claimed it enjoyed early success. His action received royal approval.[58] Despite attempts to update healthcare services in Benguela, the town officials and visiting missionaries continued to complain about a constant lack of doctors and high mortality rates. This led one captain-major to hire a surgeon from a passing ship in the 1720s.[59] During the governorship of Paulo Caetano de Albuquerque,

[56] AHU, CU, Angola, Cx. 26, Doc. 2578, Carta do governador e capitão-general de Angola, Paulo Caetano de Albuquerque, ao rei, 16 February 1728.

[57] AHU, CU, Angola, Cx. 28, Doc. 2738, Carta do governador e capitão-general de Angola, Paulo Caetano de Albuquerque, ao rei, 1 April 1731.

[58] AHU, CU, Angola, Cx. 11, Doc. 1360, Consulta do Conselho Ultramarino ao príncipe regente D. Pedro sobre a carta do governador e capitão general de Angola, Francisco de Távora, 6 October 1674; 'Carta régia sôbre a criação de hum Hospital em Benguella, 16 October 1674', *Arquivos de Angola*, First Series, 1:2 (1933): no page numbers.

[59] AHU, CU, Angola, Cx. 28, Doc. 2785, Requerimento de Maria Teresa, mulher do cirurgião Bento António, ao rei solicitando provisão, earlier than 28 February 1732.

in the same decade, another hospital was constructed.[60] According to Mariana Candido, a new hospital was added to Benguela's healing landscape in the second half of the eighteenth century. It replaced the old hospital building, which was deteriorating and did not have any doctors or medications available. However, the new hospital, primarily serving the military, operated with limited resources, occasionally employing Africans to serve as skilled workers.[61]

Governor Sousa Coutinho's correspondence reveals the administrative concerns of establishing the new hospital in the 1760s. The officials wanted the hospital to have its own pharmacy and pharmacist, arguing that the preparation of necessary medicines *in loco* would save funds. Pharmaceutical products could also be sold to the needy outside the hospital but not given freely to the poor in order to avoid 'introducing bad customs'. The hospital was to be administered by the brotherhood of the *Nossa Senhora do Populo*, as there was no Misericórdia brotherhood in Benguela. Funds derived from legacies in Luanda were used to buy the initial hospital supplies for Benguela, including clothing, tin utensils and pharmaceuticals.[62]

Officials were aware that the care offered by hospitals rarely resulted in the recovery of the patient. Thus, when Father João da Piedade was nominated as the general administrator of Luanda's military hospital, it was noted that his duties would also include the consoling of the sick and helping them to experience a good death, or in other words, ensuring the salvation of their souls. Since the hospital was run by the Misericórdia, it already had its own chaplains who assisted the sick with their spiritual needs.[63] Indeed, ensuring that the sick had made proper confession before doctors began treatment was a long-standing Catholic tradition. The care of the soul had to accompany that of the body. Ecclesiastical remedies used to combat illness included a whole battery of sacramental rites. Gentilcore has called this 'a spiritual pharmacopeia', which included making the sign of the cross and reading passages from the Bible over the sufferer. Exorcisms designed to counter the powers of the Devil to cause illness were arguably the most potent ecclesiastical

[60] AHU, CU, Angola, Cx. 26, Doc. 2637, Carta do Paulo Caetano de Albuquerque, ao rei D. João V sobre o fim do seu governo, 21 May 1729.

[61] Candido, *An African Slaving Port*, 79–80, 91, 101.

[62] BNL, Códice 8742, Correspondence of Governor Sousa Coutinho, 'Carta para Apolinario Francisco de Carvalho capitão mor de Benguela', 1r–3r (31 January 1766) and 24r–26r (27 April 1766).

[63] AHU, CU, Angola, Cx. 4, Doc. 467, Consulta do Conselho Ultramarino, ao rei, sobre o requerimento do religioso da Terceira Ordem de São Francisco, padre frei João da Piedade, 23 November 1650.

remedies. Every ecclesiastic was a possible healer because of the remedies at his disposal.[64] As discussed in Chapter 6, some Capuchin missionaries had practical experience of working in hospitals in Italy before their sojourns in Angola and Kongo. Ecclesiastics also often ran apothecary shops inside monasteries and distributed drugs to the needy. Many monks, therefore, possessed a certain degree of herbal knowledge when they arrived in West-Central Africa.

Effectiveness

Historians of medicine are often wary of estimating the effectiveness of pre-modern cures and therapies.[65] The question of whose therapies were more potent, those of African healers or European doctors, is therefore somewhat redundant. Answering the question even tentatively is made even more difficult by the nature of contemporary sources, which very rarely provide a description of what was being healed and why, or of what happened to the patients afterwards. It can be surmised that both African and European healers in Angola were at times successful and at other times unsuccessful in curing their patients. Furthermore, unsuccessful attempts to cure illnesses probably left marks in the documentation more often. Complications resulting in a person's death were occasionally mentioned in official correspondence, and requests to leave Angola because of failed attempts to treat illnesses were commonplace. Again, far more is known about Portuguese patients than about African men, women and children. The wide variety of medical conditions and diagnoses makes establishing the effectiveness of therapies all the more difficult – apparently, some diseases could be cured relatively easily while others had high mortality rates.

European medicine had an almost invisible presence in Angola. Its practitioners did not leave a constant paper trail behind them, but their agency can be discerned in sporadic archival records. One of these documents concerns the petition of a young surgeon, João Luís Leitão, who sought nomination as Angola's chief surgeon in 1654. The surgeon-major of Portugal had authorised him to assume the post. As a chief surgeon, Leitão would have been responsible for examining and granting licences to those who practised surgery or bleeding in Angola. According to the authorities, the number of people practising these arts in Angola was high, but many of them did not have an official letter proving that

---

[64] Gentilcore, *Healers and Healing*, 13–14.
[65] For a discussion on effectiveness between biomedicine and popular medicine in Africa, see Feierman, 'Struggles for Control', 105–110.

Table 5.3 *Mortality in the Misericórdia Hospital, Luanda, 1717–1720*

Year	Number of patients treated	Number of deceased patients	Notes
1717–1718	850	68	Great contagions such as measles and other diverse maladies
1719	350	35	
1720	556	42	Great contagion that killed many people

they were qualified to practise such arts. Surgeons' lack of knowledge and experience had led to many great errors and unnecessary deaths, claimed the chief surgeon of Portugal. However, Leitão's petition was met with suspicion by the Overseas Council. His young age did not command confidence. It was also pointed out that Portugal's chief surgeon did not have the authority to nominate chief surgeons to the colonies. Therefore, the president of the Council recommended sending Navy Surgeon João Sardinha to Angola instead. He was experienced in treating battle wounds and in amputating legs and hands. The council members agreed, with Salvador Correa de Sá pointing out that during his governorship of Angola (1648–1651), similar licensing of a chief surgeon or chief physician had not taken place because they put residents at risk.[66]

This important document points to the unregulated nature of medical practices in mid-seventeenth-century Angola. Unlicensed surgeons and barbers abounded and treated an array of diseases and wounds. These healers mostly remain invisible in the documentation, but they were nevertheless sought-out specialists in Angola. Authorities were concerned that self-appointed healers did more harm than good, but officials with experience of serving in Angola were not wholly convinced of the skills of those who presented some kind of authorisation letters either. While the effectiveness and extent of European medical knowledge in Angola was thrown into question, experienced military surgeons such as João Sardinha seem to have cultivated trust and respect.

A rare glimpse into diseases and their treatment in Luanda is offered in a report by the secretary of the Santa Casa da Misericórdia, who reported on the numbers of patients treated in Luanda's hospital between 1717 and 1720 (Table 5.3). Death rates in these years of 'great

[66] AHU, CU, Angola, Cx. 5, Doc. 580, Consulta do Conselho Ultramarino, ao rei, sobre o requerimento do cirurgião João Luís Leitão, 16 November 1654.

contagion' varied between 7.5 and 10 per cent. This gives an impression that the hospital was quite capable of offering great relief to the people who were admitted as patients, mainly soldiers and sailors.[67] Yet, there is no indication of the variety of the diseases these patients suffered from, and so there is no way to know whether they were cured of minor or more serious ailments and injuries. Altogether, the sample is too small to draw any conclusions on the effectiveness of hospital care, and it also stands in contrast with other evidence that points to the limitations of European health care in Angola, discussed in Chapter 7.

Yet, when reading the requests written by Portuguese soldiers to obtain permission to return to their homeland or to travel to Brazil for recovery, it becomes clear that European physicians and surgeons in Angola were well aware of the limits of the remedies they could offer. Chronic conditions were especially difficult to handle. The case of Chief Physician Manoel Andrade de Goes is telling in this regard. He had first suffered from maladies caused by the heat and effects of the climate, which had caused a fistula to form on his right cheek. Goes had sought treatment in the hands of a surgeon for close to two years without recovering his health. All the while, his patients went without medical assistance. In the end, Goes had to petition the king for permission to return to Lisbon.[68]

Doctors in Angola were sporadically involved in discussing the effectiveness of medicines and treatments. Alcohol was probably the most common medicine in Angola. Locally produced alcoholic beverages included palm wine (*malafu* or *malavu*) and beer (*ovallo* or *walo*) produced from a variety of local grains, especially millet and sorghum. Palm wine was believed to possess medicinal qualities, and seventeenth-century Portuguese priests thought it was quite healthful, especially for the stomach. Some authors were of the opinion that fresh *malavu* was a diuretic that prevented gravel and stones in the bladder. Another author remarked that as a result of drinking palm wine, no one in Kongo suffers from stones or the kidneys.[69]

In the words of Braudel, the appearance of brandy and spirits, or distilled alcohol, was a great innovation in Europe. Created in the fifteenth and sixteenth centuries, it was consolidated and popularised in the seventeenth and eighteenth centuries. It remained a popular medicine for a long time, particularly against plague, gout and loss of voice. Only slowly did its production escape the control of doctors and apothecaries.

---

[67] AHU, CU, Angola, Cx. 2413, Requerimento do físico-mor de Angola e cavaleiro fidalgo de Sua Majestade, Tomé Guerreiro Camacho Aboim, ao rei, earlier than 12 July 1725.
[68] 'Provisão autorizando o regresso'.   [69] Curto, *Enslaving Spirits*, 21–24.

The problems posed by transport, preservation and sweetening in the wine trade made the distillation of wines a lucrative business.[70] In the early modern Atlantic, the consumption of sugar-cane brandy or rum spread from the American colonies through Europe and the world, eventually also to Angola.

In contrast to wine, the introduction of sugar-cane brandy from Brazil into Angola was hotly contested. In 1678, Governor Aires de Saldanha de Menezes e Souza argued that Brazilian *gerebita* was an alcoholic beverage of very low quality, and therefore, it was extremely detrimental to the health of Portuguese soldiers and African slaves. It was claimed to have been directly responsible for the deaths of many people in and around Luanda. After deliberating the issue, the Overseas Council in Lisbon decided to recommend to the crown that *gerebita* imports at Luanda should be prohibited. Although health issues were cited as a major factor, José Curto has argued that the prohibition of *gerebita* imports was sought because sugar-cane brandy was in the process of eclipsing grape wine as the major alcohol import in Luanda. In April 1679, King Pedro II signed a royal instruction banning its importation and utilisation in Luanda and throughout the Angolan hinterland.[71]

In 1695, authorities once again debated whether the trade in sugar-cane brandy from Brazil should be allowed in Angola. One of the previous arguments against Brazilian *gerebita* was that it was dangerous to one's health and could even cause death. However, three doctors who had lived in Luanda for several years argued for the introduction of *gerebita* in Angola. They found nothing harmful in the quality of Brazilian spirits, but at the same time they admitted that drinking an excessive quantity of spirits as well as water could lead to hydropsy. Working both in the hospital and outside of it, they had witnessed that, rather than causing ailments, sugar-cane brandy could remedy certain diseases such as erysipelas. In their view, *gerebita* was a medicine rather than a toxin.[72]

Late eighteenth-century physicians Damião Cosme and José Pinto de Azeredo continued to write about the effects of alcohol on one's health. Both encouraged the moderate use of wine and spirits to prevent local illnesses. Azeredo specifically warned his readers about the immoderate use of liquor, arguing that it encouraged endemic illnesses. Moreover, he

[70] Braudel, *The Structures of Everyday Life*, 241–246.   [71] Curto, *Enslaving Spirits*, 73–75.
[72] AHU, CU, Angola, Cx. 15, Doc. 1825, Consulta do Conselho Ultramarino ao rei sobre cartas do governador de Angola, Henrique Jacques de Magalhães, e dos oficiais da câmara de Angola acerca de ser conveniente a introdução de aguardentes no reino de Angola, 17 August 1695. See also Curto, *Enslaving Spirits*, 83–84.

noted that 'the crapulence' caused by alcohol affected the strength of the entire system, disturbed the brain's function, diminished nerve sensations, caused the moving fibres to lose their strength and prevented the solids from exercising their functions.[73]

Importing Medicinals to Angola

In West-Central Africa, supplies of European medicine were constantly running out, and there were numerous and regular requests for medicinals. Occasionally, the requests were accompanied by general descriptions of the kinds of medicine needed. For example, in 1645 the governor requested some drugs for 'fevers and bubonic humours (*humores boubaticos*)'.[74] Two decades later, a surgeon in Benguela requested purgatives worth 16$000 *reis* for his pharmacy. His plea was accepted, and he received the necessary funds.[75] But even if supplies of medicine were often running out in Luanda, occasionally there was enough to send from the capital to the interior. In the 1660s, Surgeon-Major Luís Gonçalves de Andrade petitioned the governor to pay him 73$100 *reis* for two boxes of pharmaceuticals he had relayed to the interior. One box had ended up in Dande and the other had gone with Captain-Major Antonio da Silva to a military camp (*quilombo*) during the war against the Kingdom of Kongo. The medicines were therefore meant solely for the treatment of soldiers. Around the same time, another petition sent by the surgeon-major, by pharmacist Agostinho Rodrigues and by surgeon Alexandre Mogras requested 128$700 *reis* for two boxes of medicines that were given to Captain-Major Luis Lopes, who led his troops to discover mines in the interior.[76] These petitions show that Africans in the interior of Angola, and especially African soldiers in the Portuguese armed forces, continued to have contact with European medicine in the seventeenth

---

[73] Francisco Damião Cosme, 'Tractado das queixas endemicas, e mais fataes nesta Conquista', edited by Luís de Pina, *Studia* 20–22 (1967), 180; Azeredo, *Ensaios*, 55–57.

[74] AHU, CU, Angola, Cx. 4, Doc. 382, Consulta do Conselho Ultramarino ao rei sobre carta do governador de Angola, 10 February 1646.

[75] AHU, CU, Angola, Cx. 8, Doc. 913, Requerimento do cirurgião de Benguela, Pedro da Silva, before 11 August 1664; AHU, CU, Angola, Cx. 8, Doc. 918, Requerimento do cirurgião francês, Daniel de la Serra, solicitando o pagamento dos medicamentos que levaria a Benguela, before 13 August 1664.

[76] AHU, CU, Angola, Cx. 9, Doc. 1058, Requerimento do cirurgião-mor Luís Gonçalves, ao governador e capitão-general de Angola, André Vidal de Negreiros, earlier than 5 April 1666; AHU, CU, Angola, Cx. 9, Doc. 1066, Requerimento do cirurgião-mor Luís Gonçalves, do boticário Agostinho Rodrigues e do cirurgião Alexandre Mogras, ao governador e capitão-general de Angola, André Vidal de Negreiros, earlier than 17 May 1666.

century. Nonetheless, as the Portuguese in the coastal enclaves were struggling to guarantee supplies of pharmaceutical products from Europe, the contacts with European medical materials must have remained extremely limited in the interior.

It was customary that boxes of pharmaceuticals arrived with new governors, but probably in modest numbers and mainly for the personal use of colonial administrators. In 1715, Governor Noronha requested a *botica* (medicine chest) with 'competent medicines' for the purposes of the military hospital in Luanda. European pharmaceuticals were also requested for the interior fortress of Caconda, where a hospital to treat sick and injured soldiers had been built in 1721. Whether the medicines ever arrived in Caconda is unknown, but at least they were listed as necessary supplies to be sent from Lisbon in the late 1720s. Occasionally the supply of medicines was left to chance, as in 1726, when a passing ship bringing a new governor to Angola found the soldiers in Benguela dying of disease and hunger after a drought. The governor donated the ship's *botica*, along with food supplies, to the town's residents.[77]

Despite the difficulties in obtaining European medicinals, pharmacists maintained their shops in Luanda throughout the eighteenth century. In 1730, pharmacist Pedro Marques Pereira requested to be freed from other public service (as *feitor* and *depositario* of *Fazenda Real*) since he was constantly busy with preparing medicines for the poor being treated in the hospital and for the soldiers in the infantry. Governor Paulo Caetano de Albuquerque, after consulting the municipal council and the board of the Misericórdia, was ready to free Pereira from his other duties, mentioning that he gave medicines to the hospital without a charge and otherwise sold medicines at moderate prices.[78]

To avoid sending unnecessary pharmaceutical supplies to Africa, in 1734 the Overseas Council ordered the governors of Angola, São Tomé

---

[77] AHU, CU, Angola, Cx. 20, Doc. 2115, Consulta do Conselho Ultramarino ao rei D. João V sobre a carta do governador e capitão-general de Angola, D. João Manuel de Noronha, 3 April 1716; AHU, CU, Angola, Cx. 25, Doc. 2501, Carta do Paulo Caetano de Albuquerque, ao rei D. João V, 10 June 1726; AHU, CU, Angola, Cx. 25, Doc. 2561, Requerimento do capitão-mor do presídio de Caconda, João de Sousa Cabral, ao rei, earlier than 27 May 1727; AHU, CU, Angola, Cx. 27, Doc. 2646, Mapa das munições necessárias à praça de Caconda, no reino de Angola, 25 May 1729. On Caconda's hospital, see Candido, *An African Slaving Port*, 266. On the pharmaceuticals arriving with new governors, see also AHU, CU, Angola, Cx. 33, Doc. 3183, Carta do provedor-mor da Fazenda Real do Brasil, Luís Lopes Pegado Serpa, ao rei, 13 October 1738.

[78] AHU, CU, Angola, Cx. 28, Doc. 2737, Carta do governador e capitão-general de Angola, Paulo Caetano de Albuquerque, ao rei, 1 April 1731. On the practice of pharmacy in colonial Brazil, see Marques, *Natureza em Boiões*.

and Cape Verde to ask the physicians about the needed medicinals. In other words, instead of making general requests for medicines, the governors were instructed to send specific lists. This did not, however, solve the fundamental problem of drug supply, namely the preservation of plant-based medicines over the Atlantic journey. According to one pharmacist, the surgeons on board the ships sailing from Portugal and Brazil customarily sold medicines to Luanda's inhabitants, but such medicines were often lacking in quality and had resulted in numerous deaths. Strict regulation and inspections of the medicinals sold by pharmacists were proposed as solutions, but the Overseas Council does not seem to have responded to these pleas.[79]

Comprehensive data on imports of medicinals to Luanda is available for the first quarter of the nineteenth century (see Appendix B). Besides cinchona and *água de Inglaterra* (analysed in the next section), Luandan doctors and patients could draw upon a variety of remedies. In import statistics, these were usually categorised as *drogas de botica* (pharmaceutical drugs) or *remédios medicinais* (medical remedies), which usually arrived in boxes or barrels. Tin syringes (*seringas de estanho*) and cupping horns (*ventosas*)[80] were also arriving to Luanda. Finally, ointments and anise (*Pimpinella anisum*, Port. *erva doce*) were among the imported medical materials. The supplies originated in Portugal and Brazil, with Rio de Janeiro and Pernambuco as the most important sources.

Early Modern Antimalarials: Quina Bark in Angola

Quina, a medicinal tree bark harvested from various species of cinchona trees in the Andean forests of South America, spread from the Spanish Empire throughout the Atlantic world, giving rise to a distinctive geography of knowledge into which African slaving ports were also drawn. Most accounts of the history of cinchona have ignored the African dimension in the early globalisation of the bark, focusing instead on its

---

[79] AHU, CU, Angola, Cx. 30, Doc. 2942, Despacho do Conselho Ultramarino ordenando que os governadores de Angola, São Tomé e Cabo Verde, solicitassem informação dos medicamentos mais necessários aos médicos ou pessoas que curavam, 27 June 1734; AHU, CU, Angola, Cx. 33, Doc. 3141, Requerimento do boticário de Angola, Pedro Marques Pereira, ao rei, earlier than 7 November, 1737. On the preservation of medicinals, see AHU, CU, Angola, Cx. 32, Doc. 3058, Carta do governador e capitão-general de Angola, Rodrigo César de Meneses, ao rei, 9 July 1736.

[80] In Portuguese, *ventosa* refers to both cupping horns and leeches. On the use of leeches in medicine, see Robert G. W. Kirk and Neil Pemberton, 'Re-imagining Bleeders: The Medical Leech in the Nineteenth Century Bloodletting Encounter', *Medical History* 55 (2011): 355–360; Roy T. Sawyer, 'History of the Leech Trade in Ireland, 1750–1915: Microcosm of a Global Commodity', *Medical History* 57 (2013): 420–441.

introduction to Europe. Matthew Crawford has shown how epidemiological, environmental and economic developments in the Atlantic
world facilitated its transformation from a local remedy into a global
botanical commodity. Quina fundamentally confounded European science and empire in the eighteenth century, highlighting its fragility in
colonial contexts. The Spanish struggled with controlling the flows of the
bark and faced a variety of obstacles in converting nature into an imperial
natural resource. Some of these obstacles also affected the transportation
of quina to African ports. Like other plant-based medicines, the bark
became degraded and lost its medical efficacy while in transit. Quina
shipments could be adulterated by mixing cinchona bark with other
barks. Further, the medical efficacy of many different kinds of bark varied
depending on the variety of cinchona tree from which it was harvested or
whether the bark came from the trunk of the tree or its branches.[81]

As demonstrated above (see the section entitled 'Miraculous Cures,
Medical Ignorance and Colonial Scandals: The Case of Chief Physician
Aboim'), Chief Physician Camacho e Aboim administered quina to his
patients in Luanda in the 1720s. A solution called *Água de Inglaterra*, or
'water of England', a patent medicine produced from cinchona bark, was
also popular in Angola by the 1730s.[82] Governor Rodrigo César de
Meneses mentioned that experience had proven it to work well in
Angola.[83] In the following decades, it continued to be used as a treatment. In a letter dated November 1751, Chief Physician Eusébio Catela
de Lemos reported appreciatively to Jacob de Castro Sarmento, who
developed his own *Água de Inglaterra* solution and marketed it in the
Portuguese colonial world, of the success he had enjoyed with the medicine in two cases in Angola.[84] Others also reported on its use.
A Capuchin missionary suffering from intermittent fever, which he had
contracted on a trip to the Dembos region in 1754, was treated with
bloodletting, emetics and, ultimately, with two bottles of *Água de*

---

[81] Matthew James Crawford, *The Andean Wonder Drug: Cinchona Bark and Imperial Science in the Spanish Atlantic, 1630–1800* (Pittsburgh: University of Pittsburgh Press, 2016). On the use of quina in Salvador, Brazil, in the mid-eighteenth century, see Miranda, *Relação cirurgica, e medica*, 96, 104, 110.

[82] *Água da Inglaterra*, a quina solution developed by an expatriate Portuguese physician, Fernando Mendes, in the 1680s, was exported to Portugal as a treatment for malaria. See Timothy D. Walker, *Doctors, Folk Medicine and the Inquisition: The Repression of Magical Healing in Portugal during the Enlightenment* (Leiden: Brill, 2005), 114, 120.

[83] AHU, CU, Angola, Cx. 32, Doc. 3058, Carta do governador e capitão-general de Angola, Rodrigo César de Meneses, ao rei, 9 July 1736.

[84] Jacob de Castro Sarmento, *Do uso, e abuso das minhas Agoas de Inglaterra, ou directorio, e instruccam, para Se saber seguramente, quando se deve, ou não, usar dellas, assim nas enfermidades agudas; como em algumas chronicas; e em casos propriamente de Cirurgia* (London: Guilherme Strahan, 1754), 278–283.

Inglaterra. This helped him to convalesce. Two years later, Governor António Álvares da Cunha reported that he had taken *Água de Inglaterra* in addition to being treated with bloodletting. However, in his experience these measures did not provide a permanent cure for attacks of intermittent fever.[85]

Quina also continued to be used in Angola in the second half of the eighteenth century and consolidated its place as a healing material. In 1766, Governor Sousa Coutinho sent a small bottle of 'excellent quina' to Caconda's captain-major in order to smoothen the governor's request to capture a zebra and birds in the interior of southern Angola.[86] A major part of Damião Cosme's treatise was devoted to malarial fevers. The practice of phlebotomy was duly criticised and Cosme insisted that doctors in Angola should stop the practice of bleeding their patients. Instead, he was in favour of using emetics in the early stages of an illness. The use of cinchona was gradually becoming accepted in Angola. Besides naming cinchona as a medicine, Cosme mentioned that, to combat malaria, *Água de Inglaterra* continued to be used in Angola, but he criticised it as being more harmful than effective.[87]

One way to gauge the use of cinchona in Angola is to look at import statistics related to 'Água de Inglaterra' and raw quina. The most complete statistics are from the period 1799–1825. Table 5.4 shows that 'English water' (*Água inglesa*, *Água de Inglaterra*) arrived in Luanda in decreasing numbers, reaching a high of about 2,000 bottles in 1802 and 1804, but then declined to a few hundred *garrafas* a year. The highest annual number of 2,127 bottles arrived from Portugal in 1802, but by the 1810s 'English water' was being sent from Brazil.

The popularity of cinchona was guaranteed by the praise it received from José Pinto de Azeredo. His experience of easily curing intermittent fevers with large doses of Peruvian bark in Luanda convinced him of its advantages. He also gave a very detailed description of how he used it. If he saw the patient at the beginning of a remittent fever attack, he first administered an antimony emetic to reduce the fever, and then he proceeded to give an eighth of quina each hour until an ounce had been administered. This was usually sufficient to cure many fevers. If the fever

---

[85] AHU, CU, Angola, Cx. 42, Doc. 3926, Oficio de Manuel de Lemos de Vasconcelos ao governador e capitão-general de Angola, D. António Álvares da Cunha sobre a chegada do religioso capuchinho, frei Octávio, 29 June 1754; AHU, CU, Angola, Cx. 43, Doc. 4012, Oficio do governador e capitão-general de Angola, D. António Álvares da Cunha, ao secretário de estado da Marinha e Ultramar, 11 January 1756.

[86] Biblioteca Nacional de Portugal, Códice 8742, Correspondence of Governor Sousa Coutinho, f. 4v.

[87] Cosme, 'Tractado das queixas endemicas', 192–198.

Table 5.4 *Imports of* Água de Inglaterra *in Luanda*[1]

Year	Item	Quantity	Unit	Port
1802	*Água inglesa*	2,127	*Garrafas*	Portugal
1803	*Água de Inglaterra*	1,104	*Garrafas*	
1804	*Água de Inglaterra*	2,000	*Garrafas*	
1809	*Água de Inglaterra*	134	*Garrafas*	
1810	*Água inglesa*	456	*Garrafas*	Pernambuco
1812	*Água inglesa*	308	*Garrafas*	Rio de Janeiro
1813	*Água inglesa*	150	*Garrafas*	Rio de Janeiro
1813	*Água inglesa*	70	*Garrafas*	Pernambuco
1813	*Água inglesa*	266	*Garrafas*	Lisbon
1815	*Água inglesa*	200	*Garrafas*	Rio de Janeiro
1816	*Água inglesa*	300	*Garrafas*	Rio de Janeiro
1817	*Água inglesa*	650	*Garrafas*	Rio de Janeiro
1818	*Água inglesa*	830	*Garrafas*	Rio de Janeiro

[1] AHU, CU, Angola, Cx. 106, Doc. 5; Cx. 109, Doc. 54; Cx. 112, Doc. 47; Cx. 121, Doc. 6; Cx. 121A, Doc. 35; Cx. 127, Doc. 1; Cx. 128, Doc. 26; Cx. 131, Doc. 11; Cx. 132, Doc. 26; Cx. 133, Doc. 3; Cx. 134, Doc. 24. A *garrafa* was a weight unit equalling approximately five litres.

did not respond to the emetic, he administered a good dose of opium combined with the same antimony. As soon as the remission began, he administered one and a half ounces of cinchona in two-eighth doses each hour. Azeredo admitted that he had frequently used *Água de Inglaterra* but never thought it to be more effective than powdered quina. The lack of Peruvian bark in Luanda often forced Azeredo to find other means to suppress fevers. This led him to experiment with *nux vomica*, which he found to have equal, or even superior, benefits to that of quina for the treatment of quotidian intermittent fevers. During an intermission, it could be administered in doses of one-eighth of an ounce. According to Azeredo, this treatment became commonplace in Luanda. When it failed, he used white arsenic in a dose of two grains during each inter-mission for a robust man. The fevers were unfailingly defeated with the second or sometimes third repetition of this remedy.[88]

Despite Azeredo's conviction regarding the usefulness of the Peruvian bark, his successor, José Maria Bomtempo, was not easily persuaded. Remembering his first encounters with medical practices in Angola, Bomtempo referred to the 'extraordinary abuse, and consumption' of

[88] Azeredo, *Ensaios*, xiv–xv, 61–65, 87–91.

Table 5.5 *Imports of quina in Luanda*[1]

Year	Quantity	Unit	Port
1799	216	*Arráteis*	
1802	191	*Libras*	
1803	4	*Arrobas*	
1804	6	*Arrobas*	
1809	4	*Arrobas*	Rio de Janeiro
1810	211	*Libras*	Rio de Janeiro
1811	3	*Libras*	Rio de Janeiro
1812	16	*Libras*	Pernambuco
1812	150	*Libras*	Rio de Janeiro
1813	550	*Libras*	Pernambuco
1813	2	*Libras*	Lisboa
1813	103	*Libras*	Rio de Janeiro
1815	18	*Arráteis/Libras*	Pernambuco
1815	200	*Arráteis/Libras*	Rio de Janeiro
1816	20	*Arráteis*	Pernambuco
1816	150	*Arráteis*	Rio de Janeiro
1817	60	*Arráteis*	Pernambuco
1817	125	*Arráteis*	Rio de Janeiro
1818	85	*Arráteis*	Pernambuco
1818	63	*Arráteis*	Rio de Janeiro
1819	94	*Arráteis*	Rio de Janeiro
1820	94	*Libras*	Rio de Janeiro
1823–1825	723	*Libras*	Rio de Janeiro

[1] AHU, CU, Angola, Cx. 93A, Doc. 48; Cx. 106, Doc. 5; Cx. 109, Doc. 54; Cx. 112, Doc. 47; Cx. 121, Doc. 6; Cx. 121A, Doc. 35; Cx. 127, Doc. 1; Cx. 128, Doc. 26; Cx. 131, Doc. 11; Cx. 132, Doc. 26; Cx. 133, Doc. 3; Cx. 134, Doc. 24; Cx. 138, Doc. 56; Cx. 159, Doc. 13; and ANRJ, JC, Cx. 449, pacote 1. An *arroba* was a weight unit equalling thirty-two pounds (14.7 kg). The Portuguese *arrátel* equalled one *libra* (one pound or 0.45 kg).

quina and 'waters of England'.[89] As Table 5.5 shows, quina imports fluctuated greatly between 1799 and 1825, but nevertheless there was a steady inflow of the substance to Central Africa. The highest annual quantity, 655 *libras* (pounds), or 300 kilograms, reached Luanda in 1813. The lowest figures are from 1819 and 1820, when only 94 *libras*, or 43 kilograms, reached Angola. As was the case with *Água inglesa*, most of the cinchona originated in the ports of Rio de Janeiro and Recife.

[89] José Maria Bomtempo, *Trabalhos medicos offerecidos à Magestade do Senhor D. Pedro I* (Rio de Janeiro: Typographia Nacional, 1825), 50–52.

Tito Omboni recorded his experiences with quinine in Angola in the 1830s. After returning to Luanda from a two-month trip to the interior, the Italian doctor fell ill with fever. Among his initial symptoms, he reported a livid colour on his fingernails and feeling just a little bit of tiredness, which he attributed to the trip. Consulting a doctor named Ubertali, Omboni took an emetic but fell into a torpor the next day. Several doctors were now called to treat him, and a military doctor named Hordas, a Spaniard, suggested that he take quinine, which no one else had thought of at that point. While the doctors debated what course the treatment should take, the pharmacist made his own decision and independently prepared a quinine solution that helped Omboni to convalesce in a few days. Omboni concluded that 'the experience has therefore clearly shown that quinine is an effective remedy in diseases of those places, and acts much more readily if the stomach is first emptied with an emetic. Its effects are quick and the disease is cut off completely from the first invasion, or at least improves its course.' Reportedly, Doctor Hordas was suddenly so keen on the benefits of quinine that he took it every morning as a preventive, and he never had a headache while taking the remedy.[90]

These testimonies, again, show that Atlantic Africa participated in the Atlantic world medical complex not only as a distributor of knowledge to the Americas, but also as a receiver of medical knowledge and materials in the early modern period. The connections between Brazil and Angola clearly show that American medical products were desired and actively employed in Atlantic Africa.

Conclusion

This chapter has documented and identified the presence of several kinds of European medical practitioners in West-Central Africa. Medical pluralism is a fitting term to describe the context of healing in this region in the seventeenth and eighteenth centuries. In Luanda, ailing patients could theoretically go to a number of Portuguese practitioners, but in reality the number of physicians and surgeons was limited and concentrated on treating the colonial elites and soldiers serving in the military. Therefore, even in Luanda and Benguela African idioms of healing remained a potential alternative. The attempts to establish a hospital in Massangano attest to the difficulties the Portuguese had in enticing

---

[90] Omboni, *Viaggi*, 140–141.

physicians and surgeons to work in the interior – maintaining their presence in Luanda was challenging enough.

A fair number of Africans were trained as and served as barbers in Angola and Kongo, pointing to the transfer of European medical technology to Africans. Alcohol – including palm wine, grape wine and sugar-cane brandy – as medicine was part of the mutual exchanges of medical materials and knowledge, but its medical use is hard to distinguish from its recreational value as an inebriant. Experimentation, however, guaranteed the eventual success of an American plant medicine in Atlantic Africa. Quina (cinchona), or Peruvian bark, had been incorporated into Luanda's healing materials by the 1720s. It enjoyed popularity in the second half of the eighteenth century, when its use was advocated by two of Luanda's chief physicians. While continually being imported to Luanda, its status as an effective treatment against malaria was still questioned in the early nineteenth century. Local healing knowledge still reigned supreme among the Portuguese, who continued to rely on cross-cultural medical exchanges as they had done since the early days of contact.

6   Treating Their Symptoms
Limits of Humoural Medicine

Testifying to the Inquisition of Lisbon in 1757, an African freedwoman named Catarina Juliana recalled how her partner, João Pereira da Cunha, had been seriously ill (*doente*) for several months while the couple lived in Ambaca. A local African serving in the Portuguese military, Ventura Gonçalves, had come to his rescue by suggesting – and personally bringing him – the root of a local plant called *muloro* (or *mulolo*) to be used as a cure for Cunha's illness. Catarina Juliana mixed the root in cold water and administered it to her Portuguese partner. It alleviated his illness (*molestia*) and restored his health (*saúde*). Ventura Gonçalves, whose Christian name and soldier status suggest involvement in the Atlantic creole culture of Central Africa, was not denounced as a healer or diviner by any of the witnesses, although he possessed herbal knowledge of the local plants used to cure illnesses. Gonçalves, and others like him throughout Atlantic Africa, functioned as go-betweens in Afro-European interactions.[1]

The Portuguese terms used by Catarina Juliana and witnesses in Angola – *doente, doença* and *enfermidade* (disease or illness, infirmity), *molestia* and *saúde* – were very general and give no clues to what Cunha might have suffered from in modern biological terms. Other sources, however, point to the uses that the *mulolo* root might have been put. A century earlier, the Capuchin missionary Cavazzi had described *mulolo* as a plant four or five hands tall that produces a similar fruit to cedar. He described its fruit as healthy to the stomach but did not mention the medical use of its root. In the early nineteenth century, Portuguese naturalist Joaquim José da Silva described *mulolo* as 'the best succor in the fevers of the country'. Its use was identical to the remedy given to João Pereira da Cunha: a cold infusion of pieces of its trunk and roots was given to the sick person to drink. The freshest leaves could also be eaten.

---

[1] Processo 13836, f. 32v, 65r, 69r, 71v, TSO/IL, ANTT. On Atlantic creoles, see Heywood, 'Portuguese into African', Heywood and Thornton, *Central Africans, Atlantic Creoles.*

Friedrich Welwitsch, a naturalist who traversed Angola in the mid-nineteenth century, collected several samples of plants called *mulolo* (*Bauhiniu reticulata* DC.). He pointed out that its bark afforded an astringent remedy, which was used in a decoction to cleanse impure ulcers, as a wash for wounds and also in cases of intermittent fever and eruptions. It was cultivated near Luanda and was abundant near Calumguembo and Zenza do Golungo and even more frequent in the districts of Golungo Alto and from Cazengo to Ambaca (where it had been administered to João Pereira da Cunha a century earlier).[2]

West-Central African history is exceptional in providing ample primary sources for discussing health and disease in Africa prior to the nineteenth century. However, as the above examples on the uses of *mulolo* as a medicine make clear, the diseases are extremely difficult to identify from a biological standpoint. Instead, the documentation contains numerous social definitions, occasionally written by physicians or surgeons, but almost as often uttered by colonial administrators, priests, naturalists and common people. Furthermore, contemporary doctors produced few statistics on health, illness and mortality that could be used for quantitative analysis. For the most part, the sources on disease are qualitative. This chapter utilises data gleaned from botanical treatises, missionary accounts and official correspondence to approach diagnostic categories in early modern medicine in Angola. It also discusses early modern constructions of mental pathology.

African and European Bodies

Retrospective diagnostics have been widely discussed in medical history, and admittedly they represent a great challenge for historians and clinicians. This challenge is not made easier by the problem of defining disease. No definition satisfies all, and scholars even disagree about whether disease is a real entity that can be verified scientifically.[3] The diagnoses made by people living in the past (social diagnosis) differ from modern biological diagnoses. The descriptions of diseases found in the written sources are often not specific enough or sufficiently detailed, and

---

[2] Cavazzi, *Istorica descrizione*, 34; Manuel Ruela Pombo, 'Medicina indígena', *Diogo Cão*, Third Series (1935–1936): 108; Hiern, *Catalogue of the African Plants*, 193, 297. In the early twentieth century, the use of *mulolo* was documented by the Swedish missionary-linguist-ethnologist Karl Laman's Kongo catechists, who collected responses to Laman's ethnographic questionnaire among the Kamba. The plant was used in part of a *Lemba* ritual. Janzen, *Lemba*, 117.

[3] Mark Harrison, *Disease and the Modern World, 1500 to the Present Day* (Cambridge: Polity Press, 2004), 6.

some scholars have advocated a complete avoidance of retrospectively rendering a diagnosis based on modern biological labels.[4] Pablo Gómez's view on diseases in the early modern Caribbean and the use of modern biomedical epidemiological concepts of disease is instructive: 'People lived in very different bodies in the past. They also suffered differently from different illnesses (even if seemingly caused by the same agents).'[5] Given the pitfalls of retrospective diagnostics, ideally biological and epidemiological dimensions of disease history would be explored by a group of researchers or by scholars sufficiently trained in history, medicine and anthropology. This chapter stresses the social diagnoses of disease in West-Central African history because, in most cases, the list of symptoms may be compatible with a number of conditions.[6]

In the Central African case, diagnoses were often too vague to provide clues to what biological and biomedical terms would be used in the twenty-first century for common diseases. Yet, they serve as an important source for understanding early modern classifications of disease in Africa. They also reveal social views pertaining to illnesses and interactions between healers and patients. Yet, in reading the documentation and especially the quotidian paper trail on social life in the colony of Angola, it becomes clear that humoural theory had only a marginal role in local conceptualisations of disease. As Cagle has argued, seventeenth-century Portuguese physicians promoted the view that fever was a form of contagious disease, a consequence of noxious particles rather than a humoural imbalance.[7] Humoural medicine formed the basis of healing for physicians like Aleixo de Abreu and Francisco Damião Cosme, and it found its way into occasional diagnostic statements by doctors; mostly, however, doctors and patients referred to and discussed bodily symptoms, which they sometimes viewed through the prism of the Hippocratic environmentalist epistemology, a subject discussed in Chapter 7.

---

[4] Andrew Cunningham, 'Identifying Disease in the Past: Cutting the Gordian Knot', *Asclepio* 54 (2002): 13–34.

[5] Gómez, *The Experiential Caribbean*, 40. See also Cagle, *Assembling the Tropics*, 24.

[6] On the pitfalls and challenges of retrospective diagnosis, see Piers D. Mitchell, 'Retrospective Diagnosis and the Use of Historical Texts for Investigating Disease in the Past', *International Journal of Paleopathology* 1 (2011): 81–88; James L. A. Webb, *Humanity's Burden: A Global History of Malaria* (Cambridge: Cambridge University Press, 2009), 11–12. Cultural and biological definitions of illness and disease in African contexts are discussed in Megan Vaughan, 'Healing and Curing: Issues in the Social History and Anthropology of Medicine in Africa', *Social History of Medicine* 7 (1994): 283–295; Gwyn Prins, 'But What Was the Disease: The Present State of Health and Healing in African Studies', *Past & Present* 124 (1989): 159–179.

[7] Cagle, *Assembling the Tropics*, 14–15.

In the early modern world, lay beliefs about health and illness, lay self-medication and lay relations with medical practice and treatment were mapped onto varying socio-economic circumstances, religious affiliations, levels of education and literacy, class and community perceptions, the availability of skilled professional medical practitioners and other socio-cultural and personal circumstances. In the Atlantic world, skin colour would definitely have been one of these socio-cultural circumstances. Patients and healers agreed implicitly upon a range of diagnoses, therapies and services. Mutuality between sufferers and healers took place beneath the umbrella of shared knowledge, with both parties operating within overlapping, if not identical, cognitive worlds. Therefore, it would be false to draw sharp boundaries between lay and professional outlooks, oral and literate cures, and folk and learned therapeutics.[8]

Virtually all Europeans who settled in Atlantic Africa viewed the world in ways that fundamentally resembled the outlook of the peoples they encountered. They believed in the power of ghosts, monsters, witches and other creatures and thought that supernatural forces could influence the workings of the natural order. In a word, Europeans' understanding of the natural world was quite similar to that of ordinary Africans. The most decisive distinction between themselves and the peoples they encountered was not scientific but religious. While Africans rooted their belief systems in religion, they were not Christians. Therefore, Europeans devoted so much space in their accounts to pointing out differences in religious beliefs and practices.[9]

While barely visible in the documentation on West-Central Africa, religious ways of making sense of sickness were extremely relevant in the Portuguese Atlantic, where every disease had its saint. Exorcism was an important part of religious healing. Yet, lay perceptions of illness also gave much space to popular healers and herbalists, who cured with words, prayers and natural medicines. Both religious and folk ideas were compatible, at least symbolically, with African idioms of health and healing.[10] When Europeans adopted and experimented with African

---

[8] Roy Porter, 'Introduction', in *Patients and Practitioners: Lay Perceptions of Medicine in Pre-industrial Society*, edited by Roy Porter (Cambridge: Cambridge University Press, 1985), 1–22.

[9] Michael Adas, *Machines as the Measure of Men: Science, Technology, and Ideologies of Western Dominance* (Ithaca, NY: Cornell University Press, 1989), 31.

[10] On perceptions of disease and healing in Portugal, see Santos, 'O homem português perante a doença'; Walker, *Doctors, Folk Medicine and the Inquisition*, 54–66; Paiva, *Bruxaria e superstição*, 103–112; Francisco Bethencourt, *O imaginário da magia: Feiticeiras, adivinhos e curandeiros em Portugal no século XVI* (São Paulo: Companhia das Letras, 2004), 73–86.

medicines – as João Pereira da Cunha did in eighteenth-century Ambaca – they had to trust in the African healers and herbalists who possessed such medical knowledge. This was not easy, as medicines that healed could also be fatally poisonous and used for harming enemies and competitors.

A further corollary to the convergence of European and African idioms of illness and health is that Europeans stationed in Africa regarded their bodies as inherently similar to African bodies. They were only thought to differ in the sense that African bodies were acclimated to hotter climates, while European bodies were acclimated to cooler ones.[11] As Andrew Curran has demonstrated, 'facts' regarding black Africans changed over time from relatively positive to more pessimistic. The overall anatomical representation of black bodies was the product of different contexts, psychologies and geographies. The constant fear of revolt and the highly regimented racial and behavioural codes in the Americas led to extremely negative theories of 'degenerate' Africans. In Atlantic Africa, where the limited white populations mixed more freely with the local population than in the Americas, the reality was markedly different. Blackness did not unequivocally signal idolatry, savagery or a degenerate race.[12]

Another way to examine the relationship between European and African bodies is to concentrate, in addition to pharmacopoeias, on medical treatises written by Portuguese doctors. For surgeon João Cardoso de Miranda, who treated scurvy in Salvador, in the Brazilian captaincy of Bahia, African slaves became research objects not because their diseases were extraordinary but because, by treating them, he sought to find universal cures to illnesses that manifested themselves in all people regardless of ethnic origin.[13] Chief physician Azeredo, for his part, gave anatomical lectures on the human body in Luanda in 1791. There is no hint anywhere in these writings that different theories pertained to black bodies.[14] Although such views were beginning to become commonplace in European medical thought during the latter half of the eighteenth century,[15] they were not universal in the intellectual fabric of doctors writing about Atlantic Africa and the Black Atlantic.

---

[11] Sean Morey Smith, 'Seasoning and Abolition: Humoural Medicine in the Eighteenth-Century British Atlantic', *Slavery & Abolition* 36 (2015): 686.
[12] Andrew S. Curran, *The Anatomy of Blackness: Science and Slavery in an Age of Enlightenment* (Baltimore: Johns Hopkins University Press, 2011), 6–18, 38–48.
[13] Miranda, *Relação cirurgica, e medica.*   [14] Walter, *Um português carioca.*
[15] Curran, *The Anatomy of Blackness*; Rankin, *Healing the African Body*, 23–30, 38–46; Seth, *Difference and Disease*, 166–179; Rana A. Hogarth, *Medicalizing Blackness: Making Racial Difference in the Atlantic World* (Chapel Hill: University of North Carolina Press, 2017).

The logical conclusion to be drawn from these writings is that African bodies functioned the same as European bodies. Europeans and Africans were seen as variations on the same body. Environment rather than inheritable traits crucial to race shaped their differences.[16] In West-Central Africa, this meant that indigenous knowledge regarding local diseases and their cures could be trusted. This was the only way that African medicine could function and heal whites in the same way as it did Africans. European and African diagnoses were identical enough to be translated from one language to another. In a word, trust was based on obvious similarities of conceptualising diseases and human bodies.[17] Healing, therefore, functioned as a unifying rather than separating force in Afro-European interaction.

Famines, Diseases and Epidemics

Africa, the original homeland of human beings, was affected by its own indigenous medical geography long before the continent was connected to the Atlantic mercantile networks. After permanent communities began to emerge some 13,000 years ago, African settlement patterns have been quite stable and most people stayed close to home. Most Africans have lived in the consistently hospitable grasslands known as savanna, stretching from the Senegal Valley east to the Red Sea, south along the East African coast, and west again to the southern fringe of the Congo River valley. Africa's four great language groups also indicate that the peoples who speak the major modern languages have been in roughly the same place for thousands of years. Linguistic and archaeological evidence, however, shows that migrations have been an integral part of African life for millennia. Earlier images of massive migrations have given way to interpretations supporting shorter migrations, local dispersal of peoples and diffusion of languages and cultures among pre-existing populations. Frequent shorter movements over several centuries brought people into new locations, leading to the spread of existing cultural practices but also to novel innovative patterns. The *longue durée* nature of these migrations gave people time to adapt to different climates, habitats, rainfall patterns, day length and diseases. Cultural responses

---

[16] Smith, 'Seasoning and Abolition', 689.
[17] On the physiological effects of trust and expectation, essential requirements for successful healing, see David Harley, 'Rhetoric and the Social Construction of Sickness and Healing', *Social History of Medicine* 12 (1999): 407–435.

protected people from suspected environmental dangers. They learned to avoid polluted water or bushes that harboured tsetse flies.[18]

In West-Central Africa, people tended to settle in the best watered valleys of the wetter woodlands and forest-savanna mosaics. Population growth and ecological pressure drove people to move and led to migrations to marginal and less reliable farmlands. Droughts exposed the people of these marginal farming areas to famine and left them vulnerable to ensuing outbreaks of epidemic disease. As long as demographic growth and contraction alternated in this way, population levels remained relatively stable.[19] Epidemics occasionally set surviving populations on the move again and show that the medical geography of the region weighed in as a factor when pioneering people on the move sought suitable locations for permanent settlement. By the time of the Portuguese arrival, however, major settlement patterns had been in place for centuries, and they had little influence on the formation of Europeans' experience-based notions of medical geography.

Famines, droughts and diseases were interconnected and played a defining role in West-Central African history. A lack of rain meant less food and likely made the population more susceptible to sickness. These interconnections were acknowledged, for example, in the 1650s, when Governor Sousa Chichorro wrote that the lack of rain in the recent past had made the country more diseased. Discussing public health, he also referred to an ancient idea that a bissextile year caused the spread of diseases and pointed to military campaigns as a potential reason for elevated mortality rates.[20] Another glimpse into these interconnections is provided by Governor Paulo Caetano de Albuquerque, who arrived in Benguela in April 1726 and found the city in the most miserable condition imaginable. The number of soldiers was reduced to thirty because of hunger, diseases and the lack of medicine as well as doctors. Citing the great drought of previous years as the major cause for the lamentable state

---

[18] Patrick Manning, *The African Diaspora: A History through Culture* (New York: Columbia University Press, 2009), 42–48; Derek Nurse, 'The Contributions of Linguistics to the Study of History in Africa', *Journal of African History* 38 (1997): 359–391; Jared Diamond, *Guns, Germs and Steel: A Short History of Everybody for the Last 13,000 Years* (London: Vintage, 1998), 399; Oliver Ransford, *'Bid the Sickness Cease': Disease in the History of Black Africa* (London: John Murray, 1983), 46.

[19] Miller, *Way of Death*, 12–15, 21; Joseph C. Miller, 'The Significance of Drought, Disease and Famine in the Agriculturally Marginal Zones of West Central Africa', *Journal of African History* 23 (1982): 17–61; Joseph C. Miller, 'Lineages, Ideology, and the History of Slavery in Western Central Africa', in *The Ideology of Slavery in Africa*, edited by Paul E. Lovejoy (Beverly Hills, CA: Sage Publications, 1981), 41–71.

[20] AHU, CU, Angola, Cx. 6, Doc 644, Consulta do Conselho Ultramarino, ao rei, sobre a carta do governador do reino de Angola, Luís Martins de Sousa Chichorro, 3 August 1656.

of affairs, the governor pointed out that the land did not produce anything due to the lack of rain. Together with diseases, the drought also affected people in the interior. Albuquerque left medicines (*botica*) and twenty-five *arrobas* of victuals for Benguela before continuing his voyage to Luanda.[21]

People living in Central Africa were acutely aware of the connections between famines and disease. Humans had to surrender in the face of environmental and climatic forces that were far beyond their control. Governor Melo perhaps best summarised this connection. Commenting on the copious rains in April and May of 1799, he noted that while people could now await abundant harvests of cassava, beans and maize, they also suffered from the unstoppable diseases accompanying the rains. Mortality was ghastly in Luanda and in the interior. 'People living in this country', wrote Melo, 'always have these alternatives, either to die of hunger in dry years, or of diseases in rainy years.'[22]

Commenting on the connection between droughts, famines and the slave trade, Joseph Miller argued that the slave trade should be seen less as a cause of depopulation than as a consequence of it.[23] However, Mariana Candido has criticised this view as too simplistic, arguing that the colonial presence in itself, and the violence that accompanied it, constituted a major threat to the local population. The expansion of violence led to the destruction of agricultural land by raiders and, there-fore, to increased hunger. Famine cannot be disassociated from the pressures of the trans-Atlantic slave trade; rather, famine was directly linked to its expansion. Candido has also noted that diseases did not affect all inhabitants of Central Africa in the same way. Malaria and yellow fever, referred to simply as 'fevers', and gastrointestinal infections were most threatening to Europeans.[24]

The principal infectious diseases that recurred as epidemics in Central Africa included yellow fever, smallpox, measles and influenza, and they helped to limit Portuguese territorial ambitions. Epidemiological and climatological factors also had an impact on mortality and population numbers in Luanda.[25] Miller has counted sixty epidemics in West-

---

[21] AHU, CU, Angola, Cx. 25, Doc. 2501, Carta do Paulo Caetano de Albuquerque ao rei, 10 June 1726.

[22] 'De Dom Miguel Antonio de Mello sobre a communicação das duas Costas da Africa, e acerca do Plano para a Fundação da Companhia da Azia, 8 March 1800', *Arquivos de Angola*, First Series, 1:4 (1935), no page numbers. A similar refrain, or local proverb, can be found in Azeredo, *Ensaios*, 49: 'When it rains there is much food, but no one to eat it.'

[23] Miller, 'The Significance of Drought, Disease and Famine', 30.

[24] Candido, *An African Slaving Port*, 77, 84.

[25] Wheeler, 'A Note on Smallpox in Angola'; Jill R. Dias, 'Famine and Disease in the History of Angola, c. 1830–1930', *Journal of African History* 22 (1981): 349–378; Miller, 'The Significance of Drought, Disease and Famine', 17–61; José C. Curto and Raymond

Central Africa for the period between 1560 and 1830, showing that epidemic outbreaks are easier to follow in sources on Luanda and Benguela (especially in the eighteenth century) and the Kingdom of Kongo (in the seventeenth century). While sources are fairly copious for the coastal towns, much less is known about disease in the interior. Miller has linked the outbreaks of disease with the chronology of drought, arguing that 'Africans weakened by malnutrition and exhausted by dispersal into the bush or by flight into lowland became particularly vulnerable to endemic pathogens'. In other words, drought and hunger drove people to move, and these internal migrations carried them into diseased environments where they possessed little immunity. Yet, the sources do not make it possible to clearly distinguish between sickness in dense settlements and conditions in the surrounding farmlands and woods.[26]

Acknowledging that 'drought related epidemic mortality among Africans catching contagious disease followed rhythms quite different from European mortality from endemic fevers among newly arrived immigrants',[27] Miller's chronology of disease differentiates European mortality, which was the norm among newly arrived settlers in West-Central Africa, from epidemics that took a toll on the local population. It also distinguishes the higher incidence of disease and mortality that normally occurred during the rainy season. However, Miller does not problematise what constituted an epidemic. Therefore, any mention in the sources of high mortality rates becomes a reference, or at least a probable reference, to an epidemic. For example, a letter mentioning Luanda as '*muito doentio*' (very sickly) is interpreted as an epidemic for the year 1584.[28]

In sum, the question here is as follows: How reliable are sources that report high mortality rates in one location or much sickness in another? As the reports are circumstantial and subjective, it is quite a stretch to jump to the conclusion that these reports always refer to epidemics affecting the whole community, especially if they do not specify among which sections of the population diseases raged and caused elevated mortality rates. The term 'epidemic' is generally used to denote an incidence of disease that is above the statistical norm, but earlier writers in the Hippocratic tradition also used it to refer to peculiar 'constitutions' of the atmosphere that produced distinctive sets of maladies.[29]

R. Gervais, 'The Population History of Luanda during the Late Atlantic Slave Trade, 1781–1844', *African Economic History* 29 (2001): 1–59.
[26] Miller, 'The Significance of Drought, Disease and Famine', 21–23.
[27] Miller, 'The Significance of Drought, Disease and Famine', 23.
[28] Miller, 'The Significance of Drought, Disease and Famine', 37.
[29] Harrison, *Disease and the Modern World*, 6.

Portuguese officials described epidemics in Luanda in very general terms, and sometimes they even employed the term *epidemia*. When Luanda experienced great mortality between 1717 and 1728, contemporary observers used different terms to describe health conditions in the city. One officer termed them simply contagions.[30] In Governor Paulo Caetano de Albuquerque's report of 1728, one finds a reference to 'infinite diseases, [an] epidemic that continues with great damage', but no hints as to its possible causes.[31] Sometimes, even when using the word epidemic, governors specifically pointed out that it mainly affected recently arrived and temporary visitors, such as sailors.[32]

It is noteworthy that the governors' language on epidemics rarely if ever named the diseases causing elevated mortality rates. This can mean that the Portuguese simply did not understand what lay behind specific epidemics and were unable to place them within the context of European medical theory or that epidemics were chaotic events, perhaps caused by many diseases, and that the main public health measure was to bury the affected bodies as quickly as possible. However, the silences about the causes of epidemics also speak to the thinness of Portuguese medical knowledge and expertise in Angola. Chief physicians, when they were present, were in direct communication with the governors and could have easily provided medical details and their understanding of what lay behind epidemics. This kind of expert knowledge, however, is almost completely lacking in the governors' correspondence. Although not unusual in Portuguese colonial contexts, one would expect the physicians, who made their living by claiming to have very precise knowledge of diseases, to know and to be able to name them. Apparently, naming diseases was a source of tension for Portuguese physicians and surgeons practising in Luanda.

The only epidemic disease identified with some certainty was smallpox (*bexigas*, *varíola*). Mounting mortality rates in Angolan history often resulted from smallpox (*Variola major*), which was transmitted via virus-bearing moisture droplets exhaled by afflicted persons and inhaled

[30] AHU, CU, Angola, Cx. 22, Doc. 2271, Carta do ouvidor-geral e provedor-mor da Fazenda Real de Angola, Francisco de Santa Bárbara e Moura, ao rei, 14 March 1722.
[31] AHU, CU, Angola, Cx. 27, Doc. 2668, Carta do governador e capitão-general de Angola, Paulo Caetano de Albuquerque, ao rei, 20 December 1729. According to the report, 166 soldiers had fallen ill, and many of them had died. The governor had called for reinforcements from Pernambuco. Of the seventy men that had arrived with Governor Albuquerque, only seventeen were still alive 'because of the climate, and the lack of doctor contributed to the damage'. Healthcare in Luanda was left in the hands of two bad barbers.
[32] AHU, CU, Angola, Cx. 32, Doc. 3058, Carta do governador e capitão-general de Angola, Rodrigo César de Meneses, ao rei, 9 July 1736.

by those with whom they came into contact. The disease began manifesting by provoking headaches, fevers, chills and nausea. After these bodily signs subsided, a rash appeared first on the face, throat, arms and hands, and subsequently throughout the entire torso. Finally, the virus attacked the internal organs, whose eventual failure brought death to as many as one out of four sufferers. Smallpox occurred at frequent intervals in Angola and could almost be called a 'national disease'. For example, an outbreak was reported in 1627 in the interior district of Pungo Andongo.[33] A 1670 report by a Jesuit priest noted the level of decimation among the indigenous inhabitants of Angola. In the late eighteenth century, Silva Corrêa drew attention to epidemic smallpox, which took a great toll on the African population in Luanda.[34]

Smallpox was often transmitted from different parts of Atlantic Africa to Brazil and other New World destinations. Because of Brazil's low population densities, *Variola* did not become endemic there until the nineteenth century. Regular infusions of potential African carriers of the disease arrived in Brazil in rising numbers throughout the early modern period and into the nineteenth century, with conditions in Africa and on the Middle Passage favouring transmission of the infection in the bodies of enslaved Africans. Brazil witnessed several epidemics between the late sixteenth and mid-nineteenth centuries. Yet, Miller and Alden have concluded that, due to Brazil's dispersed and smaller settlements, smallpox 'may have been less devastating in Brazil than in Europe'.[35] Epidemics did not retard the number of slaves exported from Angola, which continued to increase steadily in the eighteenth century. Rather, the threat of epidemics seems to have driven slavers to dispose of their captives quickly to avoid the cost of increased mortality. Supplies of slaves in Luanda increased in times of epidemic, and this led to the selling of weakened individuals to the slave trade. This, in turn, lowered prices and resulted in the bad repute of Angolan slaves in Brazil.[36]

Smallpox prevention in the southern Atlantic had modest beginnings. Some Africans practised variolation by the early eighteenth century, and some French and British slavers experimented with the technique by the 1760s and 1770s. In the Portuguese colonial world, the possibilities of variolation were beginning to be explored in the 1790s after Francisco Arruda Câmara wrote a thesis on smallpox inoculation at the medical

---

[33] Miller, 'The Significance of Drought, Disease and Famine', 42.
[34] Wheeler, 'A Note on Smallpox', 353; Elias Alexandre da Silva Corrêa, *História de Angola* (Lisbon, 1937), I: 80.
[35] Alden and Miller, 'Out of Africa', 214.
[36] Miller, 'The Significance of Drought, Disease and Famine', 30.

school in Montpellier. According to Miller and Alden, public vaccination began in Luanda in 1819 after several unsuccessful attempts to import the vaccine live from Brazil in the first decade of the nineteenth century. By early 1821, almost 13,000 inhabitants of Luanda and about-to-embark slaves had been vaccinated. Similar progress was made in Benguela, and reports from Brazil confirmed the significant diminution in slave mortality during the Atlantic crossing.[37]

The most drastic measures against smallpox were taken with Africans who were liberated from the slave trade in Luanda in the mid-nineteenth century. They were repeatedly vaccinated between 1851 and 1854. The Foreign Office in London sent vaccine lymph to Luanda, and the chief physician, Manoel de Bastos, tested it on a representative sample of the population. However, the experiment failed. In 1864, a devastating epidemic killed at least three liberated Africans, and thirty-two of the fifty-six who were then in custody were admitted to the hospital. Remaining ignorant of the cause of failure, one British Commissioner lost 'all hopes of seeing vaccination established in this part of the world', and abandoned the project.[38]

Practising (or Ignoring) Humoural Medicine in the Tropics

Portuguese knowledge of tropical illnesses in Angola took shape fairly quickly after the settlement of Luanda. Aleixo de Abreu, who served as a physician in Angola between 1594 and 1603, wrote a comprehensive account of tropical medicine. In Luanda, he had the opportunity to become acquainted with several tropical diseases afflicting the local population.[39] Abreu worked in the hospital in Luanda with two Spanish surgeons. Besides treating illnesses, Abreu and his Spanish colleagues carried out post-mortem examinations that led to precise descriptions of scurvy, a very common disease among slaves and sailors alike. Throughout the era of the slave trade, scurvy was known as '*mal de Loanda*', or the 'Luanda disease'. It resulted from the progressive deple-tion of ascorbic acid after a diet of preserved victuals eaten during long

---

[37] Alden and Miller, 'Out of Africa', 210–213.

[38] Samuël Coghe, 'The Problem of Freedom in a Mid Nineteenth-Century Atlantic Slave Society: The Liberated Africans of the Anglo-Portuguese Mixed Commission in Luanda (1844–1870)', *Slavery & Abolition* 33 (2012): 487.

[39] F. Guerra, 'Aleixo de Abreu [1568–1630], Author of the Earliest Book on Tropical Medicine Describing Amoebiasis, Malaria, Typhoid Fever, Scurvy, Yellow Fever, Dracontiasis, Trichuriasis and Tungiasis in 1623', *Journal of Tropical Medicine and Hygiene* 71 (1968): 55–69. See also Cagle, *Assembling the Tropics*, 215–233.

periods at sea. A considerable part of Abreu's work concentrated on the doctrines and practice of phlebotomy or bleeding. This was the major form of treatment recommended for some of the ailments. In this context, Abreu also mentioned the value and usage of leeches and wet and dry cupping. For the treatment of scurvy, Abreu recommended the use of fresh milk in the diet and several syrups with plenty of vegetable ingredients. The most powerful preparation he prescribed in most of his recipes was rose syrup, one of the richest natural sources of ascorbic acid.

Abreu clearly tried to fit his observations and experience of illness in Africa into a humoural framework. It seems, however, that Abreu's interpretations were hardly disseminated among other practitioners of tropical medicine in Angola or even in Portugal. Therefore, his findings had little influence on the physicians and surgeons practising medicine in Luanda in the seventeenth and eighteenth centuries.[40] Official Portuguese medical practice remained dominated by the views of Galen and Hippocrates. Treating illness was based on humoural theory, which held that illness resulted from an imbalance in the humours or fluids, which could be redressed through diet, medicines, purging, vomiting and bleeding. This view was replaced by new medical inventions during the Enlightenment. In the early eighteenth century, Portuguese physicians began to look for texts that would convey more effective medical techniques than could be learned from the ancient texts. Instrumental in this process were expatriate Portuguese doctors, who corresponded actively with their countrymen and sought to reform medical practice in their native country.[41]

Despite the presence of Portuguese physicians in Luanda, the practical application of African medicines used to cure Europeans was mostly handled by laypeople, who had little need to explain health and illness in terms of Galenic medicine. Cadornega was one of the few to criticise the use of natural medicine among Africans on the grounds that there was little understanding of the qualities of the herbs. This criticism was clearly based on the Galenic tradition of distinguishing between the hot and cold qualities of matter. Cadornega also noted that the doses of

---

[40] Abreu's book was printed at the author's expense, and its circulation was allowed only in Portugal. Its print run probably did not exceed 200 copies. Moreover, the book was written in Spanish and Latin, giving it little chance of survival after Portugal seceded from Spain in 1640. Hence, the treatise is extremely rare and only six recorded copies exist. Guerra, 'Aleixo de Abreu'.

[41] This process is documented in Walker, *Doctors, Folk Medicine and the Inquisition*, chapter 3: 'Enlightenment Influences: The Movement toward Medical Reform in Eighteenth-Century Portugal'.

medicine were not well regulated, so that it seemed unclear how much of a certain medicine should be taken or applied as a remedy for a particular illness.[42] Nevertheless, some African remedies were adapted to a humoural framework and used as purgatives for expulsing certain humoural imbalances. For example, Afonso Mendes's mid-seventeenth-century pharmacopeia included remedies for 'frozen humours in the nerves' and 'gallic humours'.[43]

Hippocratic medicine did not survive intact when it was transferred to the tropics. Although there was common ground between African and European ways of conceptualising disease, humoural medicine was far more important to an early seventeenth-century physician like Aleixo de Abreu, who theorised about and sought to adapt it to West-Central Africa.[44] Humouralism also formed a definitive thread in the reasoning of Chief Physician Francisco Damião Cosme, who wrote his treatise on the endemic diseases of Angola in 1770.[45] The century and a half separating these two doctors demonstrates that the major influence of humoural theory was therapeutic. Bloodletting was widely administered to European patients in Central Africa.

In Portugal, as elsewhere in early modern Europe, phlebotomy was the primary therapy, and it was administered by barbers on doctors' orders.[46] In humoural medicine, the body was envisaged as supporting a number of containers that, in sickness, were pervaded by unhealthy fluids, or humours. Excess fluids could be eliminated from the body by inducing vomiting (using emetics), by inducing diarrhoea (using purgatives and enemas) or by bloodletting. However, bloodletting came to be regarded as the sovereign remedy because it was believed that all four humours were to be found, in varying proportions, in the blood. David Wootton has strongly argued that Hippocratic medicine was bad medicine – it killed when it claimed to cure.[47]

Phlebotomy was practised on European ships traversing the Atlantic and Indian oceans. A Portuguese captain bound for India wrote in the mid-seventeenth century about how, after his ship had got stuck in the calms of Guiné, he was bled ten times. After a two-month illness, he was

---

[42] Cadornega, *História geral*, III: 318.
[43] Mendes, 'Caderno que trata das ervas', 45, 303.
[44] This is evident, for example, in his detailed observations on bloodletting. Aleixo de Abreu, *Tratado de las siete enfermedades* (Lisbon: Pedro Craesbeeck, 1623), 86–102.
[45] Cosme, 'Tractado das queixas endemicas', passim.
[46] Santos, 'A Arte de Sangrar', 44–47.
[47] In other words, 'Hippocratic medicine was not a science, but a fantasy of science.' David Wootton, *Bad Medicine: Doctors Doing Harm since Hippocrates* (Oxford: Oxford University Press, 2006), 11.

barely hanging on to his life, while fifty-three people on board the ship had died. Lacking a surgeon and a barber, an imprisoned soldier meddled with bloodletting without any knowledge of medicine or pharmacy. Despite the complete medical incompetence of the soldier, the ill-fated ship managed to make landfall in Angola instead of Rio de Janeiro, where it was supposed to stop before heading to the Indian Ocean.[48]

There are few extant records of how early modern individuals in Angola experienced bloodletting. However, it is certain that it formed the core therapeutic practice in Luanda after the arrival of Paulo Dias de Novais[49] and remained in constant use well into the nineteenth century. In 1626, a Portuguese captain major wrote about how, being sick with continuous fevers, he was bled four times. He did not mention who administered the bloodletting or whether it was also practised on the sixteen soldiers under his command, who were all sick.[50] In the early eighteenth century, the Capuchin priest Lorenzo da Lucca described how bloodletting was used as a matter of course as therapy in Angola. In May 1702, he mentioned that he was bled twenty-three times. Sickness seemed to define Capuchin habitus in West-Central Africa. When Father Lorenzo arrived at the missionaries' hospice in Soyo, the Capuchins stationed there were all weakened by illness. Father Marcellino d'Atri, paralysed, inspired great compassion in Lucca, who interpreted d'Atri's sickness as a test by God to increase his merits. Two years later, when Lucca found himself in a painful convalescence after a mortal illness, and with the fever revisiting his body from time to time, he concluded that in a country where there were neither doctors nor medicine, the best remedy was 'holy patience'.[51]

Lorenzo da Lucca apparently disdained local African medicine, for he remarked more than once that Kongo was a country with no doctors and no medicine. He also claimed that bloodletting was the only conceivable and available remedy.[52] In September 1703, Father Lorenzo fell seriously ill with fever. He immediately administered a bloodletting on himself and headed to the Capuchin hospice in Soyo. After recovering, he did not remember the course of his illness, but asked Father Barletta,

---

[48] AHU, CU, Angola, Cx. 4, Doc. 463, Carta do capitão almirante do navio São Jorge, António Barreto Pereira, ao rei, relatando a viagem para o Rio de Janeiro, em companhia do vice-rei do Estado da Índia, after 20 September 1650.

[49] 'Carta de Paulo Dias de Novais', in Brásio, ed., *MMA*, IV: 423.

[50] AHU, CU, Angola, Cx. 2, Doc. 201, Ofício (cópia) do capitão-mor e tenente António Pinto, 9 April 1626.

[51] Jean Cuvelier, ed., *Relations sur le Congo du Père Laurent de Lucques (1700–1717)* (Brussels: Institut Royal Colonial Belge, 1953), 43, 48, 73.

[52] Cuvelier, ed., *Relations sur le Congo*, 88.

who had cared for him, to write a description of the disease and its treatment. Father Barletta's recollection is probably the closest one gets to a patient's perspective in Angolan history. He described the course of the disease from 8 September, when Lorenzo da Lucca arrived with a mortal pallor to his face, eyes flaming and exhaling a very strong smell, all signs of a pernicious disease that the other Capuchins deemed a mortal illness. He was immediately administered a bloodletting and many remedies (probably pharmaceutical substances brought by the Capuchins from Europe). On the fourth and fifth day of the illness, Lucca fell into a deep sleep, or a kind of lethargy, that was interpreted as a sign of approaching death. He also vomited terribly.[53]

During Father Lorenzo's illness, his fellow Capuchins could not do much beside stay by his side, pray and administer spiritual remedies and the sacrament of extreme unction when they thought that he was dying. They fed him chicken broth when he was conscious enough to eat. Local Kongo Christians also visited him and partook in his care. Father Barletta mentioned that the medicines they gave him were the 'miraculous flour of Saint Maria Magdalene of Pazzi' and the oil of Saint Felix. To monitor his condition, they took his pulse. An intermittent and weak pulse signalled imminent death. For lack of bodily help, Capuchins sought to help Lucca spiritually. Father Barletta mentioned that he had experience with treating the sick, as his training in Florence had included duties at the hospital of Santa Maria Nuova. After about ten days in the Capuchin hospice, Lorenzo da Lucca began to gradually recover. Fevers continued to assail him in the following months, but on Christmas he was able to say Mass for the first time after this bout of sickness.[54]

In addition to Lucca, Capuchin Father Marcello d'Atri documented his illnesses diligently, the first of which occurred only ten to twelve days after his initial arrival in Soyo. On this instance, he was assisted by another Capuchin priest specialising in medicine, who had served in a Capuchin infirmary in Rome but who soon ran out of remedies. D'Atri noted that it was often the case in similar situations that the sick returned to Luanda to receive treatment there, and he had to follow the same procedure. Commenting on a second bout of sickness contracted in Catumbo, d'Atri said that blood was drawn from his feet three times over a period of a day and a half, and he claimed that bleeding was an

[53] Cuvelier, ed., *Relations sur le Congo*, 103–104.
[54] Cuvelier, ed., *Relations sur le Congo*, 105–107. On the religious functions and functionaries of Florentine hospitals, see Katherine Park, *Doctors and Medicine in Early Renaissance Florence* (Princeton, NJ: Princeton University Press, 1985); John Henderson, *The Renaissance Hospital: Healing the Body and Healing the Soul* (New Haven, CT: Yale University Press, 2006).

ordinary custom and the only medical treatment in the interior of Angola. Again, he left for the healthier climate of Luanda to seek a cure. This suggests that at least some Capuchins preferred European medical practices to African remedies.[55]

If anything, Lorenzo da Lucca's patient narrative shows how the Capuchins mixed a humoural remedy (phlebotomy) with herbal and spiritual medicine. The spread of bloodletting to the interior of Angola was apparently assisted by the Capuchins and the Portuguese, who administered it as a first resort. The spread of phlebotomy, therefore, was not dependent on the presence of surgeons and physicians in the interior of Angola. African views on bloodletting, however, have largely escaped the historical record. Although taking place in Lisbon, an exceptional glimpse of an African receiving bloodletting as a treatment was documented in a letter by Dom Lourenço da Silva, the 'black prince' from Pungo Andongo. Around 1720, Dom Lourenço was visiting Portugal when he fell ill and was treated by a Portuguese doctor. He was bled six times and received various medicines. Because of high costs incurred during the treatment, he had to request financial assistance from the King of Portugal. The circumstances of Dom Lourenço's visit to Lisbon are unknown. The doctor who treated him, Francisco Teixeira Torres, diagnosed him with convulsive asthma. Lourenço also had a spurious swelling in his right hand and leg, which gave reason for bloodletting.[56]

Many Portuguese officers travelled to Brazil or Portugal to receive treatment for illnesses and recover a balance of the body. Belchior Garcia de Góis, who travelled to Bahia in July 1702 to cure maladies contracted in Angola (see Chapter 7), stayed in Salvador for one year. He was treated by a surgeon and a physician, and accordingly received both surgery and internal medicines with the goal of re-establishing a humoural balance, as the doctors put it. Apparently, the Brazilian medicines, treatments and climate had a good effect on Góis, who returned to Angola when his treatment in Bahia had ended.[57]

The diagnoses used as justifications for leave requests (Table 6.1) demonstrate that humoural theory played a minor role in defining disease. Descriptions of illness were mostly quite general, often referring

[55] Toso, *L'anarchia congolese*, 5, 14.

[56] AHU, CU, Angola, Cx. 22, Doc. 2206, Requerimento do príncipe negro do reino das Pedras, D. Lourenço da Silva, ao rei solicitando ajuda de custo, em virtude de ser pobre e estar muito doente e necessitar de muitos medicamentos, earlier than 30 July 1720.

[57] AHU, CU, Angola, Cx. 17, Doc. 1983, Requerimento do tenente de campo de Angola, Belchior Garcia de Góis, ao rei solicitando provisão para que o vedor-geral lhe pagasse os soldos do tempo em que estivera ausente para se tratar, earlier than 10 March 1704.

Table 6.1 *Diagnoses attached to leave requests of Portuguese soldiers in Angola, 1673–1806*[1]

achaques: perigosos, muitos, na garganta interiormente, alguns	malaises: dangerous, many, internal in the throat, some
apostema (abcesso) interno cirroso no peito da parte direita	cirrhotic internal abscess on the right chest
debilidade esencial do estomago, difluxo quasi continuo	essential debility of the stomach, almost continuous defluxion
diversa causa e infermidade	various causes and infirmities
doença	disease
escorbuto e outras molestias	scurvy and other illnesses
febres, varias molestias, frouxidão de nervos (cachechia)	fevers, various illnesses, laxity of nerves
freguentes attaques de febres, vicio escorbutico	frequent attacks of fever, vicious scurvy
idade, muitos achaques, mui doentio	[old] age, many malaises, very sick
irritação de estomago, grande inapetencia, continuos vomitos, exorbitante quantidade de umor fleumatico	irritation of the stomach, great inappetence, continuous vomiting, an exorbitant quantity of phlegmatic humour
molestias: grandes, graves, rheumatica, perigosas	illnesses: great, serious, rheumatic, dangerous
queixas: grandes, repetidas, várias causadas da má clima	complaints: great, continuous, various, caused by terrible climate
repetidas queixas, grande debellida de estomago	continuous complaints, great weakness of the stomach
sarna	scabies
varios achaques, huns accidentes de gota coral, espasmo universal complicado com huma melancolia e imaginação continua	various malaises, fits of epilepsy, universal spasm complicated by melancholy and continuous imagination

[1] AHU, CU, Angola, Cx. 11, Doc. 1322; Cx. 19, Doc. 1983; Cx. 22, Docs. 2200, 2226, 2238; Cx. 23, Doc. 2389; Cx. 24, Docs. 2399, 2405, 2442, 2468; Cx. 25, Doc. 2487; Cx. 26, Doc. 2628; Cx. 27, Docs. 2665, 2685; Cx. 30, Docs. 2875, 2911; Cx. 34, Doc. 3291; Cx. 35, Docs. 3327, 3335; Cx. 37, Doc. 3544; Cx. 43, Doc. 3993; Cx. 45, Doc. 4137.

to disease, illness, malaises, infirmities and complaints (*doença, molestia, achaque, infermidade, queixa*). These terms were not any different from the ones used by the African freedwoman Catarina Juliana cited at the beginning of this chapter. They were used in everyday discussions between laypersons with no training in medicine and conveyed a general sense of something not being right in the body. Sometimes illness was described in terms of bodily symptoms, such as weakness or irritation of the stomach, which suggests that both the patient and the people who were being addressed did not expect more detailed information on the nature of the disease. Although physicians and surgeons wrote the diagnoses, this would not have required specialist knowledge on health. In only a few cases was humoural theory purposely employed to demonstrate the elaborate knowledge of a doctor testifying on behalf of a soldier wanting to leave Angola. The paucity of humoural diagnoses could suggest that the colonial administration paid little attention to the physicians' detailed explanations, but it could also mean that some physicians practising in Angola disregarded humoural theory altogether, either because they were poorly educated or because humoural theory, in their experience, had little use in Africa.

The disregard for humoural medicine can also signify that the nature of European therapeutics in Africa did not call for a detailed knowledge of the medical theory taught at universities. Bloodletting was the primary form of treatment, and it could be administered by laypersons with little practical experience. Not until the second half of the eighteenth century did bloodletting begin to wane in popularity among physicians. Francisco Damião Cosme, although basing his reasoning on humouralism, argued that bloodletting was very harmful in the Angolan environment.[58] Azeredo claimed that the 'abuse' of phlebotomy ended in Angola – but not in Brazil – as the older physicians died and as new ones were trained by him personally. Here, he placed West-Central Africa at the forefront of medical advancement, arguing that it surpassed America in this sense. This claim, however, should be taken with a pinch of salt. Barber-surgeons, whose primary therapeutic approach would have been bloodletting, abounded in Angolan towns in the late eighteenth century. More specifically, Azeredo stated that 'more fevers are cured when they are completely ignored than are cured by bloodletting' and that the treatments administered by physicians make illnesses dangerous in Africa. He was especially critical of doctors who chose to cling to old diagnostic categories and an outdated healing system. Azeredo admitted to having used bloodletting to treat dysentery but had never found it to provide any benefit. Further, he advised others to avoid bloodletting in illnesses accompanied by weakness.[59]

---

[58] Cosme, 'Tractado das queixas endemicas', 220–222.

[59] Azeredo, *Ensaios*, viii–ix, 78–79, 125, 144. Azeredo was certainly not alone in his opinion on the pernicious nature of bloodletting. James Lind, *An Essay on Diseases Incidental to Europeans in Hot Climates*, 2nd ed. (London: T. Becket and P. A. De Hondt, 1771), 71–72, questioned the authority of ancient physicians and wrote that, in curing malaria, 'large and repeated bleedings are attended with fatal consequences'.

Middle Passages and New Worlds

The forced migration of Africans to the Americas caused major changes not only in the regional medical geographies of Africa but also in the Americas. Diseases and ideas about Africans' health were for a long time neglected in the Atlantic slave trade. Eighteenth-century epidemiology offered only the vaguest of clues as to why slaves died, and European maritime medicine had little to offer to make the Middle Passage more tolerable. Ship captains sought a quick loading and a quick crossing of the Atlantic in order to deliver their human cargoes alive to the New World. Just as European seamen and travellers perished on the high seas, so too did enslaved Africans die in great numbers before embarkation and during the Middle Passage.[60] Some indication of the health conditions on slave ships can be gleaned from a debate that took place in 1686, when priests in Luanda discussed the official orders of ship captains to hire chaplains on voyages to Brazil. The seriousness of the situation is apparent in the news that many priests had escaped to the countryside when a slave ship was about to embark, and an order had to be fixed on church doors for them to return to their posts. At least one priest requested royal permission to stay in Angola instead of being forced to embark on a slave ship. The ecclesiastical council cited the health conditions on slave ships and poor pay as reasons for the priests' dislike of the Atlantic crossings. They argued that, during the Middle Passage, chaplains often contracted diseases that needed to be cured in a hospital. In effect, they argued against the presence of priests on bilateral slaving voyages between Angola and Brazil that took a minimum of six months.[61]

In their deliberations, the priests in Luanda did not refer once to the conditions that awaited slaves on the ships. Yet, implicitly the 1680s discussion on Atlantic crossings demonstrates the contemporary view on the Middle Passage as an imminent threat to health. It went without saying that priests employed as chaplains would contract an illness that needed medical attention. The Middle Passage was clearly perceived as a

---

[60] For an early remark on African mortality, see AHU, CU, Angola, Cx. 1, Doc. 13, Carta do ouvidor geral de Angola, André Velho da Fonseca, ao rei, 20 November 1610; Rediker, *The Slave Ship*, 273–276; Miller, *Way of Death*, 379.

[61] AHU, CU, Angola, Cx. 13, Doc. 1624, Certidão passada pelo escrivão da auditoria eclesiástico na cidade de São Paulo de Assunção no reino de Angola, padre João Alvares Fontes, 19 November 1686; Doc. 1625, Requerimento do clérigo presbítero-mor na cidade de São Paulo de Assunção, padre Manuel Chamorro, ao rei, earlier than 27 November 1686; Doc. 1626, Certidão passada pelo cónego prebendado da sé do Congo e Angola e secretário do cabido na cidade de São Paulo de Assunção no reino de Angola, Feliciano da Vide, 27 November 1686.

great risk. The issue continued to be contested in the next decade, when the presence of clergy on board slave ships was requested for linguistic reasons. Priests were often fluent in the Kimbundu language and could serve as interpreters. In 1694, the ecclesiastical council of Luanda responded to another royal order that *escravos ladinos*, in other words 'civilised' Portuguese-speaking slaves, could serve on ships instead of priests.[62] Two decades later, the crown had relaxed its view on the issue. A request by a priest wanting to be employed as a catechist during the Middle Passage was turned down by the Overseas Council; he had argued that he wanted to serve on ships only because of his own or his brotherhood's business interests in Brazil. However, in the 1720s orders were again tightened, and a 1726 letter complained that Luanda's bishop did not allow priests to embark as chaplains on slave ships, thereby delaying their departure from Angola unless an occasional volunteer stepped in.[63]

Health was a crucial issue during the Middle Passage. It concerned both the slaves and the crew. Risks were incurred even before the Atlantic crossing began. Delays in completing loadings were common in the seventeenth-century trade; loading ships with slaves could take up to a year or longer. Fresh fruits and vegetables and meat virtually disappeared from the diet, and slaves were fed with manioc flour, beans and occasionally dried fish or meat to strengthen them after their long trek to the coast and before starting their arduous transatlantic journey. On the way to the coast, slaves drank from inadequate water supplies and developed both dietary imbalances and sheer nutritional insufficiencies.[64]

Health on slave ships was linked to hygiene, diseases and provisions. In 1664, the municipal council of Luanda requested permission from the king to appoint a municipal official to inspect the cargoes and provisions on board the ships. The Overseas Council deliberated against the interference of the municipal council but recommended that the governors and treasurers of Angola make sure that no vessel would leave Luanda without carrying at least 25 fully filled barrels of good water for every 100

---

[62] AHU, CU, Angola, Cx. 15, Doc. 1805, Carta do cabido da sé de Angola ao rei, 20 November 1694.

[63] AHU, CU, Angola, Cx. 20, Doc 2103, Consulta do Conselho Ultramarino ao rei sobre duas consultas da Junta das Missões, 21 January 1716; Angola, Cx. 25, Doc. 2482, Carta do provedor da Fazenda Real de Angola, Francisco Pereira, ao rei sobre o Bispo daquele reino não ter indicado clérigo para servir de capelão em determinado navio, 8 March 1726. See also Arlindo Manuel Caldeira, *Escravos e traficantes no império português: O comércio negreiro português no Atlântico durante os séculos XV a XIX* (Lisbon: A Esfera dos Livros, 2013), 112–113.

[64] Miller, *Way of Death*, 383–387; Caldeira, 'Angola and the Seventeenth-Century South Atlantic Slave Trade', 118.

slaves. Regulations issued by the king on 23 September 1664 stipulated against the overcrowding of ships. Following up on this ineffective legislation two decades later, the king promulgated a 'by-law on the dispatch of Black captives from Angola and other conquests, and on the tonnage of ships'. This 1684 set of laws aimed at regulating the slave trade, but its enforcement required a bureaucratic apparatus that did not exist at that time anywhere in the Portuguese Empire and least of all in Luanda.[65]

Water supplies were a critical issue in the Angolan slave trade, and thirst must have been one of the largest sources of discomfort for the enslaved. Springs of drinking water were scarce and of poor quality in the vicinity of Luanda. The fresh water drawn from *cacimbas* (wells) on the island of Luanda was often mixed with seawater, and therefore too saline for human consumption. The 1684 by-law obliged ship masters to 'carry enough water to give slaves a jug (*canada*) to drink each day without fail'. This amounted to roughly two litres of water. The Overseas Council decreed in 1694 that all slave ships calling in Luanda and Benguela had to fetch their water from the Bengo and Dande rivers, respectively. Risks of dehydration ran high among the human cargo and contributed to the distress and death of captives. Moreover, water contamination could cause illness and raise mortality rates.[66]

It was the duty of ship captains to ensure the survival of slaves. Exceptional circumstances notwithstanding, food rations were sufficient but of poor quality and minimal quantity. Manioc flour was the main staple, and it was supplemented by beans and corn flour. Manioc flour was often the return cargo of vessels transporting slaves to Brazil, and it was undoubtedly the basis of slave subsistence during the Middle Passage. Daily rations of manioc flour, cooked and seasoned with palm oil or just cooked plain, were occasionally supplemented with some dried fish.[67]

On board ships, the lack of food and water were not the only factors affecting the health of the enslaved. Parasites, sharp changes in temperature and terrible hygienic conditions fostered illnesses and infections such as dysentery. Sickness, panic and despair led many slaves to reject food. A deafening noise filled the slave ships and made rest difficult. A horrendous smell, caused by a combination of poor ventilation,

[65] Caldeira, 'Angola and the Seventeenth-Century South Atlantic Slave Trade', 130–131.
[66] AHU, CU, Angola, Cx. 15, Doc. 1808, Consulta do Conselho Ultramarino ao rei sobre carta do governador de Angola, Henrique Jacques de Magalhães, 27 November 1694. See also Caldeira, 'Angola and the Seventeenth-Century South Atlantic Slave Trade', 134–135.
[67] Caldeira, 'Angola and the Seventeenth-Century South Atlantic Slave Trade', 134–135.

humidity, faeces and filth, announced the arrival of slave ships to shore in the Americas.

Besides legislation, which was largely ineffective, medical thought on improving the conditions on slave ships began to emerge in writings during the second half of the eighteenth century. In an unpublished 1770 manuscript, Angola's chief physician, Francisco Damião Cosme, gave eight guidelines for the Middle Passage:

1. The slaves should be washed and cleaned throughout the voyage;
2. They should be well fed;
3. They should be given a sufficient amount of water, and in each portion one should add an ounce of vinegar;
4. They should be given an ounce of *gerebita* in the mornings and in the evenings;
5. The ship should be cleaned and perfumed daily;
6. The slaves should sing when they can;
7. The melancholic slaves should be called to the deck and given *gerebita* and tobacco, and they should be obliged to smile and sing when they can;
8. Those who became sick [with specific diseases] should be treated as taught by the author [in his manuscript].[68]

The documentation remains silent as to whether any of these suggestions were followed on slave ships. However, Damião Cosme's recommendation to give good food to slaves was occasionally put into actual practice on the coast when slaves were awaiting shipment. Raimundo Jalama, the administrator of the slave contract in Luanda in the 1760s, narrated a story about a woman brought to Luanda to be shipped as a slave to Brazil together with her daughter. Because of melancholy, the woman refused to eat anything, even the best food. The official in charge of loading the slaves onto the ship in Luanda began to investigate the reasons for the woman's desperation, and he found out that she and her daughter had been sold into slavery by the woman's husband. Eventually, the woman died.[69]

---

[68] Cosme, 'Tractado das queixas endemicas', 267–268.
[69] Jalama is mentioned in AHU/CU, Angola, Cx. 52, Doc. 63, Carta de D. Francisco Inocencio de Sousa Coutinho, December 2, 1768; the story is narrated in Luis Antonio de Oliveira Mendes, 'Discurso academico ao programma: Determinar com todos os seus symptomas as doenças agudas, e chronicas, que mais frequentemente accommettem os Pretos recem-tirados da Africa: examinando as causas da sua mortandade depois da sua chegada ao Brasil: se talvez a mudança do clima, se a vida mais laboriosa, ou se alguns outros motivos concorrem para tanto estragon: e finalmente indicar os methodos mais apropriados para evitalo, prevenindo-o, curando-o. Tudo isto deduzido da experiencia

West-Central Africa was the most important supply region of enslaved Africans, shipping over 5.6 million people to the Americas. Its dominance was challenged by West African slaving ports only in the first half of the eighteenth century, when the mining boom of Minas Gerais in Brazil drove the demand higher in the bights of Benin and Biafra. Brazil, in turn, was by far the most important New World destination for the slaves exported from Africa. Estimates indicate that, of the 10.5 million slaves who landed alive in the Americas between 1519 and 1867, over 4.8 million (46 per cent) of them disembarked in the land of Vera Cruz.[70]

Slave mortality in the Atlantic crossing fluctuated widely. Of the 12,331,600 slaves estimated to have been embarked from Africa, 10,538,200 (85.5 per cent) landed alive in the Americas. For the seventeenth-century Central African trade, Arlindo Manuel Caldeira has recorded mortality levels ranging between under 2 per cent to as high as 64 per cent, with the variations in shipboard mortality giving a median mortality rate of 26.4 per cent. The highest mortality rates resulted from atypical outcomes and exceptionally adverse situations, such as outbreaks of contagious disease or navigational problems.[71] On the 'floating tombs' of the Atlantic, mortality was a constant preoccupation, and it could be cut down most efficiently by loading a cargo of slaves in the shortest time possible. Tight-packing was not the primary cause of the high mortality rates: slaves were more sensitive to the provisioning of food and water on the ships.[72]

Besides the physical diseases that ravaged their bodies and caused high mortality rates on the slave ships, slaves suffered psychologically. From the late seventeenth century, slave traders acknowledged that a specific mental affliction easily took hold of slaves in the southern Atlantic. In Angola, this was expressed by the verb *banzar* (literally, a longing for home, from the Kimbundu word *banza*, meaning town or village). One can imagine how the term perhaps emerged from slaves expressing their longing verbally by crying '*banza*' as they were being taken to ships for the Atlantic crossing. A common belief among enslaved Central Africans was that they were being taken to Brazil to be killed and that the whites made oil out of their bodies. Fear and imagination, therefore, made slaves suffer mentally. As the slave traders noted, some also committed suicide.[73]

---

mais sizuda, e fiel', *Memorias economicas da Academia Real das Sciencias de Lisboa* 4 (1812): 37–38.

[70] http://slavevoyages.org/assessment/estimates

[71] Caldeira, 'Angola and the Seventeenth-Century South Atlantic Slave Trade', 123, 138–141.

[72] Miller, *Way of Death*, 314–318, 336–348.

[73] Cópia de uma petiçao que o povo e mais moradores e forasteiros fizeram ao senado, em (1698?). BML, cód. 12, fls. 89–90v. I am grateful to Roquinaldo Ferreira for sharing this

The Portuguese physicians who wrote about *banzar* or *banzo* in Angola likened it to melancholy. It has been defined as a psychological depression that overtook some Africans after they had disembarked for Brazil. Some scholars have preferred physiological explanations, attributing *banzo* to sleeping sickness. As many slaves suffering from *banzo* took their own lives, some scholars have argued for the psychopathological explanation.[74] Miller noted that it has been described as terminal lethargy, a sort of delirium, a loss of heart, losing the will to live and fixed melancholy, with it being 'ascribed variously to homesickness, despair at the circumstances in which slaves found themselves, and mental trauma at their loss of liberty'. While acknowledging these explanations, he has claimed that *banzo* 'in fact represented the primary symptom of the slaves' underlying state of malnourishment'.[75]

Historians have also tried to link *banzo* to geophagy. According to Brásio, the blacks who had been 'attacked by the madness of *banzo*' ate dirt, ashes, chalk and other earthy materials.[76] Following Brásio, Miller linked *banzo* to dirt eating, which is often associated with nutritional deficiencies, languor and loss of appetite. Finally, by noting the refusal of slaves suffering from the *banzo* to eat, he bundled together passive protest, nutritional deprivation and the fear felt by slaves to explain the condition.[77] In the Caribbean, slave owners imagined dirt eating to be a serious threat, and it was classified as a mental affliction, a conscious form of self-harm and a form of pathological nostalgia. At worst, masters warned each other, the 'mania' of dirt eating could lead to mass death on the plantations. But how real was the disease? Very few slave owners had ever witnessed dirt eating with their own eyes, and they claimed that the enslaved practised it in secret and would never admit it. The symptoms of dirt eating included tiredness, an incapacity to work, a lack of appetite, dizziness and palpitations in the neck. These symptoms rather point to deficiency diseases, the true scourge among plantation slaves. Under gruelling circumstances, dirt eating at best served as a source of nutrients, but it has rarely killed anyone. Nevertheless, slave owners put iron

source with me. On suicide and slavery, see Snyder, *The Power to Die*; Pierson, 'White Cannibals, Black Martyrs'.

[74] Clóvis Moura, *Dicionário da Escravidão Negra no Brasil* (São Paulo: Editoria da Universidade de São Paulo, 2004), 63–64.
[75] Miller, *Way of Death*, 424–425. This view is challenged in Kalle Kananoja, 'Melancholy, Race, and Slavery in the Early Modern Southern Atlantic World', in *Crises of Mind: Cultural and Institutional Approaches to Insanity*, edited by Jari Eilola, Markku Hokkanen and Tuomas Laine-Frigren (Leiden: Brill, 2019), 88–112.
[76] António Brásio, *História e missiologia: Inéditos e esparsos* (Luanda: Instituto de Investigação Científica de Angola, 1973), 747.
[77] Miller, *Way of Death*, 425–426.

masks on slaves suspected of dirt eating and physicians sought in vain an explanation for the 'disease'.[78]

Melancholy was a rare but accepted diagnosis among the Portuguese in eighteenth-century Angola. Captain Vitoriano de Faria e Melo was diagnosed with melancholy in 1724 by Chief Physician Aboim. Melo had also suffered from a range of other illnesses, including epilepsy, but it is not possible to deduce based on the doctor's statement whether melancholy had preceded or followed these other ailments. Aboim also wrote that the captain was continuously imagining things. In other words, his maladies were psychological in nature, and he had difficulties in adapting to life in Angola. Melo petitioned for permission to leave Angola, for it was thought that he could only recover his health at home in Portugal.[79]

Banzar had entered the Portuguese lexicon by the late seventeenth century, when slave traders in Angola began to refer to a specific mental affliction taking hold of slaves in the southern Atlantic. In 1698, residents of Luanda complained that many slaves took their lives because of *banzar*.[80] It was also claimed in Portugal and Brazil that *banzo* was the most common illness in Angola.[81] As early as 1707, Miguel Dias Pimenta wrote of *banzamento* and melancholic, *banzo*-like humours in Brazil. Pimenta was not trained as a physician, nor as a surgeon, but he was a prosperous merchant residing in Recife. His work described a gangrenous ulceration of dysenteric rectitis called *bicho*, which was common among enslaved Africans. Apparently, Pimenta was well read in the classical canon of medicine and he tried to place this ailment within a humoural framework. He referred to *banzamento* basically as sad thoughts and a longing for something that the individual could not reach. In a later passage, he referred to '*humores tão banzeyros*' as humours that became concentrated in the hands and feet during the night. Here, Pimenta obviously deviated from classical authorities and gave a lay interpretation to the displacements and forced migrations resulting from the Atlantic slave trade.[82]

---

[78] Kiple, *The Caribbean Slave*, 99–103; Hogarth, *Medicalizing Blackness*.

[79] AHU, CU, Angola, Cx. 24, Doc. 2399, Requerimento do capitão de Infantaria de uma companhia do terço pago da praça de Angola, Vitoriano de Faria e Melo, ao rei, earlier than 19 May 1725.

[80] Cópia de uma petiçao que o povo e mais moradores e forasteiros fizeram ao senado, em (1698?). BML, cód. 12, fls. 89–90v. I am grateful to Roquinaldo Ferreira for sharing this source with me.

[81] *Gazeta de Lisboa*, No. 32 (10 August 1719), 250, accessed 6 November 2018, http://hemerotecadigital.cm-lisboa.pt/Periodicos/GazetadeLisboa/1719/Agosto/Agosto_item1/P10.html. For examples from elsewhere in Atlantic Africa, see Postma, *The Dutch in the Atlantic Slave Trade*, 242.

[82] Miguel Dias Pimenta, *Noticias do que he o achaque do bicho, diffiniçam do seu crestameto, subimento, corrupção, sinaes, & cura ate, o quinto grao, ou intenção delle, suas differenças, & coplicações, com que se ajunta* (Lisbon: Miguel Manescal, 1707), 8, 91. On *mal do bicho*,

In 1719, the Bishop of Rio de Janeiro wrote to Lisbon about the fates of slaves arriving in the city. Demonstrating the close connections between Central Africa and Rio, he reported that although many Central Africans from Loango and Luanda arrived unbaptised, there were usually priests in the Jesuit College who could speak the Kimbundu language. They examined those who were baptised and those who were not.[83] West Africans were not similarly questioned because of a lack of interpreters. Although it was the owners' responsibility to instruct their slaves on 'the mysteries of faith', this was practically impossible to enforce. The bishop argued that proper Christian instruction would take several months, during which time 'some get the *banzo*, others get sick, and many die'. Here, one is struck by the bishop's reference to *banzo*, which was expressed as a verb: '*huns banzão*'. While Ana Maria Oda has discussed the emergence of *banzo* in Portuguese and Brazilian medical discourse in the late eighteenth and nineteenth centuries, it clearly had a much longer history in the southern Atlantic world. The bishop's letter and his casual reference to *banzo* show that it had already entered popular discourse in Brazil by the 1710s.[84]

Around the mid-eighteenth century, *banzar* started to appear with regularity in writings regarding health in Africa. The first more extensive view of this illness was included in an Italian Capuchin missionary manual in 1747, attributed to Father Giacinto da Bologna, who arrived in West-Central Africa in 1742.[85] Father Giacinto's manuscript included advice for missionaries on treating illnesses in Africa. Besides noting the most common ailments affecting Europeans in tropical Africa and listing suitable remedies for each, he argued that conserving not only physical

---

see Jaime Walter, 'A propósito de uma doença de Angola de há mais de três séculos: doença do bicho ou maculo', *Boletim clínico e estatistico do Hospital do ultramar* 7 (1957): 47–68.

[83] In another letter, the bishop who had been ordered to examine the health of the enslaved on their arrival in Brazil complained that the slaves arriving from Angola were almost completely uninstructed in the Catholic doctrine, understanding baptism only as the eating of salt. He called for the priests of Angola to take better care of their duties in converting the slaves before the Middle Passage, so that they would at least die in faith. Noting that many died during the Atlantic crossing, the bishop wanted the sick blacks to receive medical treatment immediately upon arrival in Rio de Janeiro. AHU, CU, Angola, Cx. 21, Doc. 2188, Carta do Bispo do Rio de Janeiro ao rei, 21 August 1719.

[84] AHU, CU, Angola, Cx. 21, Doc. 2185, Carta do Bispo do Rio de Janeiro ao rei, 17 July 1719; Oda, 'O banzo e outros males'.

[85] The original Italian manuscript is included in the French translation of Giacinto da Bologna, *La Pratique Missionnaire des PP. Capucins Italiens dans les royaumes de Congo, Angola et contrées adjacentes*, translated by Jacques Nothomb (Louvain: Éditions de l'Aucam, 1931). The date of Bologna's arrival in Africa is listed in P. Graziano Saccardo, *Congo e Angola con la storia dell'antica missione dei Cappuccini* (Venice-Mestre: Curia Provinciale dei Cappuccini, 1983), 3: 84–93.

but also moral health was important. Thus, one had to attempt to keep
the soul intrepid and joyful in order to avoid a certain illness that had
already claimed lives, presumably the lives of missionaries or at least
Europeans. This was the infirmity the Portuguese called *banzare*.[86]
According to Bologna, it was an illness suffered especially by timid,
apprehensive and melancholic individuals, those who were 'afraid of
danger where there exists none' and were prone to exaggerate such
dangers, making them irremediable by giving in to fear and sadness,
which in turn made them *banzare*.[87] Thus, contracting this illness was
thought to depend on a person's nature.

As can be seen, Bologna's manuscript suggests that *banzar* was an
illness that affected Europeans. As his work was primarily directed at his
fellow missionaries, it is inevitable that in Africa they were in danger of
contracting this mental illness. In order to cure it, Bologna believed
'without a doubt that the love of God can transform the soul of the timid
and the pusillanimous in intrepid and constant ... this transformation
reforms the temperament'.[88] This reflects the notion that certain mental
states – 'wrong' feelings – were seen as a threat to health. Nothing
suggests that *banzare* was conceptualised as an illness affecting
especially blacks.

If *banzo*, in the Capuchins's view, was a form of melancholy that
Europeans suffered from in Angola and adjacent regions, Central
Africans might have had a different view on the illness. A unique glimpse
into African notions of *banzo* is provided by local rulers' correspondence
in the interior of Angola.[89] In 1764, *Soba* (Chief) Damião Lopes
Caenda, or his secretary, wrote to the captain-major of Ambaca concerning a skirmish that he claimed should be resolved with recourse to a
Mbundu poison ordeal *indua*. In the letter, 'being sick of *banze*' (*estar
duente de banze*)[90] is used by the *soba* as a pretext for a missed appointment with Ambaca's captain-major. Although *banzo* is mentioned here

---

[86] The term *banzar* was Italianised by Bologna by adding an -e on the end.
[87] Bologna, *La Pratique Missionnaire*, 71.   [88] Bologna, *La Pratique Missionnaire*, 71.
[89] The spread of literacy among African populations in Angola, especially in the Dembos
region, is well known in the historiography. The correspondence has been published in
Catarina Madeira Santos and Ana Paula Tavares, eds., *Africae Monumenta:
A Apropriação da Escrita pelos Africanos, Vol. I, Arquivo Caculo Cacahenda* (Lisbon:
Centro de Estudos de História e Cartografia Antiga/ Instituto de Investigação
Científica Tropical, 2002) and *Africae Monumenta: A Apropriação da Escrita pelos
Africanos, Vol. II, Arquivos Ndala Cabassa, Mufuque Aquitupa, Pango Aluquem e Bango
Aquitamba* (Lisbon: CHAM, 2010).
[90] Colecção de Bango a Caputo, Carta de soba D. Damião Lopes Caenda, September 29,
1764. I am grateful to Eva Sebastyen for providing me with her transcription of
this document.

only in passing, it can be inferred that it was an illness recognised by Africans in Angola. Further, it was not only a slave disease but afflicted people regardless of social class. Unfortunately, there is no mention of how Soba Damião recovered from it. There was clearly a local and a mutual understanding between Africans and the Portuguese as to its meaning. Further, its mention by an Angolan *soba* makes clear that it was an illness that also afflicted free Africans, not only slaves. Only a few years later, there were clear signs that *banzo* was becoming more systematically connected to blackness and race.

This view was most clearly articulated in Chief Physician Francisco Damião Cosme's manuscript on endemic diseases in Portuguese Angola. For Damião Cosme, *banzar* meant 'to suffer from melancholy'. He argued that caring for the tranquillity or peace of one's soul was even more important than caring for one's body, and he warned his readers of a 'great passion [*paixão*] of the soul, or great melancholy'.[91] In the eighteenth century, the Portuguese word *paixão*, translated as passion, referred to anything positive or negative that disturbed both the interior and exterior of a person and diminished his or her natural tranquillity.[92] The understanding of human passions as being rooted in the biological constitution of humans had been present in Galen's thought. The theory of passions underwent several changes throughout history, including the seventeenth- and eighteenth-century theorising about human nature.[93]

Cosme continued that '[t]he constant experience in these countries has shown that death is certain in those who are preoccupied with their affliction: vulgar expression is that who goes about *banzando* goes about very sad; and that to *banzar* and to die is all the same'.[94] In this passage, Cosme likened *banzo* to melancholy. In his opinion, melancholy could

<hr/>

[91] Cosme, 'Tractado das queixas endemicas', 183.
[92] Raphael Bluteau, *Vocabulario Portuguez & Latino...* (Coimbra: Collegio das Artes da Companhia de Jesu, 1712–1728), 6: 188.
[93] Walther Riese, *La théorie des passions à la lumière de la pensée médicale du XVIIe siècle* (New York: John Wiley, 1965); See also Noga Arikha, *Passions and Tempers: A History of the Humours* (New York: Ecco, 2007); Gail Kern Paster, Katherine Rowe and Mary Floyd-Wilson, eds., *Reading the Early Modern Passions: Essays in the Cultural History of Emotion* (Philadelphia: University of Pennsylvania Press, 2004).
[94] Cosme, 'Tractado das queixas endemicas', 183.

Nada finalmente devo advertir, e recomedar mais para a conservação da vida, e utilidade da saude, que a tranquilidade ou socego da Alma, por milhor e mais bem ordenado, que seja o tratamento do Corpo; por mais perfeita, que seja a despozição de Cada hum tudo repentinamente desconporá hua grande paixão da Alma, ou grande melancolia. A constant experiençia tem mostrado nestes Paizes, como he certa a morte nos preocupados da sua afição: vulgarmente dizem, que anda banzando o que anda muy triste; e qua banzar e morrer hé tudo hum.

affect anyone, for he gave this advice to the general reader and not only to slave merchants or owners. He pointed out that *banzo* was a product of the mind. Arguing that sentiments are constantly changing and that it is pointless to try to understand their causes, Cosme advised his readers to 'let time heal' all great afflictions. Further, he wrote that '[a]ll our martyrdom is in our fantasy; that is the bottom of our melancholy, and all other passions'.[95]

While the treatise argued that *banzo* could affect anyone, its writer noted that it was a disorder that affected especially slaves. Slaves' melancholy especially is addressed in the last part of the text, which deals with the recommendations Cosme gave to merchants about the handling of slaves. First, he laid down the economic reason for treating slaves well: the loss of a slave equals or surpasses the monetary value of good treatment. Second, Cosme argued that Africans were biologically similar to Europeans: '[t]hese blacks have the nature that we have, and they are subject to same ailments and needs as we are: therefore, in order to live and to be healthy they need the same means'. Third, he went on a full-frontal attack against the cruelties practised by slave traders. Because blacks possessed 'a soul as perfect as ours', they were similarly affected by passions and many died because of them.[96] Cosme bore witness to the ever-rising number of slave exports from Luanda. The move towards a racial interpretation of *banzo* cannot be detached from the chronology of the slave trade.

Conclusion

Primary sources abound with contemporary social diagnoses of diseases in West-Central Africa. Yet, they are often of little use in determining the modern biological diagnoses. Essentially, they point out that humoural theory, although instrumental for certain physicians such as Aleixo de Abreu, was rarely a reference point when making social diagnoses. Instead, laypeople and doctors usually referred to very general symptoms and conditions. These social diagnoses were not different from the way diseases were defined among West-Central Africans. Students of local herbal remedies could easily find cures for illnesses that bothered both Africans and Europeans. Therefore, the functioning of African and European bodies was understood to be identical.

Epidemic diseases, especially smallpox, exacted a steep death toll among local populations, especially where people with no prior contact

---

[95] Cosme, 'Tractado das queixas endemicas', 183.
[96] Cosme, 'Tractado das queixas endemicas', 263.

were exposed to new pathogens. This was the case with slaves originating from deeper in the interior and with people who were forced to move due to ecological disasters. However, the Portuguese understanding of epidemic diseases remained extremely thin throughout the era of the slave trade. Physicians constantly failed to name the main causes of heightened mortality rates in human populations. European medical expertise and knowledge of local diseases was extremely limited. Physicians and surgeons, who were supposed to know, did not demonstrate a high degree of knowledge. In knowing diseases, local experience continued to play a more important role than academic medicine.

The limited success of European medicine in Atlantic Africa can also be seen in the failure of humoural theory to adapt itself to and to develop in the tropics during the early modern period. It is as if Atlantic African medical geography and the constant references to harsh climate (see Chapter 7) gave Portuguese medical doctors an excuse to remain inert. While many laypeople made use of African medicinals, trained physicians despised them, making use of only a few and almost exclusively European remedies until the nineteenth century. European medicine consisted mainly of bloodletting, which was often harmful to bodies already weakened by disease. Portuguese doctors did not abandon humoural theory completely but made very little use of it in Angola. For more than a century and half, Aleixo de Abreu remained the only physician to write a book-length treatise on the practice of medicine in Angola. Abreu's work did not exert much influence on those who followed him to Angola, meaning that each physician and surgeon coming from the outside had to figure out how to practise medicine in Angola by personally experiencing and experimenting with it in local society. Adapting theory learned in Europe was difficult, and physicians vied for patients in a medically plural society.

Although there was little medical improvement, the Portuguese administrators and officers cared considerably more about maintaining the health of Europeans than striving for decreased mortality rates of the human merchandise in the Atlantic slave trade. One is stricken by the silences pertaining to the health of local indigenous populations and slaves that traversed the Atlantic. Aside from occasional discussions on improving shipboard conditions, the first medical discussions on the Middle Passage involving Portuguese physicians emerge only in the late eighteenth century. Maritime medicine was left in the hands of surgeons, who coped poorly with outbreaks of disease on slave ships. The suggestions made by Chief Physician Damião Cosme are indicative of the tools available to care for the health of the enslaved. The best that the ship captains could do was to try to maintain good morale among slaves by providing food, water and a portion of sugar-cane brandy and giving them a chance to sing. These means were hardly enough to cure the diseases that broke out among the enslaved on the shore, on the ships and upon arrival at New World destinations.

7   Migrations
Medical Geography in the Southern Atlantic

In the closing decade of the eighteenth century, the German physician Leonhard Ludwig Finke published a comprehensive medical geography in three volumes. Finke's encyclopaedic work was in essence a global history of health and environment, which also included a substantial section on Atlantic Africa. Finke had never visited West-Central Africa but drew upon almost three centuries of popular images about it. He relied, for the most part, on the 1712 account of Capuchin Father Antonio Zucchelli, and on Abbe Proyart's 1776 description of Loango. He also drew upon James Lind's *An Essay on Diseases Incidental to Europeans in Hot Climates*. Zucchelli, however, was Finke's main primary source. This is hardly surprising, as the Capuchin accounts of Kongo and Angola circulated in numerous translations in Central and Western Europe. Modern scholarship has also recognised the Capuchins as foremost authorities on Central African natural history in the early modern period. For Finke and others citing them, Capuchin accounts, strongly rooted in local experience, became material for global analysis.[1]

Citing Zucchelli, Finke began his outline of West-Central Africa by describing Benguela's topography as being low-lying and very fertile, but with the climate and midday heat being almost unbearable. Altogether, he labelled it as one of the unhealthiest countries in the whole of Africa. Although the country produced beautiful and tasteful fruits, poisonous air made visiting Europeans pay with their health. Finke continued by claiming that local water was harmful. Cautious visitors ate only food

---

[1] Leonhard Ludwig Finke, *Versuch einer allgemeinen medicinisch-praktischen Geographie, worin der historische Theil der einheimischen Völker – und Staaten – Arzeneykunde vorgetragen wird*, 3 vols. (Leipzig: Weidmannschen Buchhandlund, 1792); on Capuchins as natural historians and on Zucchelli's descriptions of the Central African climate and environment, see Silvio Porisiensi, *Pionieri della scienza, della civiltá e della fede in Africa: I cappuccino italiani alla esplorazione del Congo, Angola e Matamba nel sec. XVII, 1645–1705: La relazioni sul congo del friuliano Antonio Zucchelli* (Udine: Chiandetti, 1981), 119–146, 214–216; Almeida, *Uma infelicidade feliz*, 207–315. For a detailed bibliography of the translated Capuchin travel accounts, see Fage, *A Guide to Original Sources*.

brought from Europe; local products were always eaten cooked, never
raw. Meat was not to be eaten because it began to stink on the second
day. He also remarked that local blacks subsisted mainly on their fruits
and millet cooked in water.[2]

Moving on to Luanda, Finke noted that it had very similar conditions
to those in Benguela, but it suffered from more rainfall. It was deemed
very dangerous to whites, who almost inevitably contracted a fever. In
Angola and Kongo, the rainy season began with little rain at the end of
October, which lasted until December. January and February were drier,
but in March the great rains began, which lasted until the end of April.
The six months from November to April were the hottest. Finke then
described the province of Soyo as populous but rural. Its people rarely ate
cooked food but relied instead on vegetables and local fruits, wine and oil
from palm trees, as well as mice and locusts for their sustenance. The
Kongolese lived long; Finke remarked that Zucchelli had encountered a
ninety-year-old woman and generally regarded the blacks from Kongo as
strong people.[3]

Finke did not have an abundance of primary sources on West-Central
Africa to draw upon. His discussion of Angola, Benguela and Kongo was
much shorter than his description of West Africa's medical geography,
for which he relied mainly on the Danish surgeon Isert's letters from the
Gold Coast. Finke was greatly interested in the nutrition of local populations. He argued that, in seeking the causes of diseases, one should follow
Hippocratic advice and notice the foodstuffs used by the inhabitants as
well as other things that may influence their health. According to Finke,
the physicians should be able to recognise the origin, development, rise
and decline of prevalent diseases by observing the nature of the soil, the
fruits and products of the land, the properties of the air and water, and
the livelihood of the people. They should also be acquainted with available medicaments, mainly botanicals and minerals, as well as with the
customary modes of treatment in each country. Therefore, it is not
surprising that he also discussed bloodletting used for treating malarial
fevers, as described in the seventeenth-century Capuchin sources, and he

[2] Finke, *Versuch*, I: 698. On Finke's work, see George Rosen, 'Leonhard Ludwig Finke and
the First Medical Geography', in *Science, Medicine and History: Essays on the Evolution of
Scientific Thought and Medical Practice, Vol. 2*, edited by E. Ashworth Underwood
(London: Oxford University Press, 1953), 186–193; Frank A. Barrett, 'Finke's
1792 Map of Human Diseases: The First World Disease Map?', *Social Science &
Medicine* 50 (2000): 915–921; Frank A. Barrett, 'A Medical Geography Anniversary',
Social Science & Medicine 37 (1993): 701–710.
[3] Finke, *Versuch*, I: 699–700.

wrote on the methods used by local folk healers in different parts of Atlantic Africa.[4]

Finke's work was important in linking disease and environment in Africa to the rest of the world and inserting them into the context of global health discussions. His short summary of Central Africa's medical topography was flawed only in the sense that his sources were quite limited. Archival sources can greatly enrich the history of Angola's medical geography. Environment played a key role in defining and dictating the migratory flows of people in the early modern Atlantic world.

This chapter examines Portuguese discourses on health, environment and migration in the context of the colonisation of West-Central Africa. It points to ideas that people from certain parts of Portugal were seen as better suited to adapt to the Angolan disease environment, or rather environments, for certain regions in the colony of Angola were seen as healthier than others. Therefore, this chapter also addresses dangerous and healing environments within West-Central Africa, some of which gained a mythical status by the end of the eighteenth century. The history of migration in, to and from Angola would be incomplete without Brazil, which was intimately connected to discourses on health and environment in the Portuguese Atlantic, first as a potential source of immigrants to Angola, and second, as a temporary healing environment for Europeans stationed in West-Central Africa. By tracing the movements of people and ideas in time and space, this chapter demonstrates the interconnectedness of environment and health in the early modern southern Atlantic world.

Ancient Ideas and Atlantic Challenges

The ideas about the relationship between environmental or geographic factors in shaping human bodies go back several millennia, but the Hippocratic treatise *Airs, Waters, and Places* is usually portrayed as laying out the crucial questions in the field. Its premise is that disease is a product of specific locales, and it portrays elements of the environment as important factors in human illness and well-being. *Airs, Waters, and Places* assumes a fundamental linkage between the four humours, or bodily fluids – namely blood, phlegm, yellow bile or choler, and black bile or melancholy – which regulated overall health, and the external forces capable of influencing the body's humoural balance. The external factors used to explain illness and humoural imbalance included the six

---

[4] Finke, *Versuch*, III: 19–21; Finke, *Versuch*, I: 721, 726–728. See also Rosen, 'Leonhard Ludwig Finke', 190–192.

non-naturals: air, food and drink, sleep, exercise, evacuations, and passions of the mind. Miasma, referring to pollution or a polluting agent, was an important concept in the medical discussions on the relationship between the environment and disease. Although the exact nature of miasmas remained undefined, the general sources contributing to the putrefaction of the air were thought to include stagnant marshes and pools, vapours from corpses of humans and animals, sick persons, excreta, spoiled foodstuffs, decaying vegetable matter and exhalations that came from the ground through ruptures or clefts.[5]

Airs, Waters, and Places was an important intellectual resource for the Portuguese, who began their Atlantic excursions to West Africa in the fifteenth century. Yet, the Hippocratic theory on *Airs, Waters, and Places* faced tremendous challenges in the local conditions of Atlantic Africa.[6] In the Portuguese case, as Hugh Cagle has shown, experiences of environment and health first took shape on the Upper Guinea Coast and the Elmina Castle on the Gold Coast over the course of the fifteenth century, where Hippocratic environmentalism came to predominate over Galenic humouralism.[7] Influences ranging from Pliny and Ptolemy to the Hippocratic corpus and Aristotelian cosmology were mixed with little-known Portuguese devotional literature, shaping questions about the relationship between climate, environment and health. While fifteenth-century authors treated West Africa as a land of health and vitality, opinions in the Latin West had begun to change radically by the opening decades of the sixteenth century. Accounts of disease, especially fever, began to predominate in descriptions of West Africa. Africa was laden with medical meaning even before Portuguese ventures to the Atlantic. A combination of contradictory classical, biblical and scholastic sources shaped Portuguese visions, which were further reinforced by popular myth and legend.[8]

Charting diagnostic shifts in Portuguese chronicles, Cagle has argued that between about 1450 and 1500, the African natural world once associated with human health and vitality came to be linked with

[5] On the six non-naturals, miasmas and *Airs, Waters, and Places*, see, e.g., Wesley D. Smith, *The Hippocratic Tradition* (Ithaca, NY: Cornell University Press, 1979); Genevieve Miller, '"Airs, Waters, and Places" in History', *Journal of the History of Medicine and Allied Sciences* 17 (1962): 129–140; Conevery Bolton Valenčius, 'Histories of Medical Geography', *Medical History* 44: S20 (2000): 3–28; Luis García-Ballester, 'On the Origin of the "Six Non-natural Things" in Galen', in *Galen and Galenism: Theory and Medical Practice from Antiquity to the European Renaissance*, edited by Jon Arrizabalaga (Aldershot: Ashgate, 2002), 105–115.
[6] On *Airs, Waters, and Places* elsewhere in the Atlantic, see Seth, *Difference and Disease*, 30–44.
[7] Cagle, *Assembling the Tropics*, 43.   [8] Cagle, 'Beyond the Senegal', 1–4.

debilitating illness and death. These views coexisted in tension with each other. The biblical legend of Prester John and its association with an earthly paradise guided early travellers to West Africa to regard it as a region of health and abundance. Only the pervasive experience of fevers challenged this view. However, a further interpretive layer was the challenge West Africa presented to Hippocratic epistemology, and especially to the treatise *Airs, Waters, and Places*. Seafarers equated unhealthy places with barrenness and viewed healthy ones as lush and teeming with abundant life. The experience of fever rendered verdant overseas landscapes suspect and prompted speculation about the causes of so much illness. The uncertainty about the reliability of the Hippocratic framework could be explained by relying on Aristotle's view of the 'torrid zone' as scorched, bleak and impassable. Travel to West Africa meant entering the torrid zone – verdant, brimming with life but at the same time plagued by heat and deadly illness.[9]

In West-Central Africa, early travellers also pointed to the prodigious fertility of the region. Jesuit reports gave an exalted picture of the fertility of Kongo and the hinterland of Luanda, and sixteenth-century reports generally underlined the natural exuberance of the region. Yet, at the same time the discourse on a pestilential climate persisted. These images continued to be displayed in Capuchin missionary literature and evoked in correspondence of the seventeenth century. Upon their arrival in Kongo, some Europeans were surprised to find that the heat was not as unbearable as they had expected. Being situated in the torrid zone did not mean that the land was uninhabitable, as writers in Antiquity had claimed. However, just like in West Africa, Europeans came to acknowledge that the same climate that sustained growth and fertility in nature also brought with it diseases and suffering.[10]

The first comprehensive medical treatise by a physician with personal experience from Angola was written by Aleixo de Abreu, who served as the personal physician of João Furtado de Mendonça, Governor of Angola, between 1591 and 1604. Despite investigating natural phenomena and the environment – climate, winds, terrain – he did not advocate the role of non-naturals, or 'airs', alone as keys to understanding illness. According to Goodyear, Abreu placed emphasis on humoural corruption, borne of improper or inadequate nutrition and extreme physical exertion. He did not conclude that latitude determined the illnesses contracted by the colonists. For example, in treating 'illness of the worm' (*enfermedad del guzano*), Abreu postulated that strenuous exercise in hot

[9] Cagle, 'Beyond the Senegal', 4–17.   [10] Almeida, *Uma infelicidade feliz*, 260–262.

weather led to humoural corruption, which generated the white whip-worms (*Tunga penetrans*) Abreu had observed when he performed autopsies on the bodies of Luandans.[11]

Yet, climate emerged and persisted as the main popular explanation for Central African diseases. By the late seventeenth century, it had become the common denominator in diagnoses. A century after Abreu, Angola's chief physician, Camacho e Aboim, put his own illness down to the harmful climate. He also testified that Captain Vitoriano de Faria e Melo, who suffered from various maladies, epileptic fits and melancholy, needed a 'change of airs' because the climate of the torrid zone provoked his sickness (*fomentado pela clima desta zona torrida*) and made it constantly worse.[12]

Although European medical theory was developing in the eighteenth century, earlier notions of medical geography continued to play an important role in the writings of chief physicians in Angola. Writing during the governorship of Sousa Coutinho in the 1760s, Francisco Damião Cosme, although giving ample instructions on hygiene and preventive medicine, had little to say on the causes of diseases. The Central African climate entered into his diagnoses when he discussed different kinds of fevers, both benign and malignant, that were common during the *caçibo* (winter) period from June to September. On the whole, however, Damião Cosme was of the opinion that people complained too much about the rigours of the climate. Although admitting that the great heat and humid climate created a pestilent environment, in his view foreigners in Angola should pay more attention to choosing and eating unspoiled food, which he considered a greater factor than climate in preserving health in the tropics.[13]

José Pinto de Azeredo, the famed and best known of Angola's chief physicians, began his work with a reference to the torrid zone, when he argued that the fevers of Angola were of the same nature as those he had observed in Rio de Janeiro, Bahia and Pernambuco in Brazil. His work

---

[11] James D. Goodyear, *Agents of Empire: Portuguese Doctors in Colonial Brazil and the Idea of Tropical Disease* (unpublished Ph.D. dissertation, Johns Hopkins University, 1982), 98–100. On Abreu's work in Angola and Brazil, see also Cagle, *Assembling the Tropics*, 215–233.

[12] AHU, Cx. 24, Doc. 2399, Requerimento do capitão de Infantaria de uma companhia do terço pago da praça de Angola, Vitoriano de Faria e Melo, ao rei, earlier than 19 May 1725; AHU, CU, Angola, Cx. 24, Doc. 2413, Requerimento do fisico-mor de Angola e cavaleiro fidalgo de Sua Majestade, Tomé Guerreiro Camacho Aboim, ao rei, earlier than 12 July 1725.

[13] Cosme, 'Tractado das queixas endemicas', 179, 184, 215–217. Literally: 'Queixão-se todos do pessimo Clima deste Pais, e não se queixão dos maus alimentos, com que se sustentão, que influem mais no estragon da sua vida e saude, que o rigor do Clima.'

was imbued with considerations of the effects of Angola's climate on the health of the people living there. He noted how new arrivals to the African coast were attacked by fevers in greater force and with greater danger to their health because they were unaware of the risks of the sun and because of the habits they were accustomed to in more benign climates. Azeredo described the medical topography of Luanda in great detail because of his conviction that endemic illness depended on a single common cause that exists in the atmosphere. After noting the location of Luanda on arid, sterile, dry and sandy land, Azeredo went on to lament the lack of fresh water in the city, which consequently led to a shortage of plants and trees. He praised, however, the abundance of locally grown fruits, such as oranges, pineapples and mangos.[14]

Climatic and environmental factors figured strongly in Azeredo's medical geography. Of the many causes that made the climate pestilent, he counted the sun as the most terrible. The heat alone was enough to provoke a fever. In Azeredo's experience, those who stayed out of the sun were the ones who remained healthy. Military campaigns were especially critical, because troops marched in the heat of the day, leading to great mortality via fevers and dysenteries. When discussing the unhealthiness of the River Bengo and the occurrence of rains, miasma also entered into Azeredo's calculations. He argued that the level of illness increased during the rainy season, but that heavy rain was not as damaging as showers, which drew vapours from the ground that were then heated by the sun, creating a thick and pestilent air impossible to breathe.[15]

In line with the Hippocratic treatise *Airs, Waters, and Places*, Azeredo did not fail to notice the winds that blew in Luanda. In his view, the city would have been wholly uninhabitable had the infallible winds ceased to blow each day. The winds cooled the air, removed the stillness and removed effluvia damaging to human life. Azeredo also remarked that the higher part of the city enjoyed healthier conditions, as it was always washed by refreshing breezes. In contrast, the people living in the lower part, where the air was more still, suffered repeated illnesses.[16]

Climate and environment figured prominently in learned expositions on health and disease in West-Central Africa. They also had a continuous presence in popular notions and experiences of illness in the three centuries preceding Damião Cosme and Azeredo. The popular consensus was that the climate was damaging and in many ways a factor in, if not the primary cause, of most diseases. Climate and environment,

---

[14] Azeredo, *Ensaios*, vii, 5, 36–46.   [15] Azeredo, *Ensaios*, 46–49.
[16] Azeredo, *Ensaios*, 51–52.

therefore, came to be employed as foundational arguments in debates about migration patterns in the southern Atlantic world and to support requests for sick leave and health travel from Angola.

Immigrants from Portugal and Brazil

In the seventeenth century, the Portuguese Empire faced a grave crisis and was definitely in decline. A shift from long-distance commerce in Asia to land-based forms of colonisation in Brazil amounted to a reconfiguration of the empire aimed at ensuring its survival. Like the Dutch maritime trading empire, Portugal had a small population compared to the extent of its empire, and both powers were constantly struggling with manning their overseas possessions. In Portugal, the 'lack of people' was observed most astutely by Manuel Severim de Faria during the first half of the seventeenth century. In his *Notícias de Portugal* (1655), Faria claimed that the primary reason for Portugal's low population had to do with its extensive colonies, which ate up manpower and hindered population growth in continental Portugal. He saw the extensive possessions in Asia as especially problematic. The longer voyages to the numerous trading posts in the Indian Ocean world occasioned much greater mortality than was experienced in the Atlantic. Therefore, little by little colonial administration and the military came to be manned by locals.[17]

In the case of Angola, this meant employing Africans and Lusoafricans as soldiers in the military. By the 1730s, some officers in Angola were even suggesting that the commanders of the interior forts should be men born in Angola, as such men were more resistant to 'the malignity of the climate' and also got along better with indigenous African rulers.[18] Several accounts demonstrate that a sizeable number of Portuguese infantrymen taken to Angola either perished or became seriously ill after arriving in Africa.[19] To a great extent, migrant flows from Portugal

---

[17] Manuel Severim de Faria, *Notícias de Portugal* (Lisbon: Officina Craesbeeckiana, 1655), 1–15. On Faria's networks, which spanned the globe and provided him with information on Africa, Asia and Brazil, see Liam Matthew Brockey, 'An Imperial Republic: Manuel Severim de Faria Surveys the Globe, 1608–1655', in *Portuguese Humanism and the Republic of Letters*, edited by Maria Berbara and Karl A. E. Enenkel (Leiden: Brill, 2012), 265–285.

[18] AHU, CU, Angola, Cx. 30, Doc. 2930, Consulta do Conselho Ultramarino ao rei sobre a nomeação de pessoas para o posto de capitão-mor do presídio de Cambambe, 2 June 1734.

[19] Roquinaldo Ferreira, *Transforming Atlantic Slaving: Trade, Warfare and Territorial Control in Angola, 1650–1800* (unpublished Ph.D. dissertation, University of California, Los Angeles, 2003), 154. When preparing for the early occupation of Benguela, Manoel Cerveira Pereira recommended that most of the requested 300 soldiers should come

consisted of orphans and banished convicts (*degredados/as*). Permanent or fixed-term exile to Angola was a common punishment for a variety of infringements. Gypsies were often targeted in deportation campaigns throughout the eighteenth century.[20] The substantial military requirements and long-term colonisation plans made Angola into a primary *degredado*-receiving region during the seventeenth century. It received convicts not only from Portugal, but also from Brazil. In the 1670s, Brazilian courts were encouraged to use Angola and only Angola for sentences of exile. The purpose was to increase manpower in Central Africa.[21] Brazilians also responded quickly to news of population loss in Angola, as in 1685, when a smallpox epidemic ravaged the population of Luanda and Pernambucan authorities hastily began preparations to empty local jails and ship criminals to Luanda. Similar situations occurred in 1710 and 1725, when large numbers of vagrants, inmates and gypsies were sentenced to exile and shipped to Luanda.[22]

In the medical hierarchy of Portuguese overseas territories, Angola was almost without exception seen as the most disease-ridden possession, although as Faria noted, Portuguese possessions in South and South East Asia, and the lengthy voyages to reach them, were not necessarily any more salubrious to Europeans. In any case, it was difficult to recruit officials and soldiers to serve in the colonial administration or the military in Africa. In the mid-seventeenth century, officials contemplating the compensation due to Angola's newly nominated chief physician noted that it should be equal to what was given to an India-bound doctor, although Angola was 'more diseased and riskier'.[23]

By the end of the seventeenth century, there were clear indications that migrants from certain regions in the Portuguese Atlantic were thought to fare better in Angola. Writing to the Overseas Council in 1696, Governor Magalhães reported on the high mortality rates experienced during the previous year. Epidemics had decimated Luanda's population and a large portion of the soldiers had died. Requesting reinforcements, the governor warned that soldiers from Madeira acclimatised poorly to Luanda. Instead, he advised the council to send troops from the

from Kongo or Angola because soldiers from Portugal tended to become sick and die. See Candido, *An African Slaving Port*, 43.

[20] On gypsies in Angola, see Carlos Couto, 'Presença cigana na colonização de Angola', *Boletim do Instituto de Investigação Científica de Angola* 8 (1971): 137–143.

[21] Timothy J. Coates, *Convicts and Orphans: Forced and State-Sponsored Colonizers in the Portuguese Empire, 1550–1755* (Stanford, CA: Stanford University Press, 2001), 77, 82.

[22] Ferreira, *Transforming Atlantic Slaving*, 148.

[23] AHU, CU, Angola, Cx. 4, Doc. 441, Consulta do Conselho Ultramarino ao rei sobre requerimento do medico licenciado pela Universidade de Coimbra, António Lopes de Oliveira, 6 May 1649.

Alentejo, Beira and Ribatejo regions. However, the Overseas Council argued that the rigours of Angola's climate were harmful to all men regardless of origins, and it therefore regarded Madeirans as being just as fit to serve in Angola as all others.[24]

Governor Magalhães's report and the debate about soldiers from Madeira that ensued in the following decades points to the important role of the island in exporting people throughout the Portuguese Empire. As Timothy Coates has argued, Madeira had become an exporter of *degredados* to Africa and Brazil by the end of the seventeenth century. For example, in March 1697, 100 soldiers were sent to Maranhão and another 200 were quickly recruited to be sent to Angola.[25] Just a few years later, the new governor, Luís César de Meneses, wrote that, of the 200 soldiers who had accompanied him to Angola, fewer than 50 were still alive. The Overseas Council now agreed that 'islanders' fared poorly in West-Central Africa, and it recommended recruiting men from the province of Ribatejo instead. However, finding volunteers to move to Angola from Portugal was difficult, and the Governor of Madeira was advised to keep men ready to embark to Africa.[26] In 1702, the municipal council of Luanda added to the debate by reminding the Overseas Council, once again, that soldiers from the Atlantic islands were of little use in Angola because they perished easily as a result of the 'disease of the land' (*doença da terra*). Moreover, many of the soldiers were young boys poorly suited to carrying arms. The council members suggested sending 'islanders' to Brazil and sending Brazilians to serve as soldiers in Angola instead. In this way, the crown could save on the expenses incurred by the poorly acclimated Madeirans, and the best soldiers who were capable of serving in the tropics would then inhabit Angola in turn.[27]

By the beginning of the eighteenth century, officials in Angola and Portugal had become increasingly aware of how the origins of colonists affected their survival rates in West-Central Africa. It is difficult to assess how accurate these assessments were, as mortality statistics do not exist for this period. Therefore, the discussion on Madeiran soldiers does not offer much beyond stereotypes. It is also easy to see where such

[24] AHU, CU, Angola, Cx. 15, Doc. 1849, Consulta do Conselho Ultramarino ao rei sobre carta do governador de Angola, Henrique Jacques de Magalhães, 26 November 1696.
[25] Coates, *Convicts and Orphans*, 77.
[26] AHU, CU, Angola, Cx. 16, Doc. 1890, Consulta do Conselho Ultramarino ao rei sobre a carta do governador e capitão-general de Angola, Luís César de Meneses, 8 November 1700. On the recruitment of 300 soldiers from Madeira to Angola in 1701, see Cuvelier, ed., *Relations sur le Congo*, 27.
[27] AHU, CU, Angola, Cx. 17, Doc. 1913, Carta dos oficiais da câmara de Angola, ao rei sobre os soldados das ilhas serem de pouca utilidade em Angola, 22 April 1702.

stereotypes originated. A shipload of soldiers made up completely of men from Madeira who experienced a 75 per cent mortality rate within a few years of arrival could easily have given rise to a popular belief regarding their weakness. However, this does not yet prove that they fared any worse than men from continental Portugal.

The early modern methodology of determining which regions produced the best colonists for Angola can be inferred from another letter by Luanda's municipal council in 1703. Reminding the Overseas Council that men from Madeira were of no use in Angola because they were 'very weak people' (*gente muita froxa*), the local council members pointed out that many of the soldiers who had arrived twelve years earlier with Governor Gonçalo da Costa Meneses from continental Portugal, and others who had been born in Angola, were still alive. They claimed that 100 men from Portugal were better than 600 from Madeira. Apparently, environmental reasoning lay behind these calculations of the fittest colonists, because the conclusion was that men from the provinces of Ribatejo, Alentejo and Algarve were the ones who survived best in Central Africa's climate. These regions were best suited to provide soldiers for Angola because they were the hottest places in Portugal. In other words, there was an imagined link between Portuguese regional environments and the West-Central African climate.[28]

The recruitment of men to Angola remained a contested issue for years to come. In 1715, Governor Noronha again touched on the issue of recruiting soldiers from Madeira. Instead of using health and survival as a measure, he argued that the crown would save money by collecting a sufficient number of men in Portugal before sailing to Angola, because finding them in Madeira was very time consuming. If anything, this shows that Madeira was still a customary collection point for manpower to serve in West-Central Africa. This was confirmed a few years later, when the Overseas Council again recommended the enlisting of soldiers in Madeira 'as was always done' (*como sempre foi estillo*).[29] The recruitment of soldiers from Madeira was still going on in the 1730s, leading Governor Rodrigo César de Meneses to once again write about how the climate destroyed the islanders completely and to request soldiers from Brazil.[30]

[28] AHU, CU, Angola, Cx. 17, Doc. 1987, Consulta do Conselho Ultramarino ao rei sobre a carta dos oficiais da câmara e governadores de Angola, 21 August 1704. Cf. Coates, *Convicts and Orphans*, 99.

[29] AHU, CU, Angola, Cx. 20, Doc. 2115, Consulta do Conselho Ultramarino ao rei sobre a carta do governador e capitão-general de Angola, D. João Manuel de Noronha, 3 April 1716; AHU, CU, Angola, Cx. 22, Doc. 2235, Requerimento do nomeado para o governo de Angola, João de Saldanha da Gama, ao rei, earlier than 4 November 1720.

[30] AHU, CU, Angola, Cx. 30, Doc. 2885, Carta do governador e capitão-general de Angola, Rodrigo César de Meneses, ao rei, 20 June 1733; AHU, CU, Angola, Cx. 32, Doc. 3088, Consulta do Conselho Ultramarino ao rei D. João V sobre carta do

The high mortality rate of Portuguese-born soldiers led to a belief that Brazilian-born individuals were better suited to withstand the Central African climate and environment. Colonial governors and the Overseas Council often turned to Bahia, Pernambuco, Rio de Janeiro and Ceará for military reinforcements, although burial records indicate that Brazilians died of 'fevers' just like other foreign settlers. In addition to soldiers, Brazilian settlers in Angola included merchants and their agents. In the late eighteenth century, many of the merchants in Benguela were individuals born in Brazil. They included criminals and political exiles as well as former crewmembers on ships sailing between Benguela and Brazil. They operated as *sertanejos* in the central highlands, were either owners or co-owners of slave ships or dealt in slaves on behalf of Brazilian commercial houses. By marrying important local women, Brazilian-born men consolidated business partnerships and established powerful families. While most members of the Benguela merchant community came from Portugal, some of them had become 'Brazilian' by way of a prolonged stay in Brazil before settling in Benguela. The most successful among them maintained property and family on both sides of the Atlantic.[31]

Humans were not the only ones whose survival in Angola's climate was a concern for colonial officials. Horses were introduced and transported from Brazil to Angola, where mounted troops were an integral component of colonial military strategy. In the seventeenth century, horses came primarily from Pernambuco and Bahia in north-eastern Brazil, and by the mid-eighteenth century horses from Pernambuco were regarded as the most suitable for the Angolan climate. Like the forced migration of humans, the transportation of horses presented a challenge well into the eighteenth century. The mortality rate for horses hovered around 30 per cent. Like human migrants, recently arrived horses were particularly affected by diseases during military operations.[32] In the 1720s, the attempts to build a cavalry in Angola caused lengthy discussions about the adaptability of horses. One officer in charge of the horses complained that no one in Angola knew about their diseases. He requested that the

governador e capitão-general de Angola, Rodrigo César de Meneses, 28 November 1736.
[31] AHU, CU, Angola, Cx. 27, Doc. 2668, Carta do governador e capitão-general de Angola, Paulo Caetano de Albuquerque, ao rei, 20 December 1729; José C. Curto, '*Americanos* in a West Central African Slaving Port: The Rise and Fall of the Brazilian Community in Benguela, c. 1650–1850', unpublished draft paper; Mariana P. Candido, 'South Atlantic Exchanges: The Role of Brazilian-Born Agents in Benguela, 1650–1850', *Luso-Brazilian Review* 50:1 (2013): 53–82; Ferreira, *Transforming Atlantic Slaving*, 127, 131, 158–159.
[32] Ferreira, *Transforming Atlantic Slaving*, 184–188.

king send two specialists from Portugal who could cure animals. However, there are no indications that specialists in veterinary medicine ever practised their trade in Luanda or elsewhere in Angola in the eighteenth century.[33]

On the Move: Medicine and Environment in Angola

By the mid-seventeenth century, Europeans in Angola had developed a systematic, experience-based classification system for Central African environments ranging from more healthy environments to diseased ones. This, in turn, led to increased mobility within the region, as Portuguese soldiers travelled from the interior back to the coast to recover from illness. Luanda was the main destination for settlers serving in the interior, and a large number of soldiers were treated in the city's hospital each year.[34] Although the interior village of Massangano had a hospital, it was next to impossible to get a physician or a surgeon to work there because of the 'malignity of the climate', as former Governor Meneses remarked in 1703.[35]

Military campaigns were key moments when the pernicious nature of environment and climate was most directly felt and experienced, and they also provided for the earliest mappings of diseased environments. Military units also employed medical personnel to continually assess the relationship between environment and health. A surgeon was usually attached to the troops and followed the soldiers on their campaigns.[36] Portuguese soldiers and their African allies often had to travel relatively long distances within short periods of time.[37] Supplies were often wanting, and troops battled against disease and hunger as much as against their human enemies. The 1641–1648 campaign to oust the Dutch from Angola was a particularly intense period of movement within the region. A military unit transporting ammunition supplies from Kikombo to Massangano in 1645 noted losing up to five or six men daily

[33] AHU, CU, Angola, Cx. 27, Doc. 2678, Requerimento do capitão de cavalos de Angola, Álvaro de Carvalho e Meneses, ao rei, earlier than 25 January 1730.
[34] E.g. AHU, CU, Angola, Cx. 15, Doc. 1818, Consulta do Conselho Ultramarino ao rei sobre carta do provedor e irmãos da Misericórdia da cidade de São Paulo de Assunção do reino de Angola, 29 January 1695.
[35] AHU, CU, Angola, Cx. 17, Doc. 1934, Consulta do Conselho Ultramarino ao rei sobre o parecer solicitado ao Luís César de Meneses, 21 May 1703.
[36] On fees paid to surgeons in military service, see, e.g., Angola, Cx. 14, Doc. 1781, Consulta do Conselho Ultramarino ao rei sobre carta do governador de Angola, 27 November 1693.
[37] For a general outline of warfare in West-Central Africa, see John K. Thornton, *Warfare in Atlantic Africa 1500–1800* (London: Routledge, 1999), 99–125.

to diseases caused by the 'malign' climate as the expedition proceeded. Governor Souto Maior described Massangano as the most harmful region in the world. In contrast, he regarded Kikombo on the coast as very healthy, which made other inconveniences more tolerable. However, this was before the onset of the rains and the diseases that came with them.[38]

A clear distinction between the coast and the interior as environmental zones with different effects on European health had clearly emerged by the mid-seventeenth century. This remained the main point of division throughout the eighteenth century. When health and the environment were discussed in the administrative letters sent to Lisbon from Angola, they almost invariably stated that any environment beyond Luanda was dangerous.[39] For example, when the Capuchins and Portuguese officials debated whether the death of a missionary in Dande should be investigated, the official view was that the missionary had died a natural death resulting from disease because the district of Dande was quite harmful.[40] The Jesuits, in turn, defended the concentration of their evangelising activities in Luanda by arguing that the Angolan *sertão* was unhealthy. However, this did not hinder the Capuchins from working inland.[41]

Officers serving in the interior *presídios* sometimes abandoned their post citing failing health. This was the case in 1720 with the captain-major of Massangano, João Quaresma de Brito, who was claimed to suffer from scabies. He had not received official permission from the governor to leave Massangano, and there were questions about whether he should receive a salary during his absence. Rumour had it that Brito had no intention of returning to Massangano. However, he continued to serve in the military, including service as the captain-major of Ambaca, and he occasionally turned up in documentation until his death was reported in 1732.[42]

[38] AHU, CU, Angola, Cx. 4, Doc. 378, Carta do governador de Angola, Francisco Souto Maior ao rei, 4 December 1645; AHU, CU, Angola, Cx. 4, Doc. 382, Consulta do Conselho Ultramarino ao rei sobre carta do governador de Angola, 10 February 1646.
[39] An early Jesuit letter giving an account of the mission in the years 1602–1603, however, alleges that Cambambe in the interior is 'one of the healthiest lands' in Atlantic Africa. Its climate was reputedly very different from that of the coast. 'Missão dos Jesuitas em Angola (1602–1603)', in Brásio, ed., *MMA*, V: 54.
[40] '... aver falecido o dito capucho de doença que lhe deu no dito destricto por ser muito nocivo'. AHU, CU, Angola, Cx. 18, Doc. 1962, Carta do ouvidor-geral de Angola, Manuel Gomes Cabral de Távora, ao rei respondendo à carta régia, 20 July 1703.
[41] AHU, CU, Angola, Cx. 22, Doc. 2305, Consulta do Conselho Ultramarino ao rei sobre o aviso do governador e capitão-general de Angola, António de Albuquerque Coelho de Carvalho, 22 March 1723.
[42] AHU, CU, Angola, Cx. 22, Doc. 2226, Carta do provedor-mor da Fazenda Real de Angola, Francisco de Santa Bárbara e Moura, ao rei sobre o capitão-mor da vila de

Although the sources abound with references to the malign environment of the Angolan interior, the movement of people to Luanda to seek treatment can also, at least partially, be explained by the fact that Luanda had practically the only permanently functioning hospital in Angola. Luanda, therefore, was perhaps not much healthier than other places in West-Central Africa. A report from the bishop in the early eighteenth century complained that many clerics in Luanda often excused themselves from Mass because of illness caused by the 'distemperance of the climate' (*destemperança do clima*).[43]

After three centuries of sporadic but uncontested documentation on the unhealthy nature of the Angolan interior, it is remarkable to see the opinion of Chief Physician José Pinto de Azeredo, who in the late eighteenth century claimed that the distant hinterlands and Benguela were healthier and more benign than Luanda. Arguing that these regions had more trees and larger forests than Luanda and its immediate environs, he based his view on environmental reasoning. Moreover, the majority of African trees produced quantities of resin and fragrant balsam that cleansed the air. Apparently, Azeredo chose not to acknowledge popular perceptions about Benguela's health or else he did not believe them.[44]

It is noteworthy that Lind, whose work Azeredo was certainly familiar with, wrote that 'the kingdom, and especially the city of Benguela, are remarkable for a pestiferous air'. This was in contrast to Luanda, which was 'said to be tolerably healthy'. Lind also raised the city of São Salvador (Mbanza Kongo) to mythical status, referring to it as 'the healthiest place, or the Montpellier, for its air', in Portuguese Africa. 'Being perfectly situated on a hill', he wrote, 'and the neighboring country being cleared of the natural woods and thickets, its inhabitants breathe a temperate and pure air, and are in a great measure exempted from all the plagues of an unhealthy climate.' How had Lind come to this conclusion? Unlike Finke, cited at the beginning of this chapter, Lind

---

Massangano, João Quaresma de Brito, 5 September 1720; AHU, CU, Angola, Cx. 26, Doc. 2604, Requerimento do ex-capitão-mor da vila de Massangano, João Quaresma de Brito, ao rei, earlier than 11 October 1728; AHU, CU, Angola, Cx. 28, Doc. 2775, Consulta do Conselho Ultramarino ao rei sobre a nomeação de pessoas para o posto de capitão-mor do presídio de Ambaca, 25 January 1732.

[43] AHU, CU, Angola, Cx. 17, Doc. 1984, Carta do Bispo de Angola, D. Luís Simão Brandão, ao rei, 10 May 1704. Distemperance generally referred to an imbalance of the four humours or of the four qualitites, or a morbid condition attributed to imbalance of the four humours. See Juhani Norri, *Dictionary of Medical Vocabulary in English, 1375–1550: Body Parts, Sicknesses, Instruments, and Medicinal Preparations* (London: Routledge, 2016); cf. Bluteau, *Vocabulario*, 3: 174.

[44] Azeredo, *Ensaios*, 42.

included references to earlier writers quite sparingly in his work, although he did cite extensively from journals kept by other surgeons. Lind's own travels as a navy surgeon took him to West Africa, where he undoubtedly discussed medical matters with other practitioners, such as a 'medical gentleman' accompanying the British troops to capture Galam from the French, and a 'surgeon, who practiced some years at Senegal'. Therefore, Lind's account must be taken as an indication of circulating popular ideas about health conditions and the environment in Central Africa.[45]

Travelling for Health: Healing Environments in the Southern Atlantic World

Medical travel was fairly common in early modern Europe. Spa towns and sanatoriums were favoured destinations for people seeking alleviation from pain and cures for diseases. In accordance with humoural theory, environment and climate were among the non-naturals that most affected an individual's constitution. Spas or thermal springs were also recognised as an important means to restored health in early modern Portugal. In his travels through Portugal in 1609, Manoel Severim de Faria drew attention to the village of Soaserra, 'a healthy place' well known for the quality of its water, which had been prescribed to Queen Dona Catherina and was regarded as a good remedy for hookworm infection.[46] In the Portuguese Empire, 'change of air' was a common expression. Medical travel emerged as an important feature of southern Atlantic migration patterns in the seventeenth century, when Portuguese soldiers began to travel from Central Africa to Brazil or Portugal for health reasons. Officers serving in Angola required permission from the king to travel. Failing health and a lack of available healthcare were often used as justifications for leave requests, and they served as an acceptable excuse for departing Africa.

---

[45] Lind, *An Essay on Diseases*, 37–38, 51–53, 55. On Lind's work, see David I. Harvie, *Limeys: The Conquest of Scurvy* (Thrupp: Sutton Publishing, 2002); Seth, *Difference and Disease*, 104–110. Lind's perception was subsequently repeated in Wadström, *An Essay on Colonization*, I: 43–44, who claimed to have 'often heard St. Salvadore mentioned as the most healthful spot on the globe, except the island of Ceylon'. Montpellier was especially renowned for its watering sites, which continue to attract patients in search of relief from chronic ills. The Eaux de Balaruc were much acclaimed and recommended by physicians. On Montpellier as a medical town in the eighteenth century, see Elizabeth A. Williams, *A Cultural History of Medical Vitalism in Enlightenment Montpellier* (Aldershot: Ashgate, 2003), 16–39.

[46] Joaquim Veríssimo Serrão, ed., *Viagens em Portugal de Manuel Severim de Faria 1604–1609–1625* (Lisbon: Academia Portuguesa da História, 1974), 79–80.

Earliest documented signs of the importance of travel for health reasons in the Portuguese Atlantic date from the 1670s, although it is likely that there were precedents to this idea. In 1673, the Overseas Council discussed Balthazar Vandunen's petition to leave Angola. Vandunen, who had served for thirty-three years in West-Central Africa, referred to his age and ailments, claiming that he was unable to find a remedy for his ailments in Angola. He argued that since the country was sickly and had no doctors, he should be allowed to return to Portugal via Brazil. The king accepted his request and granted him a licence to return to Europe.[47] Three decades later, Belchior Garcia de Góis, who had served in the *sertões* of the colonies of Angola and Benguela, travelled to Salvador, in the Brazilian captaincy of Bahia, for the treatment of serious malaise, citing a lack of medicines and surgeons in Angola as his reason for travelling.[48]

Health issues were considered an adequate reason for requesting temporary leave or a permanent exit from military service in Angola. Portugal, and more specifically Lisbon (Figure 7.1), was the most common destination. Travelling there usually implied that the patient was not going to return to Angola. Officers leaving for Brazil, on the other hand, were expected to return to Angola and assume their duties after recovering. In a few cases, the destination was left open, and leave was granted to travel either to Brazil or to Portugal. In one case, the destination was left completely open. Chief Physician Aboim and Surgeon-Major Francisco da Costa, who in 1724 had diagnosed a soldier named Manuel Rodrigues with cirrhotic internal abscess, simply wrote that Rodrigues should be transferred to a place where he would be guaranteed better air and alimentation (*melhores ares e alimentos*). Rodrigues, born in the village of Estremos, had arrived in Luanda four and half years earlier, when he was twenty-four years old. Apparently, the reasoning behind the doctors' diagnosis was that he could not be cured by eating local food in Angola's climate.[49]

For officers going on temporary leave, Brazil was thought to offer not only a more salubrious climate but also more medical expertise. It also had a much better supply of medicines compared to Angola. This was clearly expressed by Bishop Frei Manuel de Santa Catarina, who

---

[47] AHU, CU, Angola, Cx. 11, Doc. 1322, Consulta do Conselho Ultramarino ao príncipe regente D. Pedro sobre o requerimento de Balthasar van Dunen, 6 July 1673.

[48] AHU, CU, Angola, Cx. 17, Doc. 1983, Requerimento do tenente de campo de Angola, Belchior Garcia de Góis, ao rei, earlier than 10 March 1704.

[49] AHU, CU, Angola, Cx. 24, Doc. 2442, Requerimento do soldado Manuel Rodrigues, da companhia do capitão Vitoriano de Faria e Melo, ao rei, earlier than 8 November 1725.

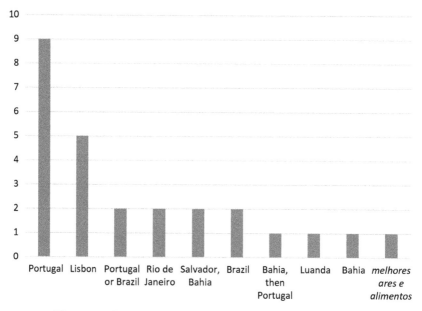

Figure 7.1 Destinations of officers granted temporary or indefinite leave from Angola, 1673–1747[50]

requested permission to travel to Bahia in 1726, where there were 'copious doctors and a multiplicity of pharmacies'.[51] Even a physician had to occasionally throw his hands up in the air and admit defeat in the face of the climate. This was the case with Physician-Major Eusébio Catela de Lemos, who wanted to leave for Brazil after serving only a year in Luanda. Citing the intemperance of the climate as a direct threat to his health, Lemos argued that he would perish if he stayed in Angola.[52] However, he was not granted leave, and seven years later Lemos renewed his request.[53]

[50] AHU, CU, Angola, Cx. 11, Doc. 1322; Cx. 19, Doc. 1983; Cx. 22, Docs. 2200, 2226, 2238; Cx. 23, Doc. 2389; Cx. 24, Docs. 2399, 2405, 2442, 2468; Cx. 25, Doc. 2487; Cx. 26, Doc. 2628; Cx. 27, Docs. 2665, 2685; Cx. 30, Docs. 2875, 2911, 2948; Cx. 34, Doc. 3291; Cx. 35, Docs. 3327, 3335; Cx. 37, Doc. 3544; Cx. 38, Doc. 3613.
[51] AHU, CU, Angola, Cx. 24, Doc. 2468, Requerimento do Bispo de Angola, ao rei, earlier than 18 January 1726.
[52] AHU, CU, Angola, Cx. 30, Doc. 2948, Requerimento do físico-mor de Angola, Eusébio Catela de Lemos, ao rei, earlier than 13 August 1734.
[53] AHU, CU, Angola, Cx. 35, Doc. 3335, Consulta do Conselho Ultramarino ao rei sobre o requerimento do físico-mor de Angola, Eusébio Catela de Lemos, 14 December 1741.

Salvador, which was the favoured destination for medical travel for officers serving in Angola, had a single general hospital administered by the Misericórdia. From the late seventeenth century onwards, it was known as the Hospital of St Christopher. While Bahia was portrayed as a healing environment, real as opposed to imagined conditions there left much to be desired. Russell-Wood has described Salvador as 'a city where sanitation was bad and disease common'. The city's municipal council failed to examine foodstuffs and medicines sent from Europe, and periodic inspections of the pharmacies, to ensure that old stock was destroyed, were not performed. Although the hygienic and medical conditions were not as perfect as they were thought to be, they were nevertheless better than in Angola.[54]

The Misericórdia hospital of Salvador had two wards, the medical ward (*enfermaria das chagas*) and the fever ward (*enfermaria das febres*). Conditions were cramped and it is unlikely that there were beds for all the patients. A madhouse and a ward for women were added in the eighteenth century. The Misericórdia employed a paid medical staff, ranging from well-qualified doctors and surgeons to male nurses and medical assistants. Their duties included visiting the hospital in the morning and evening as well as being on call at any hour of the day if summoned to the hospital. According to Russell-Wood, there are no registers of the number of patients treated in the hospital, the nature of their illness or their identity and place of origin. It is therefore unclear how many of the soldiers arriving from Angola went to be treated in the hospital. Generally, anyone who could afford the services of a doctor received treatment in his own home, and the patients of the Misericórdia mainly consisted of the poor. In the case of wealthier officers from Angola, this would have meant renting a room or staying with relatives while receiving medical attention from Bahia's doctors and surgeons. However, even Bahian soldiers usually had to rely on the hospital of the Misericórdia.[55]

Occasionally treatment in Brazil was not regarded as sufficient, and the men serving in Angola proceeded to Lisbon, some returning permanently to Portugal. This was the case with Francisco de Buitrago, who after twenty-six years of serving in Angola in various positions, travelled to Salvador in 1718 because of maladies caused by the 'adverse climate'. Not finding alleviation from his illness in Bahia, where he received

---

[54] On medical conditions, hygiene and healthcare in colonial Bahia, see Russell-Wood, *Fidalgos and Philanthropists*, 260–294, quote from page 294.

[55] Russell-Wood, *Fidalgos and Philanthropists*, 260–294.

'repetitious cures', he proceeded to Lisbon. Buitrago complained of suffering from an illness in the throat that put his life in danger.[56]

When petitioning for the right to return to Europe, Portuguese officers almost invariably referred to their own illness. Portuguese women and complete *reinol* families were few in number in Angola, but they are occasionally mentioned in documentation concerning health and travel. One of these rare glimpses is offered by acting Governor José Carvalho da Costa's letter of 1725, in which he requested that the king grant his family permission to travel to Lisbon not only because of his own illness, but because of his wife's infirmity (*huma largua infermidade*). Given that his wife could not enjoy an hour of health in Luanda, Costa argued that only the change of 'airs' (or climate) could alleviate her condition. Citing the common complaint about the lack of physicians, Costa also referred to the absence of hot springs in Luanda as a reason for returning to Lisbon. His family was granted a two-year leave, after which he was to return to Angola. Once in Lisbon, and not intending to return to Luanda, Costa renewed his petition in 1729, arguing that the climate of Central Africa was damaging to his constitution. Doctor Francisco da Fonseca Henriques wrote a letter in support of Costa that the only available remedy was the hot springs of Caldas da Rainha in Portugal.[57]

Around the same time that Costa's family requested to return to Portugal, another married couple was making plans to leave Angola. Clemente de Sousa Jácome, a resident in Luanda, complained that he had for a long time suffered from total irritation of the stomach, great inappetence and continuous vomiting. Doctor Felipe Cortes Velasco's diagnosis was that his condition was caused by an 'exorbitant quantity of phlegmatic humour', which made his constitution extremely plethoric. The sickness had debilitated his nerves and made him completely incapable of leading a normal life. Jácome's wife, Dona Catherina de Navas, was equally sick, although for a different reason. They had tried all remedies and aid available locally without finding a cure. Similar to interim Governor Costa, Jácome argued that they needed prompt and efficient medicines as well as baths in Portugal's hot springs, or otherwise they would perish shortly. The physician's medical statement was annexed to his petition. In short, his opinion summed up the fact that

---

[56] AHU, CU, Angola, Cx. 22, Doc. 2238, Consulta do Conselho Ultramarino ao rei, sobre o requerimento de Francisco de Buitrago, 11 January 1721.

[57] AHU, Cx. 23, Doc. 2389, Carta do José Carvalho da Costa ao rei, 19 April 1725; AHU, CU, Angola, Cx. 26, Doc. 2628, Requerimento do mestre de campo do terço de Infantaria paga de Angola, José Carvalho da Costa, ao rei, earlier than 27 April 1727. On the presence of Portuguese families in Angola, see Coates, *Convicts and Orphans*, 174.

the couple could not be cured so long as they remained in the Central African climate – *ratione climatis*. Therefore, they were advised to move elsewhere.[58]

Adjusting to the climate was a crucial issue for those Portuguese wanting to stay alive and not succumb to illness in Angola. In some cases, soldiers argued that their constitutions simply did not accord with life in Angola. João da Costa Rocha, who had been born near Coimbra and arrived in Angola after spending some time in Rio de Janeiro, argued in the mid-1720s that his 'temperament' was not right for the Central African climate, and having already served his term of six years in the military, he requested permission to return to Portugal. Without diagnosing his illness, Rocha simply mentioned that his health was less good than it had been before and that he suffered from repetitious maladies.[59] Yet for others, sick leave and treatment in Brazil were sufficient for recovery. Upon his return to Luanda from a one-year fixed-term leave in Rio de Janeiro, Captain Francisco Cordeiro da Silva immediately requested that the crown pay his salary for the duration of his absence. The request was granted.[60]

Maintaining Hygiene and Improving Public Health

Preventive medicine was an important part of the early modern intellectual landscape. Galen had divided medicine into hygiene and therapeutics, and the inclusion of the preventive part was thought to be necessary, although it was sometimes questioned. The six non-naturals were the main organisational principle in the field of dietetics, or hygiene. The Galenic framework continued to hold sway in early modern Europe, remaining relatively unchanged until the nineteenth century. However, the flexible theoretical framework of preventive medicine allowed for various interpretations.[61] As already alluded to above, individual physicians placed a different emphasis on environmental and climatic factors when explaining disease in Angola. Therefore, their hygienic frameworks were also different. Moreover, medical practitioners only

---

[58] AHU, Cx. 24, Doc. 2405, Requerimento de Clemente de Sousa Jácome, ao rei, earlier than 12 June 1725.

[59] AHU, CU, Angola, Cx. 25, Doc. 2487, Requerimento do soldado João da Costa Rocha, ao rei, earlier than 22 March 1726.

[60] AHU, CU, Angola, Cx. 38, Doc. 3613, Requerimento do capitão de Infantaria do terço pago de Angola, Francisco Cordeiro da Silva, ao rei, earlier than 18 March 1747.

[61] Heikki Mikkeli, *Hygiene in the Early Modern Medical Tradition* (Helsinki: Finnish Academy of Science and Letters, 1999), 8–10.

had a limited effect on Luanda's public health since their recommendations could only be put into action by governors.

In line with ancient pneumatic theories that diseases were caused by
impure air, the Portuguese occasionally made efforts to improve hygienic
conditions in Luanda. One of the early examples of this line of thought
can be found in the 1650s, when João Fernandes Vieira came to occupy
the seat of governor in Luanda. Noticing the large number of animals on
the streets, he concluded that this could cause bad odours and bring
about diseases. Vieira was informed that the municipal council had
already prohibited the keeping of these domestic animals alone on the
streets to avoid contagious diseases. Because the prohibition did not
seem to have had an effect, Vieira ordered his soldiers to kill all animals
that were roaming the streets without an apparent owner. Soon after, a
patrol observed two such animals and proceeded to slay them, but this
was interrupted by armed blacks, who not only saved the animals but left
the soldiers wounded. When the blacks were later captured, it turned out
that they belonged to the Jesuit college, which duly excommunicated
Vieira and the soldiers involved in the skirmish, causing a scandal in
Luanda and a heated argument between secular and religious authorities.
Leaving aside the ensuing scandal, this incident shows how early modern
hygienic arguments permeated colonial society. When public health was
at stake, the governor and municipal council members could call for a
stricter enforcement of hygienic measures but not necessarily without
causing ire among the residents.[62]

Portuguese physicians serving in Luanda in the second half of the
eighteenth century wrote profusely on hygienic measures and preventive
medicine. In Francisco Damião Cosme's view, it was easier to prevent
than to cure tropical maladies. He argued that it was possible to maintain
one's health in Central Africa if a person paid close attention to food,
drink, exercise, cleanliness and avoiding passions. Cosme's manuscript
on endemic diseases included detailed instructions on selecting uncor-
rupted foodstuffs, which he saw as a major factor in maintaining health
and well-being. Eating was to be accompanied by drinking moderate
amounts of wine and *aguardente,* for these were regarded as the most
efficient remedies to prevent scurvy and fevers. For people travelling to
the hinterlands, Cosme offered the advice that they should boil the

---

[62] 'Carta Régia providenciado sobre a excomunhão lançada pelos Religiosos da
Companhia de Jesus, contra o Governador João Fernandes Vieira, 9 December 1666',
Arquivos de Angola, First Series, 2:7 (1936): 13–14. Alencastro, *O Trato dos viventes,* 277;
Leandro Nascimento de Souza, *Uma experiência pernambucana em Angola: o governo de
João Fernandes Vieira, 1658 a 1661* (unpublished MA thesis, Recife, Universidade
Federal de Pernambuco, 2013), 90–93.

drinking water originating in rivers, lakes and wells before collecting it in clay pots for transportation and consumption. Further on, he pointed out that exercise, cleanliness of the body and accommodation as well as maintaining a peaceful soul were all integral to staying healthy. All this makes it clear that Damião Cosme conceptualised health and hygiene as a private matter of the individual rather than as a public health issue in colonial society.[63]

Soon after Cosme, José Pinto de Azeredo gave comprehensive descriptions of Luanda's hygiene and recommendations for improving it. The lack of fresh water was a constant cause of concern for Luandans, who mainly drank water transported from the Bengo River. Water from the Bengo, however, was corrupted by human activities; those living along the Bengo dumped the spoils from their plantations into the river. In Azeredo's view, this water was a vehicle for corrupting human bodies. The well in Maianga was used by a large number of Luandans, but its water was heavy and brackish. Besides the rainwater collected in a large cistern in the fortress of São Miguel, Azeredo found a small and completely ignored source of water on the beach at Cassandama. In his analysis, the water contained much gypsum and sulphur, but as a benign laxative it could be used daily. Azeredo had often used it successfully for certain chronic complaints.[64]

Other environmental factors also had hygienic implications. As already noted, Azeredo saw the lack of trees in Luanda as a potential cause for health problems. He insisted on their conservation and called for an increase in their numbers. Azeredo also noted the diligence of Angola's governors in ridding Luanda and its vicinity of swamps and pools of stagnant water, although some more distant ones still remained. In addition to nature, some human activities also caused Azeredo concern. The immense number of slaves brought to Luanda from all parts of the interior constituted a health risk. The large straw huts that rotted in the rain released noxious gases, and the huge numbers of cadavers that lay poorly buried around the town were all causes for alarm. Azeredo admitted that it was difficult, but not impossible, to remove them; it certainly demanded action by those responsible for the public good.[65]

Careless burial of dead bodies in and around Luanda and Benguela constituted a serious hazard to public health. The thousands of slaves dying in Luanda were dumped in a heap in a small cemetery near Luanda's commercial district or deposited in shallow graves in numbers far greater than could be covered decently. Hyenas picked over dead

[63] Cosme, 'Tractado das queixas endemicas', 178–185.   [64] Azeredo, *Ensaios*, 37–41.
[65] Azeredo, *Ensaios*, 43, 47, 50–51.

bodies during the night. At Benguela, the bodies of the slaves were simply thrown out onto the beach along with sewage until the very end of the eighteenth century. A new cemetery was laid for slaves and unbaptised Africans at the end of the eighteenth century, but even then, corpses were partially burnt and left for scavenging birds and animals. When gravediggers could not keep up with the growth of the 'mountain of semi-decomposed cadavers', they simply burned them.[66]

Very little changed in the early nineteenth century. The colonial elites and wealthier Lusoafricans were given a church burial, whereas African elites were entombed according to local rites. The vast majority of the population were either consigned to the public graveyard or buried according to local custom in tombs (*monturos*) along the side of the road. In Luanda and Benguela, hyenas and jackals continued to enter the cemetery for commoners, where the bodies lay poorly covered. The colonial administration paid more attention to the loud burial ceremonies of the blacks, which it considered heathenish and inappropriate, while neglecting public health and hygiene.[67]

Conclusion

Medical geography emerged gradually in West-Central Africa as ancient ideas gave way to practical experience in the tropics. While the majority of Portuguese settlers in Angola viewed the climate as having a major influence on health and illness, physicians who wrote about diseases had differing views that were not always in line with popular opinions. These opinions affected discourses how health and environment related to the provenance of human and animal migrants best suited to the African climate, the differences between coastal and interior regions of Angola, health travel and hygiene. Minor steps to improve the hygienic environment were taken between the seventeenth and eighteenth centuries, but these measures were extremely limited. Overall, there was minimal effort to develop public health in the colony of Angola during this period. Instead, climate emerged as the major explanatory factor for the prevalence of disease in the region. For colonial officers and settlers wanting to leave Angola behind, it became an honourable excuse for departing.

Global considerations of medical geography were not influential except in the writings of physicians, and even those remained rooted in

---

[66] Miller, *Way of Death*, 391–393.
[67] João Figueiredo, 'The City's Silent Double: Public Cemeteries in Angola from the Enlightenment to the Scramble', in *African Dynamics in a Multipolar World* (Lisbon: ISCTE-IUL, 2014), 860–879.

the Hippocratic and Galenic tradition. A local medical geography, based on directly experiencing the nature and climate of different locations in West-Central Africa, emerged and played a major role in how health and disease were conceptualised. In other words, Europeans in Angola made little use of knowledge on medical geography emerging elsewhere in the Portuguese Atlantic and Asia. A global synthesis of medical geography emerged only in the late eighteenth century. But as Finke's work (cited at the beginning of this chapter) demonstrates, even a global synthesis had to be deeply rooted in accounts describing local circumstances.

Conclusion

Maintaining health and well-being was a central concern for peoples of Atlantic Africa and for outsiders who visited or settled in the region from the mid-fifteenth century onwards. From the very beginning, cross-cultural medical interaction was the norm, not the exception, as Africans and Europeans sought to tap different sources of healing knowledge. In general, locals and newcomers were open to experimenting with different curing methods and healing materials originating on different continents, viewing these encounters as opportunities for obtaining new techniques. The mobility of people, knowledge and materials came to characterise the world of healing in the Black Atlantic.

Studying African healing knowledge in the early modern world presents a number of methodological challenges. The first is that the sources are rarely rich enough to answer all the questions a historian wants to ask, and therefore, many answers remain tentative and incomplete. The clearest obstacle to knowing the world of African healing is that textual sources were mostly produced by European colonists and describe the lives of settlers instead of autochthonous Africans. Most descriptions of African healing practices and materials remain limited because witnesses did not understand the contents and deeper meanings of ritual practices or were motivated by religious and ethnic prejudice to write derogatorily on what they regarded as pagan practices. Inquisition sources offer rare glimpses into Africans' own experiences of indigenous healing. However, even with these documents many challenges remain because Inquisitors were not necessarily interested in hearing Africans' own conceptualisations of health and medicine but wanted instead to place their testimonies within a demonic framework.

Studying the contents of ritual practices in detail, as a medical or cultural anthropologist might do, is therefore not possible in early modern Atlantic Africa. Similarly, it is impossible to know what plant medicines were used in certain rituals and why. In Inquisition trials, outsiders often mentioned only the use of roots and herbs, not their names or the local spiritual meanings attached to them.

212

Pharmacopoeias collected by European soldiers and botanists, on the contrary, mentioned the names of healing plants and tried to list their local uses, but it is likely that even they missed many local spiritual connotations either out of ignorance or disinterest. Pharmacopoeias rarely mentioned how various plants and animals were connected to local spiritual entities, although such connections must have existed.[1] A clear exception is Francisco Buitrago's manuscript on the tree of life, where he considered the Kongolese folk Catholic beliefs regarding *enkasa*.

This brings us to a second major methodological challenge, namely detecting change and innovation in Atlantic African healing knowledge in the early modern period. While more recent anthropological studies might reveal local interpretations and beliefs on the connections between spirits and natural substances, these reflect twentieth- and twenty-first-century realities. They do not reveal the ancestry of spiritual practices, nor when such beliefs were invented and introduced. By labelling African medical practices 'traditional', 'ancestral' or 'prehistoric', Africa and Africans are denied the possibility to change and evolve throughout history. Precolonial African societies changed as a result of cultural interactions with Europeans and the Islamic world, and these changes also affected health, healing and medicine.

In studying lists of medical ingredients collected in West-Central Africa between the sixteenth and eighteenth centuries, it is easy to see that new substances were from time to time added to the lists. Do these additions signal innovations or 'discoveries' that were new to both Portuguese and Africans? Or, were they medical secrets gradually revealed to Europeans? It is possible that they might simply signal the geographical expansion of Portuguese interests in the region or the increasing mobility of medical substances along slaving routes from the interior to the coast. Although not documented, it is fully possible that Africans invented local medicines to suit European needs or answer a demand. Rather than seeing African healing knowledge as a closed system, this study suggests that innovation took place in the field of health and medicine, although it is difficult to understand the full extent of these processes due to the limits of available documentation.

The third methodological issue is also connected to the nature and range of documentation. It is difficult to say how much documentation has been lost, but the lack of hospital records from Portuguese Angola is a major issue. Although some hospital statistics survive, they are mainly

---

[1] See, e.g., Allen F. Roberts, *A Dance of Assassins: Performing Early Colonial Hegemony in the Congo* (Bloomington: Indiana University Press, 2013), 72–73, 81.

from the late eighteenth century onwards. If records were kept earlier, they are still hidden in the archives somewhere. They would help clarify how many people were treated in the hospitals annually, what were the major diagnostic categories and what was the ethnic make-up of the hospital patients. Although descriptions of illness are often too vague to draw firm conclusions on biological diagnoses, the records make it possible to reconstruct contemporary social diagnoses of bodily illnesses. They also make it possible to glimpse the mental and emotional responses of Africans and Europeans in Atlantic Africa.

The spread of Atlantic slaving led to the rise of a new category of mental suffering, referred to as *banzar* or *banzamento*, and later *banzo*. Its nature and treatment were commented on by Portuguese rather than Africans, and as such the African perspective on this novel malady is harder to reach. Mental afflictions affected not only the lives of slaves destined for Brazil, but also those who stayed behind. In the southern Atlantic, the Portuguese opted to use the Kimbundu derivative *banzar* to denote melancholy. The meaning of melancholy changed dramatically in the early modern Portuguese Atlantic in the eighteenth century as *banzamento* was gradually being tied to emerging notions of race, becoming a disease of the blacks. In the southern Atlantic world of Angola and Brazil, this transformation was completed by the adoption of the Kimbundu term *banzo* to signify melancholy.

An important feature of documentation on health and medicine is the substantial number of laypeople's voices on these issues. European medical specialists writing about health and illness were rare in Atlantic Africa. Although their views can be discerned occasionally in official correspondence, only a few physicians and surgeons wrote longer treatises about tropical medicine. The foremost names in the seventeenth century, Aleixo de Abreu and Samuel Brun, wrote in completely different genres, with Abreu directing his treatise at learned physicians and Brun his travel account at general readers. Moreover, many manuscripts in the Portuguese world remained unpublished, and hence, probably had little to no influence in guiding healing practices in West-Central Africa. In the end, European physicians and surgeons were not the major specialists on matters of health in Atlantic Africa. The conceptual framework of humoural medicine was poorly adapted to tropical Africa and brought limited results in terms of recovering from illness. Physicians' inability to offer potent cures and to lower the mortality rate of Europeans on the coast might be the main reason for their relative silence in the documentary record.

In addition to lay and specialist voices, those of Africans occasionally emerge in the documentary record. Denunciations to the Inquisition in

Angola are a good place to start interpreting African views on health and medicine. Importantly, they point to the broad meaning of medicine, ranging from material to spiritual. Central Africans, who came to confess their participation in indigenous healing rituals to the Inquisitors, should be seen as good Catholics rather than as pagans who had merely been baptised but not instructed in the Catholic faith. Their confessions in front of priests show that they had not only memorised prayers but also understood quite well the sacrament of confessing sins and the concept of repentance.

Even with numerous methodological challenges, documentary evidence shows the prevalence of cross-cultural medical interaction in Atlantic Africa. Although it was often criticised by newcomers from Europe, men who wanted to survive in this region turned to local medical specialists to obtain cures and medicines. Cross-cultural exchanges moved in both directions because Africans were similarly interested in what Europeans had to offer. In Africa, obtaining new medicines was often tied to local notions of political power; those who controlled healing also controlled people. For Europeans, turning to African healers was often dictated by the practical challenges of obtaining European medicines and the lack of European practitioners in the region. However, distrust of European healing methods, especially excessive bloodletting, clearly motivated some settlers to turn to African healing knowledge.

Peak periods of cross-cultural medical interaction are difficult to identify. In Portuguese Angola, European access to local healing knowledge was a long cumulative process, one in which new medicinals were occasionally added to the arsenal of remedies. The second half of the eighteenth century, however, was a period when scientific interest in Atlantic African natural resources was especially intense. Joaquim José da Silva in Angola, Paul Erdmann Isert on the Gold Coast and Adam Afzelius in Sierra Leone stand as the best examples of European botanists' openness to the world of African natural medicines. Scientists of the eighteenth century did not shun indigenous ways of knowing but followed instead the earlier practice of employing cultural brokers, or go-betweens, to guarantee access to local knowledge. Monetary compensation was only one factor that smoothened out these exchanges. African informants possibly gained protection and established new networks by offering to assist European outsiders, who were often helpless without locals.

The search for botanical medicine in Atlantic Africa by Europeans displays a marked continuity from the sixteenth to the nineteenth centuries. The Portuguese who visited or resided in West-Central Africa documented the uses of several drugs based on their composition –

animal, vegetable or mineral. Among the most popular natural products sought and used by the Portuguese in Angola, it is possible to identify the *kikongo* tree, a redwood known locally as *takula*, *engariaria* and *enkasa*. Missionaries, military officers and merchants all played a role in disseminating ethnobotanical knowledge about these medicinals. As Africans' cultural interaction with Europeans deepened, medical practices became creolised with medicines made by mixing different ingredients.

African drugs had spread to Europe by the early seventeenth century, where they joined drugs imported from East Africa, Asia and Brazil. Information about indigenous African medicine found its way into pharmacopoeias produced in Portugal in the early eighteenth century. Knowledge may have travelled by word of mouth but also by means of written works and manuscripts. The extent to which African medicinals were exported from Atlantic Africa and moved along the Atlantic networks to the Americas and Europe remains an open question that would merit further study.

Religious and spiritual beliefs played into medical exchanges in a myriad of ways. There was both collaboration and competition, mutual interest and mutual fear. In the Kingdom of Kongo, Saint Anthony was transformed into a Kongo power object, or medicinal charm, while Italian Capuchins eagerly described plants used by local herbalists and healers. On the Gold Coast, the Danish preacher Monrad did not turn away from an African healer when he became sick; he went on to praise the work of local healers when writing his travel account of the Guinea Coast and its inhabitants. But despite these examples of positive interaction, it is worth remembering that cross-cultural medical exchanges were not always desired by the parties involved. Some individuals were suspicious of and feared the powers of the other, believing that those who could heal could also harm. Individual African healers might have felt the need to protect their knowledge and keep it secret.

Besides practical reasons regarding the lack of European medicines and doctors, perhaps a more important factor in medical interaction was openness to experimentation. This meant experimenting not only with African medicinals, but also with new materials from Asia and the Americas, such as cinchona bark, which was imported to different localities in Atlantic Africa from the beginning of the eighteenth century. Interaction was further made possible by conceptual and practical similarities in healing techniques as well as by similar European and African terms for describing health and disease. Early modern European folk beliefs connected to healing were quite similar to African spiritual ideas. Moreover, the Hippocratic-Galenic framework had little influence in daily interactions between patients and healers even before the second half of the eighteenth century, when it was openly challenged by physicians seeking to integrate new medical knowledge into their practice. Despite the efforts by physicians to introduce the newest European medical knowledge to Africa, in healthcare Europeans kept on borrowing more from locals than they gave in return.

Finally, the medical pluralism reigning in Atlantic Africa was both a precondition and a product of cross-cultural interaction in medicine. Healing and medicine in African societies was pluralistic even before the arrival of Europeans. Many kinds of healing specialists, many of them geographically mobile, offered their services to patients seeking greater health and well-being. Herbalists, healers specialising in curing certain ailments and healers devoted to certain spirits added to the African household medicine used in the daily context of treating minor illnesses. Atlantic African medical culture was open to innovative approaches and novel techniques even without the presence of Europeans, but their arrival only added to this plurality. European physicians, surgeons, pharmacists, barbers and even folk healers brought new alternatives and healing repertoires to local societies. However, the low number of European practitioners and their concentration in a few localities on the coast guaranteed that indigenous African medicines and therapies prevailed in the early modern period.

Technology transfers of medical practices were limited, but techniques were perhaps adapted to suit local needs. A good example of this is the widespread presence of black barbers in late eighteenth-century Angola. Given that lenient bloodletting and the use of cupping horns was one facet of traditional medicine in Angola before the Portuguese arrival, one should ask what was new about the presence of black barbers in this region. Perhaps there was no novelty, but nevertheless their presence speaks to cross-cultural understanding and mutual acceptance in the field of health and medicine. This was still possible in early modern Atlantic Africa before Europeans enchanted by notions of their own superiority began to shun local knowledge. Had they reflected upon their own history, they would have had to admit that African medicine and therapeutic traditions had largely sustained a European presence in the coastal settlements of Atlantic Africa for centuries.

Appendix A Francisco Buitrago's Herbal Remedies[1]

Name	Use	Buitrago's Observations
Enkasa	antidote against *feitiços*, used in indigenous poison ordeals	other virtues: can be used in curing deflux, flatus, ague, fever of the bladder, fresh wounds, colic, syphilis; also to protect its carrier from witches and *feitiços*
Pau Cobra	fever, ague, swellings, animal bites, air, gout, stomach pain, epilepsy, pains of the womb, fresh wounds, haemorrhoids, malady of Saint Lazarus	works also for large animals
Pau Musunda and its root	antidote, swellings, cordals, poisonous animals	yellow bark
Angariaria	antidote, stone, carnosity, heat, provokes urination, pain in the urinary canal, internal sores, bites of poisonous animals, chambers	experimented with it personally many times; on one occasion, gave to eight people and all were healed; kills poisonous animals and snakes
Teeth of seahorse	malign fevers, haemorrhoids, toothache	little to say about them
Genitalia of seahorse	carnosity, pleurisy	
Teeth of Angala (Engala)	fevers	
Coconut of Aflateva	cordals, fevers	originally from India, coconut of Maldives
Kiseko	fevers, headaches	white tree in Benguela, strong smell, used it personally, everybody uses it, sold in pieces and as whole trees
Kikongo	cordals	sold in the same way as Kiseko, but not as popular
Small coconuts of *misecos bravos*	stupor	comes from India, resembles small bananas (*miseko* in Kimbundu)

[1] Buytrago, *Arvore da vida*, ff. 68r–115v (see Chapter 2, fn 38 for full reference).

218

(*cont.*)

Name	Use	Buitrago's Observations
Nail of donkey, or Macoco	epilepsy	have no effect in Angola, but work well in Portugal
Eyes and tongue of viper, or tongue of São Paulo	antidote, cordals, fevers, animal bites, epilepsy	
Pepes	pain, headache, uterine accidents, epilepsy, pain in the womb, cataracts of the eye, clears eyesight	active smell; conducted many experiments with it
Kisama salt	fresh succours, reverses and cures the humour in haemorrhoids, eyes	also used in cooking
Ribs of hippopotamus	for/against air, obstructs nosebleed and bleeding in other parts, accidents and dizziness; works for fevers, pleurisies, acute and intermittent pain, and stupor	
Mundais	cordals, epilepsy, air	Experimented with this on two of my slaves, who became free of accidents
Quiseut? Quisau?	antidote, fevers	the best antidote after *enkasa*
Pau Saco (tree)	antidote	from the Kingdom of Kongo
Pau Assa (tree)	antidote	from the Kingdom of Kongo
Pau Safo (tree)	antidote	from the Kingdom of Kongo
Pau caminhaminha (tree)	antidote	from Angola
Pau Angolamuxe (tree)	antidote	from Angola
Pau Quiriato (tree)	antidote	from Angola
Pau Gungo (tree)	swellings	from Angola
Pau Paco (tree)	sores, old wounds, buboes or Gallic sores (yaws or syphilis)	from Angola
Motututo root	gout, swellings, hump, swollen testicles, provokes urination	grows abundantly in Angola
Dondolo root	sexual potency	did not have the said effect
Tumbata root	chambers	from Angola
Ensandeira (Nsanda) tree	wounds, fresh contusions, takes away pain, sores, weakness, obstructs bleedings, asthma, temples (of the head)	I tried this many times on people who did not expect to survive (when urinating blood or bleeding from the nose)

(cont.)

Name	Use	Buitrago's Observations
Elephant oil	asthma, cold pains, fevers	
Oil of Quelmes (a fish)	fresh wounds	also called the oil of São Cosme and São Damião, much used by everyone
Snake backbones	tonsillitis, seeping humours, goitre	
Maximas (big, round fava beans)	for air	
Kongo pepper	flatus	used as seasoning, imported to Angola from Kongo, much used
Irico fruit	heart chambers, carnosity, makes one urinate a lot	
Rabbit fur	pain	
Maravilhas, *Quingombo*	for air, headache	a rare flower growing in lakes, a strong scent
Porcupine teeth	fevers, colic, pain (of stone), pain (generally), womb, great antidote	
Massaa de leão	commences childbirth	
Rose of Jericho	helps in prolonged births	tried this on a slave whose life was in danger after trying to give birth for three days
Ink of China, or Nanguim	eye shadows, tripe, inflammations of the face, swellings, bloody flux	
Butua, or *Parreira Brava*	swellings, respiratory illness, kidney stones and urinary bladder, flatus, makes blood circulate better, stomach pain caused by crude humours, colic, antidote for poisonous animal bites	Kimbundu name is *Mulembuge u acanga*, much used among locals and also grows abundantly in Brazil; I always use it because it makes blood circulate and keeps the doctors and surgeons away
Almonds or nuts of sapwood	removes bones, removes pieces that get stuck in the throat	tall tree, grows abundantly in Brazil
Malice of women		a tree that grows in Bahia
Tobacco of São Domingos	headaches	
Water of the Queen of Hungary	headaches, eye sores, all kinds of scabies, phlegm and burning sensations in the throat, bladder, hearing problems, burns	

(*cont.*)

Name	Use	Buitrago's Observations
Cazango, Erva Baboza	sores in the feet	
Lemon	detergent	
Tripoli stone	detergent for cleaning silver	
Square stone	fever, carnosity, causes urination	
Root of *mugungue* tree		
Salve	removes a bad smell from the body	
Coffee	fevers, deflux, headaches	
Root of thousand men	purges the stomach	grows in the *sertão* of Bahia

Appendix B Imports of Medicinals and Medical Supplies to Luanda, 1802–1825 and 1837[1]

Year	Item	Unit	Quantity	Port	Region
1802	Rose water	Pipas	45	Portugal	Portugal
1802	Anise	Libras	78	Portugal	Portugal
1802	Ointment	Dúzias	438	Portugal	Portugal
1802	Medicinal remedies	Caixões	35		Brazil
1802	Tin syringes		76	Portugal	Portugal
1802	Brass syringes		16	Portugal	Portugal
1803	Drugs	Caixotes	4		Portugal
1803	Anise	Libras	208		Portugal
1803	Ointment	Dúzias	9,137		Portugal
1803	Medicinal remedies	Caixões	7		Brazil
1803	Tin syringes		198		Portugal
1803	Brass syringes		6		Portugal
1804	Água da Rainha	Vidros	200		Portugal
1804	Drugs	Caixões	9		Portugal
1804	Anise	Libras	409		Portugal
1804	Ointment	Dúzias	1,098		Portugal
1804	Medicinal remedies	Caixões	9		Brazil
1804	Tin syringes		220		Portugal
1804	Brass syringes		38		Portugal
1809	Pharmaceutical drugs	Caixões	6		Portugal
1809	Pharmaceutical drugs	Caixas	2		Portugal
1809	Pharmaceutical drugs	Cune	1		Portugal
1809	Pharmaceutical drugs	Caixotes	2		Portugal

[1] I would like to thank Daniel Domingues da Silva for kindly providing data on the imports of medicinals to Luanda. On the value of imported drugs, see Silva, *The Atlantic Slave Trade*, Appendix C, table C.9.

(*cont.*)

Year	Item	Unit	Quantity	Port	Region
1809	Pharmaceutical drugs	Barricas	1		Portugal
1809	Pharmaceutical drugs	Ancoretas	1		Portugal
1809	Tin syringes		6		Portugal
1810	Pharmaceutics	Caixote	1	Pernambuco	Brazil
1810	Pharmaceutical drugs	Caixas	8	Rio de Janeiro	Brazil
1810	Anise	Libras	16	Rio de Janeiro	Brazil
1810	Medical books		12	Rio de Janeiro	Brazil
1810	Ointment	Dúzias	8	Rio de Janeiro	Brazil
1810	Tin syringes		26	Rio de Janeiro	Brazil
1810	Tin syringes		11	Pernambuco	Brazil
1810	Cupping horns		40	Pernambuco	Brazil
1812	Pharmaceutical drugs	Caixote	1	Rio de Janeiro	Brazil
1812	Pharmaceutical drugs	Barris	2	Pernambuco	Brazil
1812	Pharmaceutical drugs	Caixetas	6	Pernambuco	Brazil
1812	Anise	Arrobas	2	Pernambuco	Brazil
1812	Medicinal remedies	Caixas	6	Rio de Janeiro	Brazil
1812	Medicinal remedies	Barris	2	Pernambuco	Brazil
1812	Medicinal remedies	Embro	2	Pernambuco	Brazil
1812	Tin syringes		14	Rio de Janeiro	Brazil
1812	Tin syringes		14	Pernambuco	Brazil
1812	Cupping horns	Dúzias	4	Pernambuco	Brazil
1813	Anise	Arrobas	4	Rio de Janeiro	Brazil
1813	Ointment	Dúzias	5	Bahia	Brazil
1813	Medicinal remedies	Caixotes	13	Rio de Janeiro	Brazil
1813	Medicinal remedies	Embr	2	Rio de Janeiro	Brazil
1813	Medicinal remedies	Barricas	1	Rio de Janeiro	Brazil
1813	Medicinal remedies	Caixas	4	Pernambuco	Brazil
1813	Cupping horns		200	Rio de Janeiro	Brazil

(*cont.*)

Year	Item	Unit	Quantity	Port	Region
1813	Cupping horns		66	Bahia	Brazil
1815	Pharmaceutical drugs	Caixotes	1	Rio de Janeiro	Brazil
1815	Pharmaceutical drugs	Barril	1	Pernambuco	Brazil
1815	Anise	Arrobas	3	Pernambuco	Brazil
1815	Medicinal remedies	Emb	3	Pernambuco	Brazil
1815	Medicinal remedies	Caixas	3	Rio de Janeiro	Brazil
1815	Medicinal remedies	Barris	2	Pernambuco	Brazil
1815	Tin syringes		20	Rio de Janeiro	Brazil
1815	Tin syringes		10	Pernambuco	Brazil
1815	Cupping horns	Dúzias	2	Pernambuco	Brazil
1816	Pharmaceutical drugs	Caixetinhas	3	Rio de Janeiro	Brazil
1816	Pharmaceutical drugs	Barris	2	Pernambuco	Brazil
1816	Anise	Arrobas	2	Pernambuco	Brazil
1816	Medicinal remedies	Caixas	2	Rio de Janeiro	Brazil
1816	Medicinal remedies	Barris	3	Pernambuco	Brazil
1816	Medicinal remedies	Embr	4	Pernambuco	Brazil
1816	Tin syringes		40	Rio de Janeiro	Brazil
1816	Tin syringes		20	Pernambuco	Brazil
1816	Cupping horns	Dúzias	3	Pernambuco	Brazil
1817	Pharmaceutical drugs	Caixetas	4	Rio de Janeiro	Brazil
1817	Pharmaceutical drugs	Caixetas	150	Pernambuco	Brazil
1817	Tin syringes		60	Rio de Janeiro	Brazil
1817	Tin syringes		18	Pernambuco	Brazil
1817	Cupping horns	Dúzias	1	Rio de Janeiro	Brazil
1817	Cupping horns	Dúzias	2	Pernambuco	Brazil
1818	Pharmaceutical drugs	Caixotes	3	Rio de Janeiro	Brazil
1818	Pharmaceutical drugs	Caixotes	3	Pernambuco	Brazil
1818	Anise	Arrobas	5	Rio de Janeiro	Brazil
1818	Anise	Arrobas	20	Pernambuco	Brazil

(*cont.*)

Year	Item	Unit	Quantity	Port	Region
1818	Tin syringes		35	Rio de Janeiro	Brazil
1818	Tin syringes		20	Pernambuco	Brazil
1819	Pharmaceutical drugs	Caixas	20	Rio de Janeiro	Brazil
1819	Pharmaceutical drugs	Barricas	16	Rio de Janeiro	Brazil
1819	Pharmaceutical drugs	Volumes	3	Rio de Janeiro	Brazil
1819	Pharmaceutical drugs	Caixas	5	Pernambuco	Brazil
1819	Pharmaceutical drugs	Barricas	2	Pernambuco	Brazil
1819	Pharmaceutical drugs	Caixas	2	Bahia	Brazil
1819	Pharmaceutical drugs	Volumes	2	Bahia	Brazil
1819	Pharmaceutical drugs	Volumes	3		Portugal
1819	Anise		101	Rio de Janeiro	Brazil
1819	Anise		138	Pernambuco	Brazil
1819	Syringes		219	Rio de Janeiro	Brazil
1819	Cupping horns		24		Portugal
1823	Pharmaceutical drugs	Caixas	2	Rio de Janeiro	Brazil
1823	Pharmaceutical drugs	Caixas	3	Pernambuco	Brazil
1823	Pharmaceutical drugs	Caixas	4		Portugal
1823	Tin syringes		54		Portugal
1823-1825	Drugs for the pharmacy in boxes and bundles				Brazil
1823–1825	Drugs for the pharmacy in boxes and bundles				Portugal
1837	Água de Colônia	Números	1,026		America
1837	Drugs				Portugal
1837	Drugs and herbs				America

Measurement units:

Ancoreta	anchor, approximately 36 litres
Arroba	weight unit equalling 32 pounds (14.7 kg)
Barrica	keg
Barril	barrel, approximately 85 litres
Caixa, Caixão, Caixeta, Caixote	box
Dúzia	dozen
Embrulho	bundle
Libra	pound (0.45 kg)
Pipa	cask, approximately 500 litres
Vidro	bottle

References

Archival References

Angola

Biblioteca Municipal de Luanda (BML)

Portugal

Academia das Ciências de Lisboa
 – Série Vermelha de Manuscritos
Arquivo Histórico Ultramarino (AHU)
 – Conselho Ultramarino (CU)
Arquivo Nacional da Torre do Tombo (ANTT)
 – Tribunal do Santo Ofício, Inquisição de Lisboa (TSO/IL)
Biblioteca Nacional (BNL)

Printed Primary Sources

Abreu, Aleixo de. *Tratado de las siete enfermedades* (Lisbon: Pedro Craesbeeck, 1623).
'Acerca das riquezas desta Colónia, e da possibilidade ou impossibilidade de as aproveitar, 30 July 1799', *Arquivos de Angola*, First Series, 1:4 (1935): no page numbers.
Afzelius, Adam. *Sierra Leone Journal 1795–1796*, edited by Peter Kup (Uppsala: Almqvist & Wiksells, 1967).
Almada, André Alvares d'. *Brief Treatise on the Rivers of Guinea* (Liverpool: Dept. of History, University of Liverpool, 1984).
Assis Junior, A. de. *Dicionário Kimbundu-Português: Linguístico, Botânico, Histórico e Corográfico* (Luanda: Argente, Santos & C.a, n.d.).
Atkins, John. *A Voyage to Guinea, Brasil, and the West-Indies* (London: Ward and Chandler, 1737).
Azeredo, José Pinto de. *Ensaios sobre algumas enfermidades d'Angola* (Lisbon: Regia Officina Typografica, 1799).
Beckmann, Gitte, ed. *'Man muss eben alles sammeln': Der Zürcher Botaniker und Forschungsreisende Hans Schinz und seine ethnographische Sammlung*

Südwestafrika (Zürich: Neue Zürcher Zeitung and Völkerkundemuseum der Universität Zürich, 2012).

Bentley, W. Holman. *Dictionary and Grammar of the Kongo Language* (London: Baptist Missionary Society, 1887).

Bluteau, Raphael. *Vocabulario Portuguez & Latino...* (Coimbra: Collegio das Artes da Companhia de Jesu, 1712–1728).

Bologna, Giacinto da. *La Pratique Missionnaire des PP. Capucins Italiens dans les royaumes de Congo, Angola et contrées adjacentes*, translated by Jacques Nothomb (Louvain: Éditions de l'Aucam, 1931).

Bomtempo, José Maria. *Compendios de Materia Medica* (Rio de Janeiro: Regia Officina Typografica, 1814).

Trabalhos medicos offerecidos à Magestade do Senhor D. Pedro I (Rio de Janeiro: Typographia Nacional, 1825).

Bosman, William. *A New and Accurate Description of the Coast of Guinea. Divided into the Gold, the Slave, and the Ivory Coasts* (London: Ballantyne Press, 1907 [1705]).

Brásio, António, ed. *Monumenta Missionaria Africana: Africa occidental (Série I)*. Vols. 1–11 (Lisbon: Agência Geral do Ultramar, 1952–1972). Vols. 12–14 (Lisbon: Academia Portuguesa de História, 1981, 1984–1985).

Brun, Samuel. 'Samuel Brun's Voyages of 1611–20', in *German Sources for West African History 1599–1669*, edited by Adam Jones (Wiesbaden: Franz Steiner, 1983), 44–96.

Cadornega, António de Oliveira de. *História geral das guerras angolanas*. 3 vols. (Lisbon: Agência Geral das Colónias, 1940 (vols. I and II) and 1942 (vol. III)).

Caltanissetta, P. Luca da. *Diaire Congolais (1690–1701)*, translated from Italian by François Bontinck (Louvain: Éditions Nauwelaerts, 1970).

'Relatione della missione fatta nel Regno di Congo per il Padre Fra' Luca da Caltanisetta', in *Il Congo agli inizi del settecento nella relazione di P. Luca da Caltanissetta*, edited by Romain Rainero (Florence: La Nuova Italia, 1973), 100–426.

Cannecattim, Bernardo Maria de. *Diccionario da lingua bunda, ou angolense, explicada na portugueza, e Latina* (Lisbon: Impressão Regia, 1804).

Carli, Dionigi de. *Viaggio del P Dionigi de'Carli da Piacenza, e del P. Michel Angelo de' Guatini, da Reggio Capuccini* (Reggio: Prospero Vedrotti, 1671).

Carstensen, Edward. *Closing the Books: Governor Edward Carstensen on Danish Guinea 1842–50*, translated from the Danish by Tove Storsveen (Accra: Sub-Saharan Publishers, 2010).

'Carta Régia providenciado sobre a excomunhão lançada pelos Religiosos da Companhia de Jesus, contra o Governador João Fernandes Vieira, 9 December 1666', *Arquivos de Angola*, First Series, 2:7 (1936): 13–14.

'Carta régia sôbre a criação de hum Hospital em Benguella, 16 October 1674', *Arquivos de Angola*, First Series, 1:2 (1933): no page numbers.

Cavazzi da Montecuccolo, Giovanni Antonio. *Istorica descrizione de tre regni Congo, Matamba et Angola* (Bologna: Giacomo Monti, 1687).

Cordeiro, Luciano, ed. *1617–1622: Benguella e seu sertão por um anonymo* (Lisbon: Imprensa Nacional, 1881).

Corrêa, Elias Alexandre da Silva. *História de Angola*, 2 vols. (Lisbon: Editorial Ática, 1937).

Cosme, Francisco Damião. 'Tractado das queixas endemicas, e mais fataes nesta Conquista', edited by Luís de Pina, *Studia* 20–22 (1967): 171–268.

Cuvelier, Jean, ed. *Relations sur le Congo du Père Laurent de Lucques (1700–1717)* (Brussels: Institut Royal Colonial Belge, 1953).

Dandy, J. E., ed. *The Sloane Herbarium: An Annotated List of the Horti Sicci Composing It; with Biographical Accounts of the Principal Contributors* (London: British Museum, 1958).

'De Dom Miguel Antonio de Mello acerca do Breu, da Rezina, do Enxofre e dos Uzos Médicos que, por constantes e bem provadas experiencias têm determinados Simplices, 5 June 1798', *Arquivos de Angola*, First Series, 1:1 (1933), no page numbers.

'De Dom Miguel Antonio de Mello sobre a communicação das duas Costas da Africa, e acerca do Plano para a Fundação da Companhia da Azia, 8 March 1800', *Arquivos de Angola*, First Series, 1:4 (1935), no page numbers.

Dennett, R. E. *At the Back of the Black Man's Mind or Notes on the Kingly Office in West Africa* (London: Frank Cass, 1906).

Dias, Gastão Sousa, ed. *Relações de Angola (Primórdios da ocupação portuguesa)* (Coimbra: Imprensa da Universidade, 1934).

'Do Bot.^{ro} Manoel Pereira, 11 March 1648', 'Do fizico mor L.^{do} An.^{to} Lopez de Oliveira, 26 May 1649', 'Do Surgião mor do Reino de Benguella Bernardo P.^{to}, 16 December 1649', 'Do P.^{e} M.^{tre} frei João da Fonsequa, 20 May 1650', all in *Arquivos de Angola*, First Series, 1:2 (1933): no page numbers.

Faria, Manuel Severim de. *Notícias de Portugal* (Lisbon: Officina Craesbeeckiana, 1655).

Ferreira, Luis Gomes. *Erário Mineral*. 2 vols. (Lisbon: Officina de Miguel Rodrigues, 1735).

Finke, Leonhard Ludwig. *Versuch einer allgemeinen medicinisch-praktischen Geographie, worin der historische Theil der einheimischen Völker – und Staaten – Arzeneykunde vorgetragen wird*. 3 vols. (Leipzig: Weidmannschen Buchhandlund, 1792).

Gatti, P. Evaristo, ed. *Sulle terre e sui mari: Cavalieri di S. Francesco* (Parma: Cappuccini Prov. di Parma, 1931).

Gazola, Giuseppe. *Il mondo ingannato da falsi medici* (Venice: Marino Rossetti, 1716).

Hemmersam, Michael. 'Michael Hemmersam's Description of the Gold Coast, 1639–45', in *German Sources for West African History 1599–1669*, edited by Adam Jones (Wiesbaden: Franz Steiner, 1983), 97–133.

Hepper, F. N. *The West African Herbaria of Isert & Thonning: A Taxonomic Revision and an Index to the IDC Microfiche* (Kew: Bentham-Moxon Trust & Royal Botanic Gardens, 1976).

Hiern, William Philip. *Catalogue of the African Plants Collected by Dr. Friedrich Welwitsch in 1853–61. Dicotyledons, Part I* (London: British Museum, 1896).

'Instruçõens Gerais aos Capitaens Mores, sobre a colheita, e remessa das Produçõens Naturais, que hão-de ser dirigidas ao Real Gabinete de Historia Natural, 17 October 1790', *Arquivos de Angola*, First Series, 1:4 (1935): no page numbers.

Isert, Paul Erdmann. *Letters on West Africa and the Slave Trade*, translated by Selena Axelrod Winsnes (Oxford: Oxford University Press, 1992).

Jadin, Louis. *L'Ancien Congo et l'Angola 1639–1655 d'apres les archives romaines, portugaises, néerlandaises et espagnoles* (Brussels and Rome: Institut Historique Belge de Rome, 1975).

Jones, Adam, ed. *German Sources for West African History* (Wiesbaden: Franz Steiner, 1983).

Justesen, Ole, ed. *Danish Sources for the History of Ghana 1657–1754*. 2 vols. (Copenhagen: Det Kongelige Danske Videnskabernes Selskab, 2005).

La Fleur, James D., ed. *Pieter van den Broecke's Journal of Voyages to Cape Verde, Guinea and Angola 1605–1612* (London: The Hakluyt Society, 2000).

Lind, James. *An Essay on Diseases Incidental to Europeans in Hot Climates*, 2nd ed. (London: T. Becket and P. A. De Hondt, 1771).

Marees, Pieter de. *Description and Historical Account of the Gold Kingdom of Guinea*, translated and edited by Albert van Dantzig and Adam Jones (Oxford: Oxford University Press, 1987 [1602]).

Matthews, John. *A Voyage to the River Sierra-Leone, on the Coast of Africa* (London: B. White, 1788).

Mendes, Afonso. 'Caderno que trata das ervas, raízes e outras cousas que se tem descoberto no Sertão do Reino de Angola, com várias virtudes', edited by Ruela Pombo, *Diogo Cão*, II Série, No. 10 (1934), 298–304, and III Série, No. 1 (1935–1936), 41–48.

Mendes, Luis Antonio de Oliveira. 'Discurso academico ao programma: Determinar com todos os seus symptomas as doenças agudas, e chronicas, que mais frequentemente accommettem os Pretos recem-tirados da Africa: examinando as causas da sua mortadade depois da sua chegada ao Brasil: se talvez a mudança do clima, se a vida mais laboriosa, ou se alguns outros motivos concorrem para tanto estragon: e finalmente indicar os methodos mais apropriados para evitalo, prevenindo-o, curando-o. Tudo isto deduzido da experiencia mais sizuda, e fiel', *Memorias economicas da Academia Real das Sciencias de Lisboa* 4 (1812): 1–64.

Merolla da Sorrento, P. Girolamo. *Breve, e succinta relazione del viaggio nel Regno di Congo Nell' Africa Meridionale* (Naples: F. Mollo, 1692).

Miranda, João Cardoso de. *Relação cirurgica, e médica, na qual se trata, e declara especialmente hum novo methodo para curar a infecção escorbutica, ou mal de Loanda* (Lisbon: Miguel Rodrigues, 1747).

Monrad, H. C. *A Description of the Guinea Coast and Its Inhabitants*, translated by Selena Axelrod Winsnes (Accra: Sub-Saharan Publishers, 2009).

Mota, A. Teixeira da and P. E. H. Hair. *Jesuit Documents on the Guinea of Cape Verde and the Cape Verde Islands, 1585–1617 in English Translation* (Liverpool: Dept. of History, University of Liverpool, 1989).

Müller, Wilhelm Johann. 'Müller's List of Vocabulary', in *German Sources for West African History*, edited by Adam Jones (Wiesbaden: Franz Steiner, 1983), 269–328.

Omboni, Tito. *Viaggi nell' Africa Occidentale* (Milan: Civelli, 1846).

Parco, P. Rosario dal. 'Informations sur le royaume du Congo et d'Angola du P. Rosario dal Parco, préfet des capucins en Angola et Congo, 1760', in

Louis Jadin, 'Aperçu de la situation du Congo et rite d'élection des rois en 1775, d'aprés le P. Cherubino da Savona, missionnaire au Congo de 1759 à 1774', *Bulletin de l'Institut Historique Belge de Rome* 35 (1963): 358–419.

Petiver, James. 'A Catalogue of Some Guinea-Plants, with Their Native Names and Virtues; Sent to James Petiver, Apothecary, and Fellow of the Royal Society; with His Remarks on Them. Communicated in a Letter to Dr. Hans Sloane. Secret. Reg. Soc.', *Philosophical Transactions* 19 (1695): 677–686.

Pigafetta, Filippo. *Relatione del reame di Congo et delle circonvicine contrade, tratta dalli scritti e ragionamenti di Odoardo Lopez portoghese* (Rome: Appresso Bartolomeo Grassi, 1591).

Pimenta, Miguel Dias. *Noticias do que he o achaque do bicho, diffiniçam do seu crestameto, subimento, corrupção, sinaes, & cura ate, o quinto grao, ou intenção delle, suas differenças, & coplicações, com que se ajunta* (Lisbon: Miguel Manescal, 1707).

'Provisão autorizando o regresso à Metrópole do Fisico Mor Manuel de Andrade de Goes, desde que não houvesse falecido o curandeiro Jorge Ferrer de Espinosa, 24 May 1715', *Arquivos de Angola*, First Series, 11:9 (1936): 147–148.

'Provisão determinando que, emquanto se não fizesse o Aljube, os presos da Jurisdição Eclesiastica fossem internados nas Cadêas Publicas, 20 de Maio de 1703', *Arquivos de Angola*, First Series, 2:9–10 (1936): 145–146.

Rask, Johannes. *Two Views from Christiansborg Castle. Volume I. A Brief and Truthful Description of a Journey to and from Guinea*, translated by Selena Axelrod Winsnes (Accra: Sub-Saharan Publishers, 2008).

Ratelband, Klas, ed. *Vijf Dagregisters van Het Kasteel São Jorge da Mina (Elmina) aan de Goudkust (1645–1647)* ('S-Gravenhage: Martinus Nijhoff, 1953).

'Relação de productos Naturaes, que pela Secretaria de Estado da Repartição do Ultramar vão remetidos ao Real Gabinete – Luanda, 5 November 1791', *Arquivos de Angola*, First Series, 1:1 (1933): no page numbers.

'Relação dos Productos Naturaes que pela Secretaria de Estado da Repartição do Ultramar, vão remetidos ao Real Gabinete da Ajuda, na Rela Fragata Minerva, em Cumprimento das Reaes Ordens de Sua Magestade, 18 February 1793', *Arquivos de Angola*, First Series, 1:4 (1935): no page numbers.

Reynhout, M. J. *Redevoering behelzende Kruid- en Geschiedkundige Waarnemingen omtrent de Goudkust* (unknown publisher, 1824).

Rømer, Ludewig Ferdinand. *A Reliable Account of the Coast of Guinea (1760)*, translated by Selena Axelrod Winsnes (Oxford: Oxford University Press, 2000).

Rosa, João Ferreira da. *Trattado unico da constituiçam pestilencial de Pernambuco* (Lisboa: n.p., 1694).

Santo António, D. Caetano de. *Pharmacopea lusitana augmentada: methodo pratico de prearar os medicamentos na fórma galenica, e chimica*, 4th ed. (Lisbon: Mosteiro de S. Vincente de Fóra, 1754).

Sarmento, Jacob de Castro. *Do uso, e abuso das minhas Agoas de Inglaterra, ou directorio, e instruccam, para Se saber seguramente, quando se deve, ou não, usar dellas, assim nas enfermidades agudas; como em algumas chronicas; e em casos propriamente de Cirurgia* (London: Guilherme Strahan, 1754).

Semedo, João Curvo. *Memorial de varios simplices que da India Oriental, da America e de outras partes vem ao nosso reyno* (Lisbon: Oficina de António Pedroso Galram, 1716).

Serrão, Joaquim Veríssimo, ed. *Viagens em Portugal de Manuel Severim de Faria 1604–1609–1625* (Lisbon: Academia Portuguesa da História, 1974).

Smith, Christen. 'Professor Smith's Journal', in *Narrative of an Expedition to Explore the River Zaire, Usually Called the Congo, in South Africa, in 1816, under the Direction of Captain J.H. Tuckey, R.N.* (London: John Murray, 1818), 249–346.

'Sousa Coutinho para o Exmo Sr. Francisco Xavier de Mendonça Furtado com a remessa de hum caixote em que vai huma porção de Pedra Verde – Luanda, 4 December 1769', *Arquivos de Angola*, First Series, 1:1 (1933): no page numbers.

Toso, Carlo. *L'anarchia congolese nel sec. XVII: La relazione inedita di Marcellino d'Atri* (Genoa: Bozzi, 1984).

Wadström, Carl Bernhard. *Observations on the Slave Trade and a Description of Some Part of the Coast of Guinea* (London: James Phillips, 1789).

An Essay on Colonization (London: Darton and Harvey, 1794).

Welwitsch, Frederico (Friedrich). *Synopse explicative das amostras de madeiras e drogas medicinaes e de outros objectos mormente ethnographicos* (Lisbon: Imprensa Nacional, 1862).

Wildeman, É. de. *Sur des plantes médicinales ou utiles du Mayumbe (Congo Belge) d'apres des notes du R.P. Wellens* (Brussels: Institut Royal Colonial Belge, 1938).

Winterbottom, Thomas. *An Account of the Native Africans in the Neighbourhood of Sierra Leone; to which is added an Account of the Present State of Medicine Among Them.* 2 vols. (London: Hatchard & Poultry, 1803).

Wulff, Wulff Joseph. *A Danish Jew in West Africa: Biography and Letters 1836–1842*, translated by Selena Axelrod Winsnes (Legon-Accra: Sub-Saharan Publishers, 2013).

Books, Articles, Theses

Abaka, Edmund. *Kola Is God's Gift: Agricultural Production, Export Initiatives and the Kola Industry of Asante and the Gold Coast c. 1820–1950* (Athens: Ohio University Press, 2005).

Abdalla, Ismail H. 'The Ulama of Sokoto in the Nineteenth Century: A Medical View', in *African Healing Strategies*, edited by Brian M. du Toit and Ismail H. Abdalla (Owerri: Trado-Medic Books, 1985), 8–19.

'Diffusion of Islamic Medicine into Hausaland', in *The Social Basis of Health and Healing in Africa*, edited by Steven Feierman and John M. Janzen (Berkeley: University of California Press, 1992), 177–194.

Abreu, Laurinda. 'O papel das Misericórdias dos "lugares de além-mar" na formação do Império português', *História, Ciências, Saúde – Manguinhos* 8 (2001): 591–611.

Adams, C. D. 'Activities of Danish Botanish Botanists in Guinea 1783–1850', *Transactions of the Historical Society of Ghana* 3 (1957): 30–46.

Adas, Michael. *Machines as the Measure of Men: Science, Technology, and Ideologies of Western Dominance* (Ithaca, NY: Cornell University Press, 1989).

Ahlskog, Jonas. 'The Political Economy of Colonisation: Carl Bernhard Wadström's Case for Abolition and Civilisation', *Sjuttonhundratal* 7 (2010): 145–167.

Akyeampong, Emmanuel Kwaku. 'Disease in West African History', in *Themes in West Africa's History*, edited by Emmanuel Kwaku Akyeampong (Athens: Ohio University Press, 2006), 186–207.

Alden, Dauril and Joseph C. Miller. 'Out of Africa: The Slave Trade and the Transmission of Smallpox to Brazil, 1560–1831', *Journal of Interdisciplinary History* 18 (1987): 195–224.

Alencastro, Luiz Felipe de. *O Trato dos viventes: Formação do Brasil no Atlântico Sul* (São Paulo: Companhia das Letras, 2000).

Almeida, Carlos José Duarte. *Uma infelicidade feliz: A imagem de África e dos Africanos na Literature Missionária sobre o Kongo e a região Mbundu (meados do séc. XVI – primeiro quartel do séc. XVIII)* (unpublished Ph.D. thesis, Faculdade de Ciências Sociais e Humanas, Universidade de Lisboa, 2009).

Arikha, Noga. *Passions and Tempers: A History of the Humours* (New York: Ecco, 2007).

Arrizabalaga, Jon, John Henderson and Roger French. *The Great Pox: The French Disease in Renaissance Europe* (New Haven, CT and London: Yale University Press, 1997).

Barrera-Osorio, Antonio. *Experiencing Nature: The Spanish American Empire and the Early Scientific Revolution* (Austin: University of Texas Press, 2006).

Barrett, Frank A. 'A Medical Geography Anniversary', *Social Science & Medicine* 37 (1993): 701–710.

'Finke's 1792 Map of Human Diseases: The First World Disease Map?', *Social Science & Medicine* 50 (2000): 915–921.

Beckmann, Gitte, ed. *'Man muss eben alles sammeln': Der Zürcher Botaniker und Forschungsreisende Hans Schinz und seine ethnographische Sammlung Südwestafrika* (Zürich: Neue Zürcher Zeitung and Völkerkundemuseum der Universität Zürich, 2012).

Bender, Gerald J. *Angola under the Portuguese: The Myth and the Reality.* (Berkeley and Los Angeles: University of California Press, 1978).

Bethencourt, Francisco. *O imaginário da magia: Feiticeiras, adivinhos e curandeiros em Portugal no século XVI* (São Paulo: Companhia das Letras, 2004).

Bilby, Kenneth M. and Jerome S. Handler. 'Obeah: Healing and Protection in West Indian Slave Life', *The Journal of Caribbean History* 38 (2004): 153–183.

Bossard, Eric. *La medecine traditionnelle chez les Ovimbundu* (Neuchâtel: Institut d'Ethnologie, Université de Neuchâtel, 1987).

La medecine traditionnelle au centre et a l'ouest de l'Angola (Lisbon: Instituto de Investigação Científica Tropical, 1996).

Boxer, Charles R. *Two Pioneers of Tropical Medicine: Garcia d'Orta and Nicolás Monardes* (London: The Hispanic & Luso-Brazilian Councils, 1963).

Braidwood, Stephen J. *Black Poor and White Philanthropists: London's Blacks and the Foundation of the Sierra Leone Settlement, 1786-1791* (Liverpool: Liverpool University Press, 1994).

Brásio, António. 'As Misericórdias de Angola', *Studia* 4 (1959): 106–149.

História e missiologia: Inéditos e esparsos (Luanda: Instituto de Investigação Científica de Angola, 1973).

Braudel, Fernand. *Civilization and Capitalism, 15th–18th Centuries, Vol. I: The Structures of Everyday Life: The Limits of the Possible*, translated by Siân Reynolds (London: Collins, 1981).

Breen, Benjamin. 'The Flip Side of the Pharmacopoeia: Sub-Saharan African Medicines and Poisons in the Atlantic World', in *Drugs on the Page: Pharmacopoeias and Healing Knowledge in the Early Modern Atlantic World*, edited by Matthew James Crawford and Joseph M. Gabriel (Pittsburgh: University of Pittsburgh Press, 2019), 143–159.

Brixius, Dorit. 'From Ethnobotany to Emancipation: Slaves, Plant Knowledge, and Gardens on Eighteenth-Century Isle de France', *History of Science* 58 (2019): 51–75.

Brockey, Liam Matthew. 'An Imperial Republic: Manuel Severim de Faria Surveys the Globe, 1608-1655', in *Portuguese Humanism and the Republic of Letters*, edited by Maria Berbara and Karl A. E. Enenkel (Leiden: Brill, 2012), 265–285.

Brooks, George E. *Eurafricans in Western Africa: Commerce, Social Status, Gender, and Religious Observance from the Sixteenth to the Eighteenth Century* (Athens: Ohio University Press, 2003).

Brothwell, Don R. 'Yaws', in *The Cambridge World History of Human Disease*, edited by Kenneth F. Kiple (Cambridge: Cambridge University Press, 1993), 1096–1100.

Brown, Christopher Leslie. 'Empire without America: British Plans for Africa in the Era of the American Revolution', in *Abolitionism and Imperialism in Britain, Africa, and the Atlantic*, edited by Derek R. Peterson (Athens: Ohio University Press, 2010), 84–100.

Cagle, Hugh Glenn. 'The Botany of Colonial Medicine: Gender, Authority, and Natural History across Iberian Empires', in *Women of the Iberian Atlantic*, edited by Sarah E. Owens and Jane E. Mangan (Baton Rouge: Louisiana State University Press, 2012), 174–195.

'Beyond the Senegal: Inventing the Tropics in the Late Middle Ages', *Journal of Medieval Iberian Studies* 7 (2015): 1–21.

Assembling the Tropics: Science and Medicine in Portugal's Empire, 1450–1700 (Cambridge: Cambridge University Press, 2018).

Calainho, Daniela Buono. *Metrópole das Mandingas: Religiosidade negra e inquisição portuguesa no Antigo Regime* (Rio de Janeiro: Garamond, 2008).

Caldeira, Arlindo Manuel. *Escravos e traficantes no império português: O comércio negreiro português no Atlântico durante os séculos XV a XIX* (Lisbon: A Esfera dos Livros, 2013).

'Angola and the Seventeenth-Century South Atlantic Slave Trade', in *Networks and Trans-cultural Exchange: Slave Trading in the South Atlantic, 1590–1867*, edited by David Richardson and Filipa Ribeiro da Silva (Leiden: Brill, 2015), 101–142.

Candido, Mariana P. 'Different Slave Journeys: Enslaved African Seamen on Board of Portuguese Ships, c. 1760–1820s', *Slavery & Abolition* 31 (2010): 395–409.

An African Slaving Port and the Atlantic World: Benguela and Its Hinterland (Cambridge: Cambridge University Press, 2013).

'South Atlantic Exchanges: The Role of Brazilian-Born Agents in Benguela, 1650–1850', *Luso-Brazilian Review* 50:1 (2013): 53–82.

Canny, Nicholas. 'Atlantic History and Global History', in *Atlantic History: A Critical Appraisal*, edited by Jack P. Greene and Philip D. Morgan (Oxford: Oxford University Press, 2009), 317–335.

Carney, Judith A. and Richard Nicholas Rosomoff. *In the Shadow of Slavery: Africa's Botanical Legacy in the Atlantic World* (Berkeley: University of California Press, 2009).

Chakrabarti, Pratik. *Medicine and Empire 1600–1960* (Basingstoke: Palgrave Macmillan, 2014).

Chandler, David L. 'Health Conditions in the Slave Trade of Colonial New Granada', in *Slavery and Race Relations in Latin America*, edited by Robert B. Toplin (Westport, CT: Greenwood Press, 1974), 51–88.

Health and Slavery in Colonial Colombia (New York: Arno Press, 1981).

Coates, Timothy J. *Convicts and Orphans: Forced and State-Sponsored Colonizers in the Portuguese Empire, 1550–1755* (Stanford, CA: Stanford University Press, 2001).

Coghe, Samuël. 'The Problem of Freedom in a Mid Nineteenth-Century Atlantic Slave Society: The Liberated Africans of the Anglo-Portuguese Mixed Commission in Luanda (1844–1870)', *Slavery & Abolition* 33 (2012): 479–500.

Coleman, Deirdre. *Romantic Colonization and British Antislavery* (Cambridge: Cambridge University Press, 2005).

Henry Smeathman, the Flycatcher: Natural History, Slavery, and Empire in the Late Eighteenth Century (Liverpool: Liverpool University Press, 2018).

Cook, Harold J. *Matters of Exchange: Commerce, Medicine, and Science in the Dutch Golden Age* (New Haven, CT: Yale University Press, 2007).

Cooper, Frederick. 'African History/Global History', *Perspectives on History* 50 (December 2012).

Couto, Carlos. 'Presença cigana na colonização de Angola', *Boletim do Instituto de Investigação Científica de Angola* 8 (1971): 137–143.

Crawford, Matthew James. *The Andean Wonder Drug: Cinchona Bark and Imperial Science in the Spanish Atlantic, 1630–1800* (Pittsburgh: University of Pittsburgh Press, 2016).

Cunningham, Andrew. 'Identifying Disease in the Past: Cutting the Gordian Knot', *Asclepio* 54 (2002): 13–34.

Curran, Andrew S. *The Anatomy of Blackness: Science and Slavery in an Age of Enlightenment* (Baltimore: Johns Hopkins University Press, 2011).

Curtin, Philip D. '"The White Man's Grave": Image and Reality, 1780–1850', *The Journal of British Studies* 1 (1961): 94–110.

Disease and Empire: The Health of European Troops in the Conquest of Africa (Cambridge: Cambridge University Press, 1998).

Curto, José C. '*Americanos* in a West Central African Slaving Port: The Rise and Fall of the Brazilian Community in Benguela, c. 1650–1850', unpublished draft paper.

Alcoól e Escravos: O comércio luso-brasileiro do alcoól em Mpinda, Luanda e Benguela durante o tráfico atlântico de escravos (c. 1480–1830) e o seu impacto nas sociedades da África Central Ocidental (Lisbon: Editora Vulgata, 2002).

Enslaving Spirits: The Portuguese-Brazilian Alcohol Trade at Luanda and Its Hinterland, c. 1550–1830 (Leiden: Brill, 2004).

Curto, José C. and Raymond R. Gervais. 'The Population History of Luanda during the Late Atlantic Slave Trade, 1781–1844', *African Economic History* 29 (2001): 1–59.

Dandy, J. E., ed. *The Sloane Herbarium: An Annotated List of the Horti Sicci Composing It; with Biographical Accounts of the Principal Contributors* (London: British Museum, 1958).

Delbourgo, James. *Collecting the World: The Life and Curiosity of Hans Sloane* (London: Penguin, 2017).

Delumeau, Jean. *Sin and Fear: The Emergence of a Western Guilt Culture, 13th–18th Centuries* (New York: St. Martin's Press, 1990).

Denbow, James. *The Archaeology and Ethnography of Central Africa* (Cambridge: Cambridge University Press, 2013).

Denis, Adrián López. 'Melancholy, Slavery, and Racial Pathology in Eighteenth-Century Cuba', *Science in Context* 18 (2005): 179–199.

Dewhurst, Kenneth. *John Locke (1632–1704), Physician and Philosopher: A Medical Biography – with an Edition of the Medical Notes in His Journals* (London: Wellcome Historical Medical Library, 1963).

Diamond, Jared. *Guns, Germs and Steel: A Short History of Everybody for the Last 13,000 Years* (London: Vintage, 1998).

Dias, Jill R. 'Famine and Disease in the History of Angola, c. 1830–1930', *Journal of African History* 22 (1981): 349–378.

Dias, José Pedro Sousa. 'Índice de drogas medicinais angolanas em documentos dos séculos XVI a XVIII', *Revista Portuguesa de Farmácia* 45 (1995): 174–184.

'Bibliografia sobre a farmácia e a material médica da expansão e da colonização portuguesa (séculos XVI a XVIII)', *Mare Liberum* 11–12 (1996): 165–207.

Dongen, Bart E. van, Sharon E. Fraser and Timothy Insoll. 'The Composition and Origin of Ghana Medicine Clays', *Anthropology & Medicine* 18 (2011): 285–302.

Douglas, Starr. 'The Making of Scientific Knowledge in an Age of Slavery: Henry Smeathman, Sierra Leone and Natural History', *Journal of Colonialism and Colonial History* 9 (2008). DOI: 10.1353/cch.0.0029.

Douglas, Starr and Felix Driver. 'Imagining the Tropical Colony: Henry Smeathman and the Termites of Sierra Leone', in *Tropical Visions in an Age of Empire*, edited by Felix Driver and Luciana Martins (Chicago: University of Chicago Press, 2005), 91–112.

Drayton, Richard. *Nature's Government: Science, Imperial Britain, and the 'Improvement' of the World* (New Haven, CT: Yale University Press, 2000).

Emmer, Pieter C. *The Dutch Slave Trade 1500–1850* (New York: Berghahn Books, 2006).

d'Ésaguy, Augusto. 'A abertura da Escola Médica de Luanda (duas obras inéditas do dr. José Pinto de Azeredo)', *Imprensa Médica* 15:3 (1951): 31–37. *Breve notícia sobre a Escola Médica de Luanda (Documentos)* (Lisbon: Ed. Império, 1951).

Fabian, Johannes. *Out of Our Minds: Reason and Madness in the Exploration of Central Africa* (Berkeley: University of California Press, 2000).

Fage, J. D. *A Guide to Original Sources for Precolonial Western Africa Published in European Languages: For the Most Part in Book Form* (Madison: African Studies Program, University of Wisconsin – Madison, 1994).

Farelo, Mário Sérgio. 'On Portuguese Medical Students and Masters Travelling Abroad: An Overview from the Early Modern Period to the Enlightenment', in *Centres of Medical Excellence? Medical Travel and Education in Europe, 1500–1700*, edited by Ole Peter Grell, Andrew Cunningham and Jon Arrizabalaga (Farnham: Ashgate, 2010), 126–147.

Feierman, Steven. 'Change in African Therapeutic Systems', *Social Science and Medicine* 13:4 (1979): 277–284.
'Struggles for Control: The Social Roots of Health and Healing in Modern Africa', *African Studies Review* 28 (1985): 73–147.

Feinberg, Harvey M. 'New Data on European Mortality in West Africa: The Dutch on the Gold Coast, 1719–1760', *Journal of African History* 15 (1974): 357–371.
'Africans and Europeans in West Africa: Elminans and Dutchmen on the Gold Coast during the Eighteenth Century', *Transactions of the American Philosophical Society* 79:7 (1989): 1–186.

Ferreira, Roquinaldo. *Transforming Atlantic Slaving: Trade, Warfare and Territorial Control in Angola, 1650–1800* (unpublished Ph.D. dissertation, University of California, Los Angeles, 2003).
Cross-Cultural Exchange in the Atlantic World: Angola and Brazil during the Era of the Slave Trade (Cambridge: Cambridge University Press, 2012).

Fett, Sharla M. *Working Cures: Healing, Health, and Power on Southern Slave Plantations* (Chapel Hill: University of North Carolina Press, 2002).

Field, M. J. *Religion and Medicine of the Gã People* (London: Oxford University Press, 1937).

Figueiredo, João. 'The City's Silent Double: Public Cemeteries in Angola from the Enlightenment to the Scramble', in *African Dynamics in a Multipolar World* (Lisbon: ISCTE-IUL, 2014), 860–879.

Fromont, Cécile. *The Art of Conversion: Christian Visual Culture in the Kingdom of Kongo* (Chapel Hill: University of North Carolina Press, 2014).

Fuller, Dorian Q. and Chris J. Stevens. 'Sorghum Domestication and Diversification: A Current Archaeobotanical Perspective', in *Plants and People in the African Past: Progress in African Archaeobotany*, edited by Anna Maria Mercuri et al. (New York: Springer, 2018), 427–452.

Furtado, Júnia Ferreira. 'Tropical Empiricism: Making Medical Knowledge in Colonial Brazil', in *Science and Empire in the Atlantic World*, edited by James Delbourgo and Nicholas Dew (London: Routledge, 2007), 127–151.

García-Ballester, Luis. 'On the Origin of the "Six Non-natural Things" in Galen', in *Galen and Galenism: Theory and Medical Practice from Antiquity to the European Renaissance*, edited by Jon Arrizabalaga (Aldershot: Ashgate, 2002), 105–115.

Geertz, Clifford. *Local Knowledge: Further Essays in Interpretive Anthropology* (New York: Basic Books, 1983).

Geest, Sjaak van der. 'Is There a Role for Traditional Medicine in Basic Health Services in Africa? A Plea for Community Perspective', *Tropical Medicine and International Health* 2 (1997): 903–911.

Geissler, Paul Wenzel. 'Studying Trial Communities: Anthropological and Historical Inquiries into Ethos, Politics and Economy of Medical Research in Africa', in *Evidence, Ethos and Experiment: The Anthropology and History of Medical Research in Africa*, edited by P. Wenzel Geissler and Catherine Molyneux (New York: Berghahn Books, 2011), 1–28.

Geissler, Paul Wenzel, Guillaume Lachenal, John Manton and Noémi Tousignant, eds. *Traces of the Future: An Archaeology of Medical Science in Africa* (Bristol: Intellect, 2016).

Gentilcore, David. *Healers and Healing in Early Modern Italy* (Manchester: Manchester University Press, 1998).

Golinski, Jan. *Making Natural Knowledge: Constructivism and the History of Science* (Chicago: University of Chicago Press, 2005).

Gómez, Pablo F. 'The Circulation of Bodily Knowledge in the Seventeenth-Century Black Spanish Caribbean', *Social History of Medicine* 26:3 (2013): 383–402.

The Experiential Caribbean: Creating Knowledge and Healing in the Early Modern Atlantic (Chapel Hill: University of North Carolina Press, 2017).

Goodyear, James D. *Agents of Empire: Portuguese Doctors in Colonial Brazil and the Idea of Tropical Disease* (unpublished Ph.D. dissertation, Johns Hopkins University, 1982).

Gossweiler, John. *Flora exótica de Angola: nomes vulgares e origem das plantas cultivadas ou subespontâneas*. Separata of *Agronomia Angolana* (Luanda: Repartição Central dos Serviços de Agricultura de Angola, 1950).

Green, Toby. *Inquisition: The Reign of Fear* (Basingstoke: Macmillan, 2007).

The Rise of the Trans-Atlantic Slave Trade in Western Africa, 1300–1589 (Cambridge: Cambridge University Press, 2012).

A Fistful of Shells: West Africa from the Rise of the Slave Trade to the Age of Revolution (London: Allen Lane, 2019).

Green, Toby. ed. *Brokers of Change: Atlantic Commerce and Cultures in Pre-colonial Western Africa* (Oxford: Oxford University Press, 2012).

Greenblatt, Stephen. *Marvelous Possessions: The Wonder of the New World* (Oxford: Oxford University Press, 1991).

Grimaldi, Ilaria Maria. 'Taro across the Oceans: Journeys of One of Our Oldest Crops', in *News from the Past: Progress in African Archaeobotany*, edited by Ursula Thanheiser (Groningen: Barkhuis, 2016), 67–82.

Grossi, Ramon Fernandes. 'O caso de Ignácio Mina: tensões sociais e práticas "mágicas" nas minas', *Varia Historia* 20 (1999): 118–131.

Grove, Richard. *Green Imperialism: Colonial Expansion, Tropical Island Edens and the Origins of Environmentalism, 1600–1860* (Cambridge: Cambridge University Press, 1995).

Guerra, F. 'Aleixo de Abreu [1568–1630], Author of the Earliest Book on Tropical Medicine Describing Amoebiasis, Malaria, Typhoid Fever, Scurvy, Yellow Fever, Dracontiasis, Trichuriasis and Tungiasis in 1623', *Journal of Tropical Medicine and Hygiene* 71 (1968): 55–69.

Guthrie, Malcolm. *Comparative Bantu: An Introduction to the Comparative Linguistics and Prehistory of the Bantu Languages*. 4 vols. (Farnborough: Gregg Press, 1967–1971).

Handler, Jerome. 'Slave Medicine and Obeah in Barbados, circa 1650 to 1834', *New West Indian Guide–Nieuwe West-Indische Gids* 74 (2000): 57–60.

Harley, David. 'Rhetoric and the Social Construction of Sickness and Healing', *Social History of Medicine* 12 (1999): 407–435.

Harms, Robert. *Africa in Global History with Sources* (New York: W. W. Norton, 2018).

Harrison, Mark. *Disease and the Modern World, 1500 to the Present Day* (Cambridge: Polity Press, 2004).

   Medicine in an Age of Commerce and Empire: Britain and Its Tropical Colonies, 1660–1830 (Oxford: Oxford University Press, 2010).

   'A Global Perspective: Reframing the History of Health, Medicine, and Disease', *Bulletin of the History of Medicine* 89 (2015): 639–689.

Harvie, David I. *Limeys: The Conquest of Scurvy* (Thrupp: Sutton Publishing, 2002).

Havik, Philip. 'Hybridising Medicine: Illness, Healing and the Dynamics of Reciprocal Exchange on the Upper Guinea Coast (West Africa)', *Medical History* 60 (2016): 181–205.

Hayden, Cori. *When Nature Goes Public: The Making and Unmaking of Bioprospecting in Mexico* (Princeton, NJ: Princeton University Press, 2003).

Heintze, Beatrix. 'Historical Notes on the Kisama of Angola', *Journal of African History* 13 (1972): 407–418.

Henderson, John. *The Renaissance Hospital: Healing the Body and Healing the Soul* (New Haven, CT: Yale University Press, 2006).

Herschtal, Eric. *The Science of Antislavery: Scientists, Abolitionism, and the Myth of Slavery's Backwardness* (unpublished Ph.D. thesis, Columbia University, 2017).

Heywood, Linda M. 'Portuguese into African: The Eighteenth-Century Central African Background to Atlantic Creole Cultures', in *Central Africans and Cultural Transformations in the American Diaspora*, edited by Linda M. Heywood (Cambridge: Cambridge University Press, 2002), 91–113.

   Njinga of Angola: Africa's Warrior Queen (Cambridge, MA: Harvard University Press, 2017).

Heywood, Linda M. and John K. Thornton. 'Central African Leadership and the Appropriation of European Culture', in *The Atlantic World and Virginia, 1550–1624*, edited by Peter C. Mancall (Chapel Hill: University of North Carolina Press, 2007), 194–224.

   Central Africans, Atlantic Creoles, and the Foundation of the Americas, 1585–1660 (Cambridge: Cambridge University Press, 2007).

Hilton, Anne. *The Kingdom of Kongo* (Oxford: Clarendon Press, 1985).

Hodacs, Hanna. 'Local, Universal, and Embodied Knowledge: Anglo-Swedish Contacts and Linnaean Natural History', in *Global Scientific Practice in an Age of Revolutions, 1750–1850*, edited by Patrick Manning and Daniel Rood (Pittsburgh: University of Pittsburgh Press, 2016), 90–104.

Hogarth, Rana A. *Medicalizing Blackness: Making Racial Difference in the Atlantic World* (Chapel Hill: University of North Carolina Press, 2017).

Hokkanen, Markku. 'Imperial Networks, Colonial Bioprospecting and Burroughs Wellcome & Co.: The Case of *Strophanthus Kombe* from Malawi (1859–1915)', *Social History of Medicine* 25 (2012): 589–607.

Medicine, Mobility and the Empire: Nyasaland Networks, 1859–1960 (Manchester: Manchester University Press, 2017).

Hopkins, Daniel. 'Danish Natural History and African Colonialism at the Close of the Eighteenth Century: Peter Thonning's "Scientific Journey" to the Guinea Coast, 1799–1803', *Archives of Natural History* 26 (1999): 369–418.

Horta, José da Silva. 'Africanos e portugueses na documentação inquisitorial, de Luanda a Mbanza Kongo (1596–1598)', in *Actas do Seminário Encontro de povos e culturas em Angola* (Lisbon: Comissão Nacional para as Comemorações dos Descobrimentos Portugueses, 1997), 301–321.

Horton, Robin. 'African Traditional Thought and Western Science', *Africa* 37 (1967): 50–71, 155–187.

Hunt, Nancy Rose. 'Health and Healing', in *The Oxford Handbook of Modern African History*, edited by John Parker and Richard Reid (Oxford: Oxford University Press, 2013), 378–395.

Ipsen, Pernille. *Daughters of the Trade: Atlantic Slavers and Interracial Marriage on the Gold Coast* (Philadelphia: University of Pennsylvania Press, 2015).

Jacobson-Widding, Anita. *Red–White–Black as a Mode of Thought: A Study of Triadic Classification by Colours in the Ritual Symbolism and Cognitive Thought of the Peoples of the Lower Congo* (Uppsala: Acta Universitatis Upsaliensis, 1979).

Janzen, John M. *The Quest for Therapy: Medical Pluralism in Lower Zaire* (Berkeley: University of California Press, 1978).

Lemba, 1650–1930: A Drum of Affliction in Africa and the New World (New York: Garland Publishing, 1982).

Ngoma: Discourses of Healing in Central and Southern Africa (Berkeley: University of California Press, 1992).

Jensen, Niklas Thode. *For the Health of the Enslaved: Slaves, Medicine and Power in the Danish West Indies, 1803–1848* (Copenhagen: Museum Tusculanum Press, 2012).

Kananoja, Kalle. 'Healers, Idolaters and Good Christians: A Case Study of Creolization and Popular Religion in Mid-Eighteenth Century Angola', *International Journal of African Historical Studies* 43 (2010): 443–465.

Central African Identities and Religiosity in Colonial Minas Gerais (unpublished Ph.D. thesis, Åbo Akademi University, 2012).

'Pai Caetano Angola, Afro-Brazilian Magico-Religious Practices, and Cultural Resistance in Minas Gerais in the Late Eighteenth Century', *Journal of African Diaspora Archaeology and Heritage* 2 (2013): 19–39.

'Bioprospecting and European Uses of African Natural Medicine in Early Modern Angola', *Portuguese Studies Review* 23 (2016): 45–69.

'Infected by the Devil, Cured by Calundu: African Healers in Eighteenth-Century Minas Gerais, Brazil', *Social History of Medicine* 29 (2016): 490–511.

'Melancholy, Race, and Slavery in the Early Modern Southern Atlantic World', in *Crises of Mind: Cultural and Institutional Approaches to Insanity*, edited by Jari Eilola, Markku Hokkanen and Tuomas Laine-Frigren (Leiden: Brill, 2019), 88–112.

Kiple, Kenneth F. *The Caribbean Slave: A Biological History* (Cambridge: Cambridge University Press, 1984).

Kirk, Robert G. W. and Neil Pemberton. 'Re-imagining Bleeders: The Medical Leech in the Nineteenth Century Bloodletting Encounter', *Medical History* 55 (2011): 355–360.

Koivunen, Leila. *Visualizing Africa in Nineteenth-Century British Travel Accounts* (London: Routledge, 2009).

Kubik, Gerhard. *Angolan Traits in Black Music, Games and Dances of Brazil: A Study of African Cultural Extensions Overseas* (Lisbon: Junta de Investigações Científicas do Ultramar, 1979).

Lachenal, Guillaume. *The Lomidine Files: The Untold Story of a Medical Disaster in Colonial Africa*, translated by Noémi Tousignant (Baltimore: Johns Hopkins University Press, 2017).

Langwick, Stacey A. *Bodies, Politics, and African Healing: The Matter of Maladies in Tanzania* (Bloomington: Indiana University Press, 2011).

'Healers and Scientists: The Epistemological Politics of Research about Medicinal Plants in Tanzania', in *Evidence, Ethos and Experiment: The Anthropology and History of Medical Research in Africa*, edited by P. Wenzel Geissler and Catherine Molyneux (New York: Berghahn Books, 2011), 263–295.

Langwick, Stacey A., Hansbjörg Dilger and Abdoulaye Kane. 'Introduction: Transnational Medicine, Mobile Experts', in *Medicine, Mobility, and Power in Global Africa: Transnational Health and Healing*, edited by Hansbjörg Dilger, Abdoulaye Kane and Stacey A. Langwick (Bloomington: Indiana University Press, 2012), 1–27.

Lindroth, Sten. 'Adam Afzelius. En linnean i England och Sierra Leone', *Lychnos* (1944–1945): 1–54.

'Adam Afzelius: A Swedish Botanist in Sierra Leone', *Sierra Leone Studies*, New Series, 4 (1955): 194–207.

Loth, Heinrich. *Altafrikanische Heilkunst* (Leipzig: Verlag Philipp Reclam, 1984).

Lovejoy, Paul E. *Caravans of Kola: The Hausa Kola Trade 1700–1900* (Zaria: Ahmadu Bello University Press, 1980).

Transformations in Slavery: A History of Slavery in Africa (Cambridge: Cambridge University Press, 1983).

Manning, Patrick. *The African Diaspora: A History through Culture* (New York: Columbia University Press, 2009).

Marcussi, Alexandre Almeida. 'Estratégias de mediação simbólica em um calundu colonial', *Revista de História* 155 (2006): 97–124.

Marques, Vera Regina Beltrão. *Natureza em Boiões: Medicina e boticários no Brasil setecentista* (Campinas: Editora da UNICAMP, 2000).

Martin, Phyllis. *The External Trade of the Loango Coast, 1576–1870: The Effects of Changing Commercial Relations on the Vili Kingdom of Loango* (Oxford: Clarendon Press, 1972).

McCaskie, Tom C. '"The Art or Mystery of Physick" – Asante Medicinal Plants and the Western Ordering of Botanical Knowledge', *History in Africa* 44 (2017): 27–62.

Megenney, William W. 'Sub-Saharan Lexicon in Afro-Brazilian Cantigas de Pretos Velhos (Umbanda) as Clues to Slave Demography', *Iberoromania* 45 (1997): 27–43.

Metcalf, Alida C. *Go-Betweens and the Colonization of Brazil: 1500–1600* (Austin: University of Texas Press, 2005).

Meuwese, Mark. *Brothers in Arms, Partners in Trade: Dutch-Indigenous Alliances in the Atlantic World, 1595–1674* (Leiden and Boston: Brill, 2012).

Mignolo, Walter D. 'The Geopolitics of Knowledge and the Colonial Difference', *South Atlantic Quarterly* 101 (2002): 56–96.

Mikkeli, Heikki. *Hygiene in the Early Modern Medical Tradition* (Helsinki: Finnish Academy of Science and Letters, 1999).

Miller, Genevieve. '"Airs, Waters, and Places" in History', *Journal of the History of Medicine and Allied Sciences* 17 (1962): 129–140.

Miller, Joseph C. 'Lineages, Ideology, and the History of Slavery in Western Central Africa', in *The Ideology of Slavery in Africa*, edited by Paul E. Lovejoy (Beverly Hills, CA: Sage Publications, 1981), 41–71.

'The Significance of Drought, Disease, and Famine in the Agriculturally Marginal Zones of West-Central Africa', *Journal of African History* 23 (1982): 17–61.

Way of Death: Merchant Capitalism and the Angolan Slave Trade 1730–1830 (Madison: University of Wisconsin Press, 1988).

'History and Africa/Africa and History', *American Historical Review* 104 (1999): 1–32.

Mitchell, Piers D. 'Retrospective Diagnosis and the Use of Historical Texts for Investigating Disease in the Past', *International Journal of Paleopathology* 1 (2011): 81–88.

Mott, Luiz. 'O calundu-angola de Luiza Pinta: Sabará, 1739', *Revista do Instituto de Arte e cultura, Ouro Preto* 10 (1994): 73–82.

Moura, Clóvis. *Dicionário da Escravidão Negra no Brasil* (São Paulo: Editoria da Universidade de São Paulo, 2004).

Mouser, Bruce L. 'Women Slavers of Guinea-Conakry', in *Women and Slavery in Africa*, edited by Claire C. Robertson and Martin Klein (Madison: University of Wisconsin Press, 1983), 320–339.

Mustakeem, Sowande' M. *Slavery at Sea: Terror, Sex, and Sickness in the Middle Passage* (Urbana, Chicago and Springfield: University of Illinois Press, 2016).

Neill, Deborah. *Networks in Tropical Medicine: Internationalism, Colonialism, and the Rise of a Medical Specialty, 1890–1930* (Stanford, CA: Stanford University Press, 2012).

Nelson, Philip K. *Carl Bernhard Wadström: Mannen bakom myten* (Nörrköping: Föreningen Gamla Nörrköping, 1998).

Neumann, Katharina and Elisabeth Hildebrand. 'Early Bananas in Africa: The State of the Art', *Ethnobotany Research & Applications* 7 (2009): 353–362.

Nogueira, André. 'Relações sociais e práticas mágicas na capitania do ouro: o caso do negro angola Pai Caetano (Vila Rica – 1791)', *Estudos Afro-Asiáticos* 27 (2005): 181–203.

Norri, Juhani. *Dictionary of Medical Vocabulary in English, 1375–1550: Body Parts, Sicknesses, Instruments, and Medicinal Preparations* (London: Routledge, 2016).

Nurse, Derek. 'The Contributions of Linguistics to the Study of History in Africa', *Journal of African History* 38 (1997): 359–391.

Oda, Ana Maria Galdini Raimundo. 'O banzo e outros males: o pathos dos negros escravos na Memória de Oliveira Mendes', *Revista Latinoamericana de Psicopatologia Fundamental* 10 (2007): 346–361.

'Escravidão e nostalgia no Brasil: o banzo', *Revista Latinoamericana de Psicopatologia Fundamental* 11 (2008): 735–761.

Olsen, William C. and Carolyn Sargent. 'Introduction', in *African Medical Pluralism*, edited by William C. Olsen and Carolyn Sargent (Bloomington: Indiana University Press, 2017), 1–27.

Osseo-Asare, Abena Dove. *Bitter Roots: The Search for Healing Plants in Africa* (Chicago and London: University of Chicago Press, 2014).

Packard, Randall M. *A History of Global Health: Interventions into the Lives of Other Peoples* (Baltimore: Johns Hopkins University Press, 2016).

Paiva, José Pedro. *Bruxaria e superstição num país sem "caça as bruxas" 1600–1774* (Lisbon: Editorial Notícias, 1997).

Pantoja, Selma. 'Personagens entre mares atlânticos: Visões de Luanda setecentista', *Revista de História Comparada* 7 (2013): 136–148.

Park, Katherine. *Doctors and Medicine in Early Renaissance Florence* (Princeton, NJ: Princeton University Press, 1985).

Parrish, Susan Scott. 'Diasporic African Sources of Enlightenment Knowledge', in *Science and Empire in the Atlantic World*, edited by James Delbourgo and Nicholas Dew (London: Routledge, 2007), 281–310.

Paster, Gail Kern, Katherine Rowe and Mary Floyd-Wilson, eds. *Reading the Early Modern Passions: Essays in the Cultural History of Emotion* (Philadelphia: University of Pennsylvania Press, 2004)

Paton, Diana. *The Cultural Politics of Obeah: Religion, Colonialism and Modernity in the Caribbean World* (Cambridge: Cambridge University Press, 2015).

Pearson, Michael N. 'First Contacts between Indian and European Medical Systems: Goa in the Sixteenth Century', in *Warm Climates and Western Medicine: The Emergence of Tropical Medicine, 1500–1900*, edited by David Arnold (Amsterdam: Rodopi, 1996), 20–41.

Peterson, Mark A. '*Theopolis Americana*: The City-State of Boston, the Republic of Letters, and the Protestant International, 1689–1739', in *Soundings in Atlantic History: Latent Structures and Intellectual Currents, 1500–1830*, edited by Bernard Bailyn and Patricia L. Denault (Cambridge, MA: Harvard University Press, 2009), 329–370.

Pierson, William D. 'White Cannibals, Black Martyrs: Fear, Depression, and Religious Faith as Causes of Suicide among New Slaves', *Journal of Negro History* 62 (1977): 147–159.

Pimenta, Tania Salgado. 'Barbeiros-sangradores e curandeiros no Brasil (1808–28)', *História, Ciências, Saúde – Manguinhos* 2 (1998): 349–372.

Pina, Luiz de. 'Notas para a medicina indígena angolense no século XVIII', *Boletim Geral das Colónias* 151 (1938): 12–26.

Pombo, Manuel Ruela. 'Medicina indígena', *Diogo Cão*, Third Series (1935–1936): 105–112.

Porisiensi, Silvio. *Pionieri della scienza, della civiltá e della fede in Africa: I cappuccino italiani alla esplorazione del Congo, Angola e Matamba nel sec. XVII, 1645–1705: La relazioni sul congo del friuliano Antonio Zucchelli* (Udine: Chiandetti, 1981).

Porter, Roy. 'Introduction', in *Patients and Practitioners: Lay Perceptions of Medicine in Pre-Industrial Society*, edited by Roy Porter (Cambridge: Cambridge University Press, 1985), 1–22.

Postell, William Dosite. 'Mental Health among the Slave Population on Southern Plantations', *The American Journal of Psychiatry* 110 (1953): 52–54.

Postma, Johannes Menne. *The Dutch in the Atlantic Slave Trade, 1600–1815* (Cambridge: Cambridge University Press, 1990).

Prins, Gwyn. 'But What Was the Disease: The Present State of Health and Healing in African Studies', *Past & Present* 124 (1989): 159–179.

Purseglove, John W. 'The Origins and Migrations of Crops in Tropical Africa', in *Origins of African Plant Domestication*, edited by Jack R. Harlan, Jan M. J. de Wet and Ann B. L. Stemler (The Hague and Paris: Mouton Publishers, 1976), 291–309.

Rankin, John. *Healing the African Body: British Medicine in West Africa 1800–1860* (Columbia: University of Missouri Press, 2015).

Ransford, Oliver. *'Bid the Sickness Cease': Disease in the History of Black Africa* (London: John Murray, 1983).

Rediker, Marcus. *The Slave Ship: A Human History* (New York: Penguin, 2007).

Reis, João José. *Domingos Sodré, um sacerdote africano: Escravidão, liberdade e candomblé na Bahia do século XIX* (São Paulo: Companhia das Letras, 2008).

Rhine, Kathryn. 'Introduction', in *Medical Anthropology in Global Africa*, edited by Kathryn Rhine et al. (Lawrence: University of Kansas, 2014), 3–7.

Ribas, Oscar. *Ilundo: Divindades e ritos angolas* (Luanda: Museu de Angola, 1958).

Ribeiro, Márcia Moises. *A ciência dos trópicos: A arte médica no Brasil do século XVIII* (São Paulo: Editora HUCITEC, 1997).

   Exorcistas e demônios: Demonologia e exorcismos no mundo luso-brasileiro (Rio de Janeiro: Campus, 2003).

Riese, Walther. *La théorie des passions à la lumière de la pensée médicale du XVIIe siècle* (New York: John Wiley, 1965).

Roberts, Allen F. *A Dance of Assassins: Performing Early Colonial Hegemony in the Congo* (Bloomington: Indiana University Press, 2013).

Roberts, Jonathan. 'Medical Exchange on the Gold Coast during the Seventeenth and Eighteenth Centuries', *Canadian Journal of African Studies* 45 (2011): 480–523.

Rodney, Walter. 'The Guinea Coast', in *The Cambridge History of Africa*, Vol. 4, edited by Richard Gray (Cambridge: Cambridge University Press, 1975), 223–324.

Rönnbäck, Klas. 'Enlightenment, Scientific Exploration and Abolitionism: Anders Sparrman's and Carl Bernhard Wadström's Colonial Encounters in Senegal, 1787–1788 and the British Abolitionist Movement', *Slavery & Abolition* 34:3 (2013): 425–445.

'The Idle and the Industrious – European Ideas about the African Work Ethic in Precolonial West Africa', *History in Africa* 41 (2014): 117–145.

Rosen, George. 'Leonhard Ludwig Finke and the First Medical Geography', in *Science, Medicine and History: Essays on the Evolution of Scientific Thought and Medical Practice*, Vol. 2, edited by E. Ashworth Underwood (London: Oxford University Press, 1953), 186–193.

Russell-Wood, A. J. R. *Fidalgos and Philanthropists: The Santa Casa da Misericórdia of Bahia, 1550–1755* (London: Macmillan, 1968).

The Portuguese Empire, 1415–1808: A World on the Move (Baltimore and London: Johns Hopkins University Press, 1998).

Rutten, A. M. G. *Dutch Transatlantic Medicine Trade in the Eighteenth Century under the Cover of the West India Company* (Rotterdam: Erasmus Publishing, 2000).

Saakwa-Mante, Norris. 'Western Medicine and Racial Constitutions: Surgeon John Atkins' Theory of Polygenism and Sleepy Distemper in the 1730s', in *Race, Science, and Medicine, 1700–1960*, edited by Waltraud Ernst and Bernard Harris (London and New York: Routledge, 1999), 28–57.

Saccardo, P. Graziano. *Congo e Angola con la storia dell'antica missione dei Cappuccini*, 3 vols. (Venice-Mestre: Curia Provinciale dei Cappuccini, 1983).

Santos, Catarina Madeira and Ana Paula Tavares, eds. *Africae Monumenta: A Apropriação da Escrita pelos Africanos*, Vol. I, *Arquivo Caculo Cacahenda* (Lisbon: Centro de Estudos de História e Cartografia Antiga/ Instituto de Investigação Científica Tropical, 2002).

Santos, Catarina Madeira and Ana Paula Tavares, *Africae Monumenta: A Apropriação da Escrita pelos Africanos*, Vol. II, *Arquivos Ndala Cabassa, Mufuque Aquitupa, Pango Aluquem e Bango Aquitamba* (Lisbon: CHAM, 2010).

Santos, Eugénio dos. 'O homem português perante a doença no século XVIII: Atitudes e receituário', *Revista da Faculdade de Letras: História, II série*, 1 (1984): 187–201.

Santos, Georgina Silva dos. 'A Arte de Sangrar na Lisboa do Antigo Regime', *Tempo* 10 (2005): 43–60.

Santos-Stubbe, Chirly dos. 'Banzo: Uma nostalgia afro-brasileira', *Journal of Psychology in Africa* 1 (1989): 8–14.

Savage, John. 'Slave Poison/Slave Medicine: The Persistence of Obeah in Early Nineteenth-Century Martinique', in *Obeah and Other Powers: The Politics of Caribbean Religion and Healing*, edited by Diana Paton and Maarit Forde (Durham, NC and London: Duke University Press, 2012), 149–171.

Savitt, Todd L. *Medicine and Slavery: The Diseases and Health Care of Blacks in Antebellum Virginia* (Urbana and Chicago: University of Illinois Press, 1978).

Sawyer, Roy T. 'History of the Leech Trade in Ireland, 1750–1915: Microcosm of a Global Commodity', *Medical History* 57 (2013): 420–441.

Schiebinger, Londa. *Plants and Empire: Colonial Bioprospecting in the Atlantic World* (Cambridge, MA: Harvard University Press, 2004).

'Scientific Exchange in the Eighteenth-Century Atlantic World', in *Soundings in Atlantic History: Latent Structures and Intellectual Currents, 1500–1830*, edited by Bernard Bailyn (Cambridge, MA: Harvard University Press, 2009), 294–328.

Secret Cures of Slaves: People, Plants, and Medicine in the Eighteenth-Century Atlantic World (Stanford, CA: Stanford University Press, 2017).

Schoenbrun, David Lee. *A Green Place, A Good Place: Agrarian Change, Gender, and Social Identity in the Great Lakes Region to the 15th Century* (Oxford: James Currey, 1998).

Schwartz, Marie Jenkins. *Birthing a Slave: Motherhood and Medicine in the Antebellum South* (Cambridge, MA: Harvard University Press, 2006).

Seth, Suman. *Difference and Disease: Medicine, Race, and the Eighteenth-Century British Empire* (Cambridge: Cambridge University Press, 2018).

Sheridan, Richard B. *Doctors and Slaves: A Medical and Demographic History of Slavery in the British West Indies, 1680–1834* (Cambridge: Cambridge University Press, 1985).

Silva, Daniel B. Domingues da. *The Atlantic Slave Trade from West Central Africa, 1780–1867* (Cambridge: Cambridge University Press, 2017).

Simon, William. 'A Luso-African Formulary of the Late Eighteenth Century: Some Notes on Angolan Contributions to European Knowledge of Materia Medica', *Pharmacy in History* 18 (1976): 103–114.

Scientific Expeditions in the Portuguese Overseas Territories (1783–1808) and the Role of Lisbon in the Intellectual-Scientific Community of the Late Eighteenth Century (Lisbon: Instituto de Investigação Científica Tropical, 1983).

Simonsen, Gunvor. 'Magic, Obeah and Law in the Danish West Indies, 1750–1840s', in *Ports of Globalisation, Places of Creolisation: Nordic Possessions in the Atlantic World during the Era of the Slave Trade*, edited by Holger Weiss (Leiden: Brill, 2016), 245–279.

Smith, Sean Morey. 'Seasoning and Abolition: Humoural Medicine in the Eighteenth-Century British Atlantic', *Slavery & Abolition* 36 (2015): 684–703.

Smith, Wesley D. *The Hippocratic Tradition* (Ithaca, NY: Cornell University Press, 1979).

Snyder, Terri L. *The Power to Die: Slavery and Suicide in British North America* (Chicago and London: University of Chicago Press, 2015).

Soares, Mariza de Carvalho. 'African Barbeiros in Brazilian Slave Ports', in *The Black Urban Atlantic in the Age of the Slave Trade*, edited by Jorge Cañizares-Esguerra, Matt D. Childs and James Sidbury (Philadelphia: University of Pennsylvania Press, 2013), 207–230.

Souza, Laura de Mello e. *O diabo e a terra de Santa Cruz* (São Paulo: Companhia das Letras, 1986).

Souza, Leandro Nascimento de, *Uma experiência pernambucana em Angola: o governo de João Fernandes Vieira, 1658 a 1661* (unpublished MA thesis, Universidade Federal de Pernambuco, Recife, 2013).

Sparks, Randy J. *Where the Negroes Are Masters: An African Port in the Era of the Slave Trade* (Cambridge, MA: Harvard University Press, 2014).

Sundelin, Robert. *Svedenborgianismens historia i Sverige under förra århundradet* (Uppsala: W. Schultz, 1886).

Sutton, Elizabeth A. *Early Modern Dutch Prints of Africa* (Farnham: Ashgate, 2012).

Sweet, James H. *Recreating Africa: Culture, Kinship, and Religion in the Portuguese World, 1441–1770* (Chapel Hill: University of North Carolina Press, 2003).

Domingos Álvares, African Healing, and the Intellectual History of the Atlantic World (Chapel Hill: University of North Carolina Press, 2011).

Thornton, John K. *Africa and Africans in the Making of the Atlantic World, 1400–1800*, 2nd ed. (Cambridge: Cambridge University Press, 1998).

The Kongolese Saint Anthony: Dona Beatriz Kimpa Vita and the Antonian Movement, 1684–1706 (Cambridge: Cambridge University Press, 1998).

Warfare in Atlantic Africa 1500–1800 (London: Routledge, 1999).

Tilley, Helen. 'Global Histories, Vernacular Science, and African Genealogies; or, Is the History of Science Ready for the World', *Isis* 101 (2010): 110–119.

Tilley, *Africa as a Living Laboratory: Empire, Development, and the Problem of Scientific Knowledge, 1870–1950* (Chicago: University of Chicago Press, 2011).

Turner, Victor W. *The Forest of Symbols: Aspects of Ndembu Ritual* (Ithaca, NY and London: Cornell University Press, 1967).

The Drums of Affliction: A Study of Religious Processes among the Ndembu of Zambia (Oxford: Oxford University Press, 1968).

Valenčius, Conevery Bolton. 'Histories of Medical Geography', *Medical History* 44: S20 (2000): 3–28.

van Dantzig, Albert. 'Willem Bosman's "New and Accurate Description of the Coast of Guinea": How Accurate Is It?', *History in Africa* 1 (1974): 101–108.

'English Bosman and Dutch Bosman: A Comparison of Texts', *History in Africa* 2 (1975): 185–216.

Vansina, Jan. *How Societies Are Born: Governance in West Central Africa before 1600* (Charlottesville: University of Virginia Press, 2004).

Vaughan, Megan. 'Healing and Curing: Issues in the Social History and Anthropology of Medicine in Africa', *Social History of Medicine* 7 (1994): 283–295.

Vicente, Filipa Lowndes. 'Travelling Objects: The Story of Two Natural History Collections in the Nineteenth Century', *Portuguese Studies* 19 (2003): 19–37.

Voeks, Robert A. *Sacred Leaves of Candomblé: African Magic, Medicine, and Religion in Brazil* (Austin: University of Texas Press, 1997).

Walker, James St. G. *The Black Loyalists: The Search for a Promised Land in Nova Scotia and Sierra Leone 1783–1870* (Toronto: University of Toronto Press, 1992).

Walker, Timothy D. *Doctors, Folk Medicine and the Inquisition: The Repression of Magical Healing in Portugal during the Enlightenment* (Leiden: Brill, 2005).

'Acquisition and Circulation of Medical Knowledge within the Early Modern Portuguese Colonial Empire', in *Science in the Spanish and Portuguese Empires*, edited by Daniela Bleichmar, Paula de Vos, Kristin Huffine and Kevin Sheehan (Stanford, CA: Stanford University Press, 2009), 247–270.

'The Medicines Trade in the Portuguese Atlantic World: Acquisition and Dissemination of Healing Knowledge from Brazil (c. 1580–1800)', *Social History of Medicine* 26 (2013): 403–431.

'Global Cross-Cultural Dissemination of Indigenous Medical Practices through the Portuguese Colonial System: Evidence from Sixteenth to Eighteenth-Century Ethno-Botanical Manuscripts', in *The Globalization of Knowledge in the Iberian Colonial World*, edited by Helge Wendt (Berlin: Max Planck Institute for the History of Science, 2016), 161–192.

Walter, Jaime. 'A propósito de uma doença de Angola de há mais de três séculos: doença do bicho ou maculo', *Boletim clínico e estatístico do Hospital do ultramar* 7 (1957): 47–68.

Um português carioca professor da primeira escola médica de Angola 1791 (as suas lições de anatomia) (Lisbon: Junta de Investigações do Ultramar, 1970).

Watkins, Case. *An Afro-Brazilian Landscape: African Oil Palms and Socioecological Change in Bahia, Brazil* (unpublished Ph.D. dissertation, Louisiana State University, 2015).

Watson, Gilbert. *Theriac and Mithridatium: A Study in Therapeutics* (London: Wellcome Historical Medical Library, 1966).

Watts, Sheldon. *Epidemics and History: Disease, Power and Imperialism* (New Haven, CT and London: Yale University Press, 1997).

Weaver, Karol K. *Medical Revolutionaries: The Enslaved Healers of Eighteenth-Century Saint Domingue* (Urbana and Chicago: University of Illinois Press, 2006).

Webb, James L. A. *Humanity's Burden: A Global History of Malaria* (Cambridge: Cambridge University Press, 2009).

Weiss, Holger. 'Tanskalaiset alusmaat Länsi-Afrikassa ylirajaisena yhteisönä', in *Pohjola, Atlantti, maailma: Ylirajaisen vuorovaikutuksen historiaa 1600–1900-luvuilla*, edited by Kalle Kananoja and Lauri Tähtinen (Helsinki: Finnish Literature Society, 2018), 142–177.

Westerlund, David. *African Indigenous Religions and Disease Causation: From Spiritual Beings to Living Humans* (Leiden: Brill, 2006).

Wheeler, Douglas L. 'A Note on Smallpox in Angola, 1670–1875', *Studia* 13–14 (1964): 351–362.

Whyte, Susan Reynolds. 'The Power of Medicines in East Africa', in *The Context of Medicines in Developing Countries: Studies in Pharmaceutical Anthropology*, edited by Sjaak van der Geest and Susan Reynolds Whyte (Dordrecht: Kluwer, 1988), 217–233.

Whyte, Susan Reynolds, Sjaak van der Geest and Anita Hardon. *Social Lives of Medicines* (Cambridge: Cambridge University Press, 2002).

Williams, Elizabeth A. *A Cultural History of Medical Vitalism in Enlightenment Montpellier* (Aldershot: Ashgate, 2003).

Wimberly, Fayette. 'The Expansion of Afro-Bahian Religious Practices in Nineteenth-Century Cachoeira', in *Afro-Brazilian Culture and Politics: Bahia, 1790s to 1990s*, edited by Hendrik Kraay (Armonk: M. E. Sharpe, 1998), 74–89.

Wootton, David. *Bad Medicine: Doctors Doing Harm since Hippocrates* (Oxford: Oxford University Press, 2006).

Index

www.ingramcontent.com/pod-product-compliance
Ingram Content Group UK Ltd.
Pitfield, Milton Keynes, MK11 3LW, UK
UKHW022002190125
453752UK00007B/54

9 781108 491259